To: Dr. Kate Richardson

From:
Barbara Scr [D0745628]
Microbiology 234
Fall 2001

Cholera

CURRENT TOPICS IN INFECTIOUS DISEASE

Series Editors:

William B. Greenough III
The Johns Hopkins University
Baltimore, Maryland

Thomas C. Merigan
Head, Division of Infectious Disease
Stanford University Medical Center
Stanford, California

A Continuation Order Plan is available for this series. A continuation order will bring delivery of each new volume immediately upon publication. Volumes are billed only upon actual shipment. For further information please contact the publisher.

Cholera

Edited by
Dhiman Barua
Formerly of the School of Tropical Medicine
Calcutta, India
and Formerly of the Diarrhoeal Diseases
    Control Programme
World Health Organization
Geneva, Switzerland

and
William B. Greenough III
The Johns Hopkins University
Baltimore, Maryland
Formerly of the International Centre for Diarrhoeal
    Disease Research
Dhaka, Bangladesh

PLENUM MEDICAL BOOK COMPANY
New York and London

Library of Congress Cataloging-in-Publication Data

Cholera / edited by Dhiman Barua and William B. Greenough III.
        p.   cm. -- (Current topics in infectious disease)
     Includes bibliographical references and index.
     ISBN 0-306-44077-6
     1. Cholera.   I. Barua, Dhiman.   II. Greenough, William B.
   III. Series.
     [DNLM: 1. Cholera.   WC 262 C5463Q]
   RC126.C522   1992
   616.9'32--dc20
   DNLM/DLC
   for Library of Congress   92-14365
                                                                  CIP

ISBN 0-306-44077-6

© 1992 Plenum Publishing Corporation
233 Spring Street, New York, N.Y. 10013

Plenum Medical Book Company is an imprint of Plenum Publishing Corporation

Printed in the United States of America

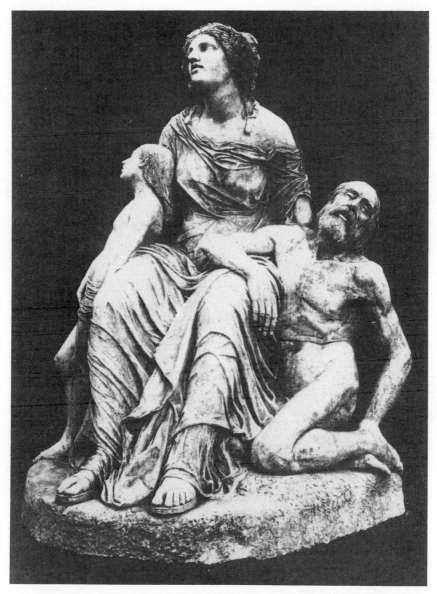

City of Paris, 1851. Statue imploring heaven to take away plague of Cholera.

Contributors

Mary M. Baldini, Center for Vaccine Development, Division of Geographic Medicine, Department of Medicine, University of Maryland School of Medicine, Baltimore, Maryland 21204

Dhiman Barua, Formerly of the School of Tropical Medicine, Calcutta, India, and formerly of the Diarrhoeal Diseases Control Programme, World Health Organization, Geneva, Switzerland.

Robert E. Black, Department of International Health, School of Hygiene and Public Health, The Johns Hopkins University, Baltimore, Maryland 21205

Rita R. Colwell, Department of Microbiology, Maryland Biotechnology Institute, College Park, Maryland 20742

Richard A. Finkelstein, Department of Microbiology, School of Medicine, University of Missouri-Columbia, Columbia, Missouri 65212

J. A. Frost, WHO Collaborating Center for Phage Typing and Resistance of Enterobacteria, Division of Enteric Pathogens, Central Public Health Laboratory, London NW9 5HT, United Kingdom

Eugene J. Gangarosa, Professor of International Health, School of Public Health, Robert W. Woodruff Health Sciences Center, Emory University, Atlanta, Georgia 30087

Roger I. Glass, Division of Viral Diseases, Center for Infectious Diseases, Centers for Disease Control, Atlanta, Georgia 30333

William B. Greenough III, The Johns Hopkins University, Baltimore, Maryland 21205; formerly of the International Centre for Diarrhoeal Disease Research, Dhaka, Bangladesh.

Jan Holmgren, Department of Medical Microbiology, University of Goteborg, Guldhedsgatan 10, S-41346, Goteborg, Sweden

James B. Kaper, Center for Vaccine Development, Division of Geographic Medicine, Department of Medicine, University of Maryland School of Medicine, Baltimore, Maryland 21201

Myron M. Levine, Center for Vaccine Development, Division of Geographic Medicine, Department of Medicine, University of Maryland School of Medicine, Baltimore, Maryland 21201

Dilip Mahalanabis, International Centre for Diarrhoeal Disease Research, Dhaka, Bangladesh

Michael H. Merson, Diarrhoeal Diseases Control Programme, World Health Organization, Geneva, Switzerland

A. M. Molla, Department of Pediatrics, Aga Khan University, Karachi, Pakistan

Sudhir Chandra Pal, National Institute of Cholera and Enteric Diseases, Beliaghata, Calcutta 700 010, India

Nathaniel F. Pierce, Diarrhoeal Diseases Control Programme, World Health Organization, Geneva, Switzerland

G. H. Rabbani, International Centre for Diarrhoeal Disease Research, Dhaka, Bangladesh

B. Rowe, WHO Collaborating Centre for Phage Typing and Resistance of Enterobacteria, Division of Enteric Pathogens, Central Public Health Laboratory, London NW9 5HT, United Kingdom

David A. Sack, Department of International Health, School of Hygiene and Public Health, The Johns Hopkins University, Baltimore, Maryland 21205

R. Bradley Sack, Department of International Health, School of Hygiene and Public Health, The Johns Hopkins University, Baltimore, Maryland 21205

Riichi Sakazaki, Enterobacteriology Laboratories, National Institute of Health, Kamiosaki, Shinagawa-ku, Tokyo, Japan

S. C. Sanyal, Department of Microbiology, Institute of Medical Sciences, Banaras Hindu University, Varanasi 221 005, India

William M. Spira, Department of International Health, School of Hygiene and Public Health, The Johns Hopkins University, Baltimore, Maryland, 21205

Robert V. Tauxe, Chief, Epidemiology Section, Enteric Diseases Branch, Division of Bacterial and Mycotic Diseases, National Center for Infectious Diseases, Centers for Disease Control, Atlanta, Georgia 39333

Foreword

When cholera attacked St. Louis in 1849, over 10% of the population of that city died, as did over half of the individuals who developed acute diarrheal illness. When cholera attacked Peru in 1991, over 300,000 people, or 1% of the population, developed clinical manifestations of cholera, but less than 1% of affected individuals died.

The basis for this remarkable achievement is described in this comprehensive volume, which deals with all aspects of cholera and is written by individuals intimately involved with developing the current simple, inexpensive, but remarkably effective approach to the treatment of this disease.

Key to the current successful management of cholera is the development of oral rehydration therapy, a remarkable achievement of multinational teams of clinical investigators in Calcutta and Dhaka in the mid-1960s. Since oral rehydration therapy (ORT) requires only ingredients (sugar and salt) that are available to almost all individuals throughout the world, and since it can be administered by knowledgeable family members under the most primitive conditions, this therapeutic innovation, described by the *Lancet* as perhaps the most important innovation of twentieth century medicine, has empowered mothers throughout the world to administer simple but lifesaving treatment to children with cholera and other acute diarrheal illnesses.

The development of oral rehydration therapy involved the application of a basic physiologic observation of the late 1950s: that intraluminal glucose enhanced the absorption of sodium in the mammalian gut. This observation was made by basic scientists who had not considered the application of this principle to patients with acute diarrheal illness. The transfer of this basic observation to the clinical practice of medicine occurred within less than a decade, a truly remarkable achievement.

This volume also describes our less successful approach to developing a vaccine that confers effective immunity against cholera. Although several promising new approaches to cholera vaccine development are currently under way, the need is somewhat less urgent than in 1960, when the mortality rate from cholera exceeded 50% in many parts of the world.

The authors of this volume also acknowledge the embryonal state of our knowledge of the epidemiology of *Vibrio cholerae* infection. Although certain fundamentals are understood (e.g., fecal–oral transmission, the importance of the gastric acid barrier in protection), our experience with the seventh cholera pandemic, especially the unprecedented rapid spread of cholera in Peru in 1991–1992, has made it abundantly clear that current knowledge is not sufficient to predict when cholera will attack a new geographic area or precisely what circumstances determine whether cholera will become endemic in a newly infected region.

The remarkable achievements of the Peruvian medical profession in the treatment of the largest documented outbreak of cholera since 1945 have provided a magnificent example to the rest of the world. The authors of this volume illuminate the scientific background upon which this achievement has been based.

Charles C. J. Carpenter, M.D.

Professor of Medicine
Brown University

Preface

It has been more than 30 years since the first monograph on cholera, by Pollitzer, was published (1959), and more than 17 years since the first multiauthored comprehensive volume was produced, by Barua and Burrows (1974).

During these 30 years, the world has been experiencing the seventh cholera pandemic and has seen many advances of major import in understanding almost all aspects of this and other diarrheal diseases. There have been major advances in the classification and in understanding the bacterial genetics, bacteriology, epidemiology, pathogenesis, and immunology of cholera, and in the development of vaccines and therapy. A great deal has been learned by both scientists and public health communities, particularly during the last two decades. As cholera remains a global endemic and epidemic problem with no evident retreat, however, many students of cholera have expressed the need for a current book reviewing the available knowledge and experience to permit more rational and effective handling of cholera and to provide a stepping-stone for the scientist. We, however, realize that many areas of research are progressing rapidly, and that by the time of publication, there may have been some advances that the present volume does not cover.

We attempt in this book to present the recent advances in a more complete historical perspective and to bring the practical aspects into prominence. Each author was encouraged to write from his or her personal point of view. We have not edited the style or the opinions and views of the authors, in the hope that this will add variety and individuality to the text. For the same reason, we have preferred to allow a certain amount of repetition. We are pleased with and grateful for the cooperation of our contributors, each of whom writes with authority in his or her given field of research. Each of the contributors has a long-sustained interest and research experience with cholera. We hope that this book will have lasting value for those interested in cholera and diarrheal diseases, which remain some of the most important causes of illness and death globally.

The knowledge gained by research on cholera has been a key that has unlocked the door not only to our understanding of diarrheal illnesses in general, but also to the fundamental ways in which cells communicate with one another and process the humoral signals that produce integrated responses such as fluid and electrolyte secretion and absorption by the intestinal tract. Cholera toxin is presently one of the best understood of all bacterial toxins, and because of its unique mode of action, it serves as an important biologic probe.

The editors express their deep appreciation to Dr. Nyunt-Nyunt-Wai for her assistance in completing the editorial tasks and to Dr. Khin-Maung-U for his useful suggestions in producing the manuscript for this book. Without the enthusiastic support and capable assistance of

Charlene Dale and of the International Child Health Foundation (ICHF), the book could not have been completed. The patience and sustained interest of the staff of the Plenum Medical Book Company have enabled the work on this book to continue and encouraged its completion. The ICHF's Clifford Pease Tribute Fund provided the financial support to enable us to complete the book.

William B. Greenough III
Dhiman Barua

Baltimore and Geneva

Contents

Chapter 8
CHOLERA ENTEROTOXIN (CHOLERAGEN):
A HISTORICAL PERSPECTIVE 155
Richard A. Finkelstein

Chapter 9
COLONIZATION AND PATHOLOGY 189
R. Bradley Sack

Chapter 12

LABORATORY DIAGNOSIS   229
Sudhir Chandra Pal

Chapter 13

CLINICAL MANAGEMENT OF CHOLERA   253
Dilip Mahalanabis, A. M. Molla, and David A. Sack

Chapter 14
IMMUNITY AND VACCINE DEVELOPMENT 285
Myron M. Levine and Nathaniel F. Pierce

Chapter 15
PREVENTION AND CONTROL OF CHOLERA 329
Dhiman Barua and Michael H. Merson

1

History of Cholera

Dhiman Barua

1. INTRODUCTION

What is cholera? How and where did it start? How did and does it spread? There is a lack of agreement about the early history of cholera. Confusion arose because it was difficult to define cholera precisely (which has a broad clinical spectrum) and to distinguish it from many other diseases associated with diarrhea and vomiting.

There is also not agreement on the etymology of the term "cholera." The term, first seen in the works of Hippocrates, was believed to have been derived from the Greek words *chole* (bile) and *rein* (to flow), thus meaning flow of bile.[1-3] Alexander Trallianus, however, said in 1622 that the word had come from *cholades* which means intestine, as the evacuations were often serous and not bilious. In 1872, an eminent philologist, Emile Littre, expressed the opinion that the term originated from the Greek word *cholera,* which means gutter (of a roof), probably because the discharges in cholera flow as from a spout. He reaffirmed his conviction again in 1878.[4] Thomas Sydenham, the "English Hippocrates" of the 17th century, is given the credit[3] for coining the term *cholera morbus* to distinguish cholera, the disease, from cholera, the state of anger. Haeser has been quoted[2] as maintaining that the later Greek writers added the word *nousos* (which means sickness) after cholera to distinguish the illness from the building structure, i.e., roof gutter. McLeod[5] thought the Hippocratic term cholera meant bilious diarrhea. However, it is difficult to agree after reading the description of cholera cases by Hippocrates, as will be seen later.

In India, the Sanskrit word believed to denote cholera is *visuchika,* which found a place in the *Sushruta Samhita.*[6] The age of the *Sushruta Samhita* is difficult to ascertain but it is estimated to have been written about 500–400 BC, or around the time of Lord Buddha. The word *visuchika* literally may mean an abnormal bowel movement or merely a disturbance of the stomach and intestine. However, the description of a case of *visuchika* in the Sanskrit literature, as will be seen later, agrees very closely with a typical case of cholera.

Cholera, edited by Dhiman Barua and William B. Greenough III. Plenum Medical Book Company, New York, 1992.

There are different words for cholera in different Indian languages. In Bengali, it is *ola-utha* (*ola* = an act of descending or purging and *utha* = act of coming up or vomiting); in the Marathi language, the word is *mordeshim* or *mordezin,* the word which also was used by early Portuguese writers; in Urdu it is *heidja,* by which cholera is now generally recognized in India (as has always been so by the Mohammedans). The word *haida* was used in AD 900 by Rhazes of Baghdad[1] as he described cholera. *Haida* literally means shattered or broken. This word is rarely used by the common people now. The Arabic word for cholera is *haida* or *heyda* and seems quite close to the Urdu word used in India. The Arabic word *wuba* or *el wuba* means an epidemic, the same as the word *mahamari* in India; they both mean epidemic or "a great killer." These words also are sometimes used to mean a major cholera epidemic. For over 2000 years in China, cholera has been called *fok lun,* a term meaning something huddled up in a confused manner inside the body and which is expressed by vomiting and purging.[7] The present Chinese word for cholera seems to be *huo luon* which also is found in old Chinese chronicles, but it appears to have been used to cover a group of affections of the gastrointestinal tract.[7]

McPherson[1] did a careful search for various names under which cholera has been described in different places. He came to the conclusion that cholera must have been a very familiar disease all over the world for in almost every country in Europe and in every language in India had a popular name for it as do Chinese and Arabic languages. In recent years, Howard-Jones[3] did a similar but limited survey and observed that the term cholera has been used for defining gastrointestinal derangements of diverse etiology for more than 2000 years. There is little doubt that confusion on terminology has added considerably to the difficulties in studying the history of cholera.

2. CHOLERA BEFORE 1817

There is no disagreement among cholera historians about the presence of choleralike diseases in Asia, including China, and in Europe during ancient times. The main dispute is about whether the disease known as cholera today, i.e., true cholera caused by *Vibrio cholerae* 01, was present in Europe before 1817 when the first pandemic was supposed to have spread out of India. This debate cannot be solved now by scientific means, but it is possible to review the clinical and epidemiologic descriptions of the similar diseases present in those days in Europe and try to make a reasonable deduction.

Although there is almost no recorded evidence of the presence of cholera in India (except for the description in *Sushruta Samhita*) before the writings of the Portuguese settlers in the early 16th century, there is little doubt that the disease was present there from very early days.

MacNamara[8] of the Indian Medical Services, a leading British authority on cholera, who had studied under Koch himself, wrote "while we have numerous treatises on the works of Sushruta and Avicenna, we have literally no clue in the oriental languages as to the history of epidemic cholera in India." While the description of the disease in the translated *Sushruta Samhita* agrees closely with that of cholera as is known today, it has been described as a sporadic condition. In *Charaka Samhita,* a slightly later publication in India, there is a chapter on epidemics which also does not mention visuchika.*

---

*As density of population is an important factor in the causation of cholera epidemics, it is possible that cholera did not cause epidemics in India at the time of Sushruta until later, when the population density became favorable. A progressive change in the virulence of the causative agent could have been a theoretical possibility as well.

De,[9] one of the most eminent scientists in the field of cholera, collected strong evidence from published literature to show that true cholera was present in Europe before the extension of the pandemics of the 19th century, as did MacPherson[1] in 1872 and 1884, but others disagreed.[3,8,10,11]

Howard-Jones[3] quoted Hirsch saying at the fourth International Sanitary Conference in Vienna in 1874 that it is "indisputable that before 1817 all countries of the globe, except India and Ceylon, were free of cholera."

It may, therefore, be useful to quote some of the typical case descriptions collected by MacPherson,[1] who was Inspector General of Hospitals, H.M. Bengal army in India, as they are not easily available to readers for their own appraisal. One example of a case recounted in the works of Hippocrates ran thus:

> At Athens a man was seized with cholera. He vomited, and was purged and was in pain, and neither the vomiting nor the purging could be stopped; and his voice failed him, and he could not be moved from his bed, and his eyes were dark and hollow, and spasms from the stomach held him, and hiccup from the bowels. But the purging was much more than the vomiting. This man drank hellebore with juice of lentils; and he again drank juice of lentils, as much as he could, and after that he vomited. He was forced again to drink, and the two (vomiting and purging) were stopped; but he became cold.

A later famous Greek writer on medicine, Aretaeus of Capdadocia, described cholera as follows:

> Cholera is an inverted movement of everything in the whole body to the stomach, to the belly, and to the intestines—a very sharp malady. For the matters collected in the stomach escape by vomiting, and the fluid matters in the belly and intestines run through by the lower passage. What is first vomited is like water, but what passes by stool is stercoraceous fluid and of ill odour. For continued bad digestion has been the cause of this. But what is washed away is first like phlegm, afterwards like bile. At the beginning the disease is free from pain, but after that, there are tension of the stomach and tormina of the belly; but if the disease increases, the tormina are augmented, there is syncope, the limbs are unknit, there is helplessness, loathing of food; and if they swallow anything, yellow bile rushes out unceasingly by vomiting with sickness, and the dejections are like. There are spasms, and drawing together of the muscles of the calves of the legs and of the arms. The fingers are twisted; there is vertigo and hiccup; the nails are livid; there is cold refrigeration of the extremities, and the whole body becomes rigid; but if the malady runs on to its end, then the man is covered with perspiration; black bile bursts out upwards and downwards. There is retention of urine from spasm of the bladder; but indeed, much water is not collected in it, owing to the pouring out of the fluids into the intestines. There is loss of voice; the pulse becomes very small and frequent, as in syncope; there are constant fruitless attempts at vomiting, desire to evacuate with tenesmus, but dry and without fluid; death, full of pains and miserable, with spasms and suffocation, and fruitless vomiting. . . . But if he rejects everything by vomiting, and a perpetual perspiration flows, and the patient becomes cold and ash-coloured, and the pulse approaches extinction, and the patient becomes speechless, it is well, under such circumstances, (for physician) to make a graceful (becoming) retreat.

Aretaeus also observed that the disease prevailed "most in Summer, next most in Autumn, less in Spring and least in Winter."

Quoting from Sanskrit accounts of cholera from *Ayurveda of Sushruta,* Calcutta, 1835, Vol. II, p.518, MacPherson[1] added:

> "Visuchika chiefly attacks those who are timid or immoderate in their living. . . . Along with convulsions, the patient has intellectual torpor, diarrhoea, vomiting, thirst, giddiness, restlessness, tenesmus, yawning, feeling of heat, lividity, shivering, pain in the head and at the praecordia. The belly is retracted; the patient, whose voice is lost, is in a state of extreme agitation. The gases contained in the belly rise. When the faeces and the air remain shut up in the belly, the patient grows weak, loses power of moving, then come hiccup and eructations. . . . When the patient's gums are livid, his nails and lips pale, when he vomits abundantly, and loses consciousness of his acts, when his eyes become hollow, when his voice is lost, when his joints are all relaxed, one ought to have

recourse to the instructions of the sacred books," or as Dr. Wise translates it, "such a person may be taken out to be burnt, he will not recover."

The similarity between the clinical features, particularly the last sentences in the case descriptions of Aretaeus and *Sushruta,* is remarkable. Although the writers on Indian medicine, MacPherson[1] added, "do not give nearly so clear and distinct account of cholera as the Greek and Roman ones, they afford no indication of any particularly virulent or epidemic form of the disease being known to them."

MacPherson[1] cited an account of *Ho Luan* (Chinese word for cholera) from a Chinese book, *Ching-che-chin-shing* printed in 1790, which described most of the usual symptoms and some very characteristic ones:

> Sometimes the patient is hot and restless, and desires to throw off every covering. When there are spasms, vomiting and purging, cold perspiration, giddiness in the head, and confused vision, the disease becomes incurable.

Rhazes, the Arab author from Baghdad earlier, gave the following description of *heyda* in about AD 900:

> It begins with nausea and diarrhoea, or one of the two, and when it reaches the stomach it goes on multiplying itself. The pulse fails, and the breathing is attenuated; the face and the nose become thin; the colour of the skin of the face is changed, and the countenance of the dead succeeds. The extremities become cold and there is cold perspiration, and there are spasms in the hands and feet and legs. There is urgent thirst, which cannot be satisfied, as the patient immediately rejects what he drinks.

About a century later, Avicenna repeated Rhazes' description while writing about *heyda.* Avicenna appears to be the author who first used the Arabic word indicating milky or rice-water evacuations.[1]

A very lively description of the *trousse-galant,* or *flux de ventre,* French expressions sometimes used for *cholera morbus,* written by the Belgian physician Van der Heyden in 1643 ran as follows:[1]

> The furious onset of *trousse-galant* in a short time takes away from the body so much of its substance and of its force, and occasions in it so much mischief and change, that in seven hours their domestics would not recognise in such a sufferer a master or a relative, unless they knew it could be none else, for they encounter the true Hippocratic expression, which indicates the extreme of debility and the image of death. Once when I was called to see a patient, only five hours after his attack, I found him in a condition giving the most unfavourable prognosis, to wit, without pulse or speech, passing in his evacuations only a fluid resembling clear milk. Along with this, his eyes were so sunk that one could scarcely see them, and his legs and arms so drawn back by convulsions, that one saw no movement in them, and so cold from the moisture of a cold and clammy perspiration adhering to them, that the patient seemed more dead than alive.

In 1649, Riverus of Montpellier, France, also gave a full account of cholera, mainly sporadic, but of very considerable intensity.[1]

MacPherson[1] cited more reports on the presence of cholera in: Brazil (1658), Ghent (1665), Montpellier (1649), and England in the second half of the 17th century. Thomas Sydenham, a famous name that has been mentioned earlier, drew attention to the regularity of the occurrence of cholera in London in late summer and early autumn by comparing it to the coming of the swallows in spring and of the cuckoo in early summer.[11]

Faber in his classic monograph,[12] while describing the work of Sydenham in London mentioned that in 1667 2000 people in London (out of the city's population of 500,000) died of cholera. MacNamara,[8] however, refutes Sydenham's claim that these cases were due to cholera because Dr. Willis, a contemporary physician of Sydenham, thought the cases were of an aggravated form of dysentery and because the outbreak did not extend beyond a distance of three miles from the city. Therefore, it will be interesting to examine Willis's own description of the cases[1]:

> The disease invading suddenly and frequently without any manifest occasion, did reduce those labouring with it by great vomiting, frequent and watery stools (excretory convulsions, with tormenting perturbation of the whole body), quickly to a very great debility, to horrid failure of the spirits, and loss of all strength. I knew some, the day before well enough, and very strong, in twelve hours' space so miserably cast down by the tyranny of this disease, that with a weak and small pulse, cold sweat, short and quick breath, they seemed just ready to die; and truly not a few to whom fit remedies or opportunity of cure were wanting, were suddenly killed by it. This sickness, raging for a whole month, began to decrease about the middle of October, and before the beginning of November was almost wholly vanished. Very few in that time had bloody stools, and not many bilious, but very many had vomits, and watery, almost clear, and plentiful stools. Whilst that popular dysentery raged in the city so cruelly, in the country or at least three miles beyond the city, almost none was sick of it.

There were reports of cholera and dysentery in Nuremberg in 1689, cholera in Breslaw in 1701, in Tubingen in 1711, and in several other parts of Europe during this period.

Another contemporary physician, Dr. Morton, mentioned that during the first cholera and dysentery season in the year 1666, the whole town was seized and between 300 to 500 persons died of the disease in a week.[9]

Van Swieten, a great authority in medicine, spoke briefly about cholera in his commentaries on the period of 1742–1747 in this way[1]:

> In cholera morbus, of a sudden and in a few hours' time, there is so great a discharge of the humors both by vomiting and by stool, that the whole body is exhausted, the face is pale and collapsed. All the strength is destroyed, and even convulsions are observed from so profuse and sudden an inanition, even though not so much as a drop of blood is discharged either upwards or downwards. This I have often observed with great astonishment, and especially in the case of a strong girl, who in the space of three hours had her face so altered and collapsed, that her most intimate acquaintances could not know her, all the humors being dissolved as it were by a poisonous force, and violently expelled by vomiting and purging.

It is possible that both cholera and dysentery (griping of the gut) were present in that period, but the Willis and Van Swieten descriptions of cases leave little doubt about the presence of severe cholera at that time. Creighton[11] mentioned that choleraic disease and dysentery were having "great seasons" all over Europe during the 16th century, beginning in 1539–1540, and the descriptions by Willis of cases in London in 1669–1670 "serve to show the prevalence of cholera nostras among adults in London in former times." The descriptions of cases quoted here would indicate that *cholera morbus* was no different from true cholera, having also the same potential to cause epidemics.

C.E.A. Winslow,[13] dean of American historians of epidemiology, also included cholera as one of the diseases that assumed epidemic proportions in Europe in the 15th century. René Dubos[14] wrote in 1950 that "there had been well-identified cases of cholera in Europe before the 19th century, in Nimes in 1654, in London in 1669, in Vienna in 1768."

Howard-Jones,[10] writing brilliantly in 1972 on various aspects of the history of cholera, disregarded these eminent writers because their statements were based on a "superficial symptomatic resemblance." He felt that the name cholera "was a blunderbuss epithet for almost all acute gastrointestinal disturbances, except the one that we now call cholera." This statement is only partially acceptable as it would be difficult for any student of cholera to agree that true cholera was not present in Europe in those days along with other types of acute diarrheas after an unemotional, critical review of the case descriptions. Only those who have never seen a case of cholera and have not had a chance to compare it with other diarrheas, could disregard these case descriptions presented here.

There is little disagreement about the existence of true cholera in India in early times, despite the absence of any account of the disease after that of *Sushruta*. Written accounts of cholera in India, however deficient, began to appear after the Portuguese settled in Goa in about 1502. The first report, that of an outbreak of cholera during the war between the settlers and the ruler of Calicut in 1503, was written by Gaspar Correa in *Lendas da India,* and was translated into English by Gaskoin[15] in 1867. Before this report, outbreaks due to cholera in Delhi[1] in 1325 and among the troops of Ahmed Shah at Merwah[2] in 1438 had been recorded. Reference to this disease in Goa was again made in 1563 by Garcia da Orta,[16] who described a varied clinical picture of the disease. In the 17th century, reports of cholera in Goa and Surat in India and in neighboring countries such as Java were recorded.[1,8]

MacNamara[8] described at length a longstanding custom of the people of Bengal of worshipping the goddess of cholera called *Ola Beebee* as evidence of cholera being present for a long time and of the seriousness of the problem caused by it. He could not determine when this custom began, but he was told that originally the deity was in a bamboo shed; a temple was provided early in the 18th century, probably about 1720, which was moved to a more convenient site in Calcutta around 1750. De,[9] who spoke the local language, talked to the family of the priest owning the temple and consulted the *Asiatic Journal* of 1818 (Vol 5, pp 446–54) referred to by MacPherson, and found that the temple was a hoax. It was built by an unscrupulous family of Brahmin as a means of earning money, probably some time after 1817 when Jessore became famous as the district where the first pandemic was supposed to have begun and where cholera is called *ola*.

Similar tales of the goddess of cholera being worshipped in various other parts of India were mentioned[1] as evidence of the presence of cholera from antiquity, but the story cited above indicates that these tales neither prove nor disprove the contention.

Howard-Jones[3] commented on the ambiguities of the reports of cholera in India in the 17th century by Dellon (1685), a French physician, and by Fryer (1698), an English physician. However, he described at length the report of Sonnerat, a French traveler in India, of an epidemic in 1769 near Pondicherry, South India, which claimed 60,000 victims suffering from watery stools, vomiting, extreme feebleness, ardent thirst, and suppression of urine. They were often pulseless, with cold extremities and sunken orbits. Howard-Jones[3] wrote "it was difficult not to believe that he was writing about true Asiatic cholera," but failed to notice the similarity between the description of these cases in India and those in Europe.

Accounts of choleralike diseases in South India and Bengal are to be found in the reports of Jesuit missionaries and travelers during the first decade of the 18th century, but a 1736 publication on diseases of India by Paxman, who lived for 9 years in Bengal, did not make any special comments about cholera or choleralike diseases, or about epidemics in that part of India.[1] In the later part of that century, reports were recorded of cholera in Arcot near Vellore, in Pondicherry, in the English fleet in India, and in Arabia. The first large outbreak since the British occupation of India was described by MacNamara.[8] The outbreak which traveled widely to different areas of the country, began in Ganjam (South India) in 1781 among a division of Bengal troops while proceeding toward Madras on their way to Calcutta.[1,8] Reports were that "men in perfect health dropped down in dozens." The epidemic found its way to Calcutta where it caused "a great mortality" and then proceeded northward to Sylhet. It also broke out "with great violence in Hardwar" at the time of *Kumbh mela* (pilgrimage) in 1783. Southward, the epidemic was "most deadly along the whole of the eastern coast" in 1782, raged among the Mahratta army fighting with Tipo Sultan, visited Madras in October 1782, and then appeared among the men of the British fleet in Trincomalee, Ceylon (Sri Lanka). The existence of cholera in Burma in July 1783 was also recorded. MacNamara[8] gave the following reasons for not possessing clearer indications of the course of the disease: the malady was not recognized by English medical men,* no official reports of the sick were made until 1786 and then only irregularly until 1802, and the British possessions in India prior to 1781 were surrounded by large provinces about which very little could be found out.

Cholera was again rampant in Vellore and Arcot in 1787–1789, in Ganjam in 1790, and in Malabar and Coromandel in 1796, although the disease was described by some as intestinal colic.[1] The Madras Medical Board,[1] in 1787, opined that the epidemic raged "under the appearance of dysentery, cholera morbus or mordezin." It is again apparent from this description that a similar confusion in differentiating cholera from dysentery existed both in India and in Europe in those days.

In addition to the reports of cholera in different parts of South India during the last decade of the 18th century, the Bengal Medical Board reported a large epidemic in Lower Bengal, where cholera apparently had reappeared after an absence of some 20 years.[1]

The early years of the 19th century were evidently a period of quiescence, although occasional reports of the disease were received in the summer. MacPherson[1] described the cholera situation in Bengal and in the rest of India during 1817 as normal, excepting the summer exacerbations in the northern parts of the province, which later reached Calcutta and Jessore. He was surprised that Jessore ever came to be considered as the center from which the disease spread as a pandemic in 1817. He considered different possible factors that could have favored an explosive situation and wrote "no great change of any kind, no new palpable cause or class of causes came into operation about the year 1817 as has been inferred to have been the case by the Constantinople Cholera Conference." He added "Increased facilities of communication sprang up very gradually in India and this commencement can be referred to no particular date and certainly not to so early a period as the year 1817." Pollitzer,[2] however, wrote "in 1817 cholera began to show an unusual virulence in India." MacNamara[8] narrated elaborately the march of cholera from the east to the west of India in 1817–1820; he thought it then reached Oman in 1821 from Bombay, accompanying the British and native troops sent there to assist the Imam. Van Heyningen and Seal[17] have recently reviewed various accounts of this extraordinary situation in 1817. The germ concept was not yet known at that time and, hence, the possibility of any change in the causative agent was not considered, but, in retrospect, this cannot be excluded. Selwyn[18] writing in 1977 thought that a subtle genetic change in the vibrio might have led to the birth of a new disease around 1781, as before that time there were no authentic reports on epidemics.

3. THE SIX PANDEMICS (1817–1923)

The history of cholera in the period 1817–1923 is generally described as the history of the six pandemics caused by cholera during this period, although there is a lack of agreement among different writers[2,19] about the dates of these pandemics, as can be seen in Table 1. Pollitzer's dates will be followed in this narration as they appear to be more widely known. The intervals between the individual pandemics were not always clear; that between the second and third was particularly obscure.

---

*It is possible that the disease gradually became infrequent in Europe and England during the later years of the 18th century as descriptions of it do not seem to appear in contemporary literature. If that was so, young English medical men probably had no opportunity to learn about the disease and, therefore, had difficulty in recognizing it.

TABLE 1
Cholera Pandemics (1817–1923/5)

Pandemic	Haesser[2] (1882)	Hirsch[2] (1883)	Sticker[2] (1912)	Kolle and Priggs[2] (1928)	Pollitzer[2] (1959)	Wilson and Miles[19] (1975)
				According to		
1	(a)1816–1823	1817–1823	1817–1838	—	1817–1823	1817–1823
	(b)1826–1837	—	—	—	—	—
2	1840–1850	1826–1837	1840–1864	—	1829–1851	1826–1837
3	1852–1860	—	1863–1875	—	1852–1859	1846–1862
4	1863–1873	1865–1875	1881–1896	—	1863–1879	1864–1875
5	—	—	1899	1883–1896	1881–1896	1883–1896
6	—	—	—	1902–1923	1899–1923/5	1899–1923

3.1. First Pandemic (1817–1823)

When cholera appeared in Oman in 1821 after a large war in which soldiers from Bombay took part, it was considered to have come with the troops.

From Muscat, cholera traveled to Bahrain, the Persian Gulf, parts of Iran, Iraq, and Turkey, knocked on the doors of Astrakhan and Tbilisi in Russia, and overran Syria as far as the border with Egypt. MacNamara[8] described how cholera affected the war between Persia (Islamic Republic of Iran) and Turkey and how the returning troops helped to disseminate the disease in Persia. In 1823, cholera broke out in Alexandretta, and reappeared in most of the places it had visited in the preceding years, especially along the borders of the Mediterranean, but disappeared almost entirely from all these areas at the end of the year.

In the other direction, cholera invaded Nepal in 1818, Ceylon (now Sri Lanka), and Burma (Myanmar) in 1819, and Siam (Thailand), Malacca, Penang, and Singapore almost at the same time in 1820. Java, Borneo, and other islands of the Indonesian archipelago and in the Philippines were also affected in 1820. China was probably reached in 1817 by land, and again by sea from Burma and Bangkok in 1820, causing a large outbreak in Peking (Beijing) in 1822–1824. Japan was invaded in 1822 via Nagasaki through a ship from Java.

In addition, Mauritius and Réunion were infected through shipping, probably from Ceylon (Sri Lanka) in 1819, Zanzibar during 1820–1821 by dhows (Arabian sailing ships) plying between Arabia and the east coast of Africa (though some writers thought Zanzibar was affected in 1836–1837), and Somalia in 1833–1834.

In India, "1822 was marked by almost absolute rest as regards cholera" said Mac-Namara,[8] who was also struck by the difference in case–fatality rates among the European and native troops, which were 21 per 1000 in the former and 10 per 1000 in the latter.

3.2. Second Pandemic (1829–1851)

It was believed that cholera appeared in Astrakhan (USSR) in 1830 due to a recrudescence of infection, which had persisted from the time of the first pandemic, although some thought the disease had traveled from India anew via Afghanistan (where cholera was rampant in 1829) and Persia (now Iran) to Orenburg (now called Chaklov) in the southeast corner of European Russia where the epidemic was discovered in August, 1829. "Though every possible effort was made by the authorities to stem the tide with the aid of cordons and other rigid quarantine measures," wrote Pollitzer,[2] "cholera steadily advanced into Russia and reached Moscow by the autumn of 1830."

In Moscow, a chemist named Herman, working in the Institute for Artificial Mineral Waters, conceived the idea of injecting fluid into the veins of cholera victims as he had observed hemoconcentration in them. In 1830, at Herman's suggestion, Jaehnichen, his clinician colleague, injected six ounces of fluid into the vein of a patient. The patient's pulse returned, but he eventually died. During the next two years when cholera arrived in Great Britain, O'Shaughnessy, an Irish physician followed this lead, studied the chemical pathology of cholera and concluded that the objective of treatment should be to restore the specific gravity of blood and to replace the deficient saline matter. His idea was later followed up by Latta of Scotland in 1832 when he treated 15 moribund patients by intravenous saline infusions; as only five survived, he had to face severe criticism, although the *Lancet* considered the treatment life-saving. These brilliant observations were however completely ignored by contemporary physicians, who preferred prescribing venesection, leeching, emetics, and cathartics, etc., until the last decade of the 19th century when Rogers, in Calcutta,[20,21] demonstrated convincingly the effectiveness of intravenous fluid. Rogers used hypertonic saline; alkali and potassium were added during 1905–1910 and case–fatality was reduced from 60–70% to around 30%. The treatment was further improved during 1958–1964 when normal saline replaced the hypertonic saline and antibiotics came into routine use and case fatality was reduced to around 1% in the treatment centers.[20,21] Oral rehydration with glucose–electrolyte solution (ORS) was developed in 1964–1968; this ORS further simplified the treatment and came into use in the 1970s (see Chapter 13).

To the south of Russia, cholera extended further westward into Bulgaria. In the spring of 1831, it advanced through Leningrad into Finland and Poland, where infection among the Polish troops helped the further dispersal of the disease in Poland and Austria. Hungary was affected in June, 1831 and Vienna in August. Despite "most rigid quarantine measures," cholera appeared in Prussia (Germany), reaching Berlin, Hamburg, and the Rhine province. In October, 1831, cholera appeared in the port of Sunderland, England, favored by the close shipping connections with German ports. The disease soon after appeared in various cities of England and Scotland, including London in February, 1832, and reached Ireland and Calais, France, in March, 1832.

There was a widespread cholera outbreak in Paris on March 24, 1832; of the first 98 cases, 96 perished. Belgium was affected near the French border in the spring of 1832, the Netherlands in June and Norway in the autumn, but a severe epidemic occurred there only in 1834.

Cholera existed in epidemic form in Arabia in 1828 and 1831, and a violent epidemic raged among the pilgrims assembled in Mecca. The governors of Mecca and Jeddah, the Pasha accompanying the Syrian caravan, and numerous other distinguished people were among the many victims of the epidemic when, it is said, the "living ceased to bury the dead singly." The returning pilgrims carried the disease to Syria, Palestine, Egypt (Cairo, Alexandria, Suez), Tunisia, and Istanbul, and then to Romania, Bulgaria, and Warsaw.

Cholera also crossed the Atlantic to reach the distant shores of America in 1832, accompanying the ships carrying Irish immigrants. Quarantine could not prevent the importation of cases, because not all ships could be quarantined and not always equally rigidly. Cholera broke out in Quebec on June 8 and on the 10th in Montreal, and then spread very fast along the St. Lawrence River and its tributaries into the interior of Canada. At about the same time, cholera appeared in New York (June 23) and Philadelphia (July 5). Despite all the dire warnings and the advice given by the newspapers in various cities[22,23] to prevent cholera by leading a "moral and temperate life," the disease continued its inexorable spread, reaching New Orleans, where it caused heavy casualties, and the west coast; the epidemics lasted for three to six weeks in most cities, killing so many people that mass burials were held. The ravage continued in New York, Louisiana, and elsewhere until about 1834. A further invasion seemed to have occurred in 1835 via New Orleans, extending across the south and up to Charleston, South Carolina; then the disease mysteriously disappeared for nearly 15 years.[22,23]

In Europe, Portugal, and Spain escaped invasion for a long time. However, a merchant steamer from England landed her passengers at Oporto and Foz in January 1833, bringing cholera into Portugal at the same time. Spain imposed draconian quarantine measures for travelers from infected areas; anyone entering Spain without going through quarantine was liable to be punished with the death sentence and to have his apparel burned; the same punishment was threatened to those who received such a person. Despite these precautions, cholera raged with great violence in many provinces during the summers of 1833 and 1834. Reports of cholera in Peru and Chile in 1832 remained unconfirmed, but it caused a severe epidemic in Cuba in February, 1833 and later in the year appeared in Mexico. In 1837, besides a coastal outbreak in Guyana and a severe epidemic in Nicaragua, cholera prevailed in Guatemala.

In 1834, the disease reached Morocco, probably from Spain. It reached Sweden, Toulon, Nice, Cannes, Turin, and Genoa in April, 1835 and traveled to Venice and Trieste and throughout the north of Italy in November. In 1836, cholera appeared in Prague, Milan, Sicily, Rome, Switzerland (via the Tessin) and Yugoslavia, and in 1837 in Malta and Algeria. During 1835–1837, the disease invaded Libya, Sudan, and Ethiopia, besides being very active in Egypt and Tunisia.

Although cholera broke out in epidemic form in Mecca during the 1835 pilgrimage, it was difficult to ascertain how much of the cholera problem in the world outside India in 1835–1837 was due to a reactivation of the earlier foci or to fresh importations from India. In 1839–1846, cholera appeared to be rather quiescent in Europe.

To the east of India, cholera appears to have persisted in Indonesia and the Philippines until 1830, and to have reached the Swan river region in Australia in 1832. There was a newspaper report of cholera on the west coast of Australia. Cholera was reported in the Straits Settlements and China in 1826, and there was a large epidemic in Canton in 1835. Japan was apparently reinfected in 1831. In 1840, troops from India were sent to Chusan, an island near Shanghai, where cholera broke out, spread to the mainland, and caused "one of the most frightful visitations."[8] Pollitzer[2] described at length how cholera found its way back from Canton in China eastwards to Rangoon in Burma, the Philippines, etc., and westward to Afghanistan and then back to the Punjab, Karachi, Delhi, Teheran, and towns on the Caspian Sea in 1845. He[2] also narrated a new wave of cholera from Bengal in 1845 that reached Madras, Ceylon, Bombay, and then Arabia again in 1846, and led to a reinvasion of Persia and Mesopotamia and further spread along the Euphrates and Tigris. In 1846, a large outbreak started from the port of Jeddah on the Red Sea and killed about 15,000 people near Mecca. In April, 1847, cholera spread along the Caspian shore to Astrakhan and then up the Volga, caused an epidemic in Tbilisi and progressed along the Black Sea coast and northeastwards across the Caucasus mountains into the interior of Russia.

After a lull in 1847 through early 1848, cholera continued to spread in Europe, reaching Norway in the North, the Balkan countries in the south, England, Scotland, and Ireland in the northwest, Spain in the southwest.

Cholera reached the United States again through Staten Island outside New York and New Orleans in 1848 despite strict quarantine measures, and continued for 7 years.[22] It spread along the Mississippi, reached Texas, and continued to flare up in New Orleans every year through 1855, and thereafter, in the form of scattered cases until 1866, when a large epidemic broke out.[22] Egypt was also affected seriously at this time by pilgrims returning from Mecca. The disease also reappeared in Istanbul and spread to Syria, Palestine, and neighboring areas.

In the spring of 1849, cholera reappeared all over France, Italy, and North Africa; the epidemic in England is said to have taken 53,293 lives. It is during this epidemic in London that one of the greatest discoveries in cholera epidemiology was made by John Snow,[24] a London anaesthetist and amateur epidemiologist, who demonstrated the role of water in the transmission of cholera, long before the causative agent was discovered; more definitive proof came from him again in 1855.[25]

Cholera was designated as "America's greatest scourge"[26] after its widespread ravages in 1849 from New York, as well as from New Orleans, the infection overran practically the whole land and reached Canada, which was also directly invaded by sea routes from Europe. The epidemic reached Mexico, and also Panama, by a ship from New Orleans.

In 1850, a violent epidemic appeared in Egypt and progressed along the coastal routes to North Africa. The problem reappeared in most areas of Europe affected earlier, and also the Maltese and Ionian islands in the south and Sweden in the north. Denmark was probably affected for the first time. The mainland of Greece was not affected at this time nor in 1832 and 1837.

Areas affected by cholera also expanded in the United States in 1850, when a ship from Panama introduced it to San Francisco, whence it spread by land to Sacramento, California. In South America, cholera reached Colombia and perhaps also Ecuador. In 1850 and 1851, it is reported to have caused a very severe epidemic in Cuba and Jamaica (affected for the first time) and also in Grand Canary Island (1851). Morocco faced a severe epidemic in the same year but cholera appeared to be quiescent in most of the countries of Europe, although there was evidence of a persistence of infection in Poland.

3.3. Third Pandemic (1852–1859)

Pollitzer[2] observed that the third pandemic was the combined result of recrudescences and importations, which may have been the case during all the pandemics after the first. Experience during the seventh pandemic (to be described later) has shown that it is often very difficult to determine when an outbreak in an endemic area is due to a recrudesence or is caused by an importation from outside the country.

International cooperation in health began for fear of cholera. The first international meeting was held in Paris in 1851, followed by 14 international sanitary conferences between 1851–1938. An International Sanitary Convention was signed in Paris in 1903, according to which all the signatories would inform each other of epidemics in their territories. In 1907, the Office International d'Hygiene, the first international health organization, was established in Paris. After the First World War, in 1920, the Health Organization of the League of Nations was established[21,27] and began to issue weekly reports on cholera and other epidemic diseases, an activity that has been continued by the World Health Organization (WHO), established in 1948. A comprehensive set of International Health (then called Sanitary) Regulations were approved on May 25, 1951 by the Fourth World Health Assembly; according to these, every member nation is required to notify WHO as soon as cholera appears in its territory. The 26th World Health Assembly in 1973 amended the Regulations on cholera as dictated by the new knowledge (see Chapter 15).

Cholera was rampant in 1853–1854 in Persia, Mesopotamia, Northern Europe, including England, the United States, Mexico, the West Indies, Colombia, and Canada. Troops moving from southern France during the Crimean War may have brought cholera to Greece and Turkey. In the Near East, cholera prevailed in Arabia, Syria, Asia Minor, Sudan, and Egypt, whence it spread along the coast to Morocco. Cape Verde was affected for the first time; cholera broke out in Venezuela and Brazil and also affected parts of Italy, Austria, and Switzerland in Europe. In 1856–1858, it caused problems only in Spain and Portugal.

When cholera occurred in Tuscany in Italy, Filippo Pacini examined the intestinal contents of some cadavers of cholera victims and found a large number of curved bacteria, which he called *Vibrio cholera*. This was a great discovery, but remained obscure as the finding was published in a little-known local journal in 1854; moreover, the etiological relationship was not convincingly demonstrated.[21]

In the East, beyond India, cholera was present in Indonesia in 1852; China and Japan were affected in 1854, but more seriously in 1857–1859 when the Philippines and Korea were also involved. In East Africa, cholera caused four outbreaks in Mauritius (1854–1862) and one in Réunion (1859). The infection spread from Zanzibar along the coast to Mozambique and from there to Madagascar, the Comoros Islands, and inland to Uganda. Epidemics also recurred in 1853, 1855, and 1858 in Ethiopia. In the Americas, cholera was recorded in various parts of Central America in 1856 and in Guyana in 1857.

The prevalence of cholera increased again in 1859 in Persia, Arabia, Mesopotamia, Russia, Sweden, Denmark, Western Prussia, the Netherlands, Spain, Morocco, and Algeria. In 1860, Gibraltar was also affected. Apart from the infection that apparently persisted in Leningrad until 1864, Europe seemed to remain free from cholera from the end of 1859.

3.4. Fourth Pandemic (1863–1879)

The Mecca pilgrimage in 1865 was the scene of a major epidemic. According to MacNamara,[8] about 30,000 deaths occurred out of 90,000 pilgrims. The after-effects of the epidemic were also disastrous, as the routes of spread changed from the ancient paths to Europe through Persia and the Caspian Sea ports to new traffic routes over Arabia to Egypt (Alexandria), Istanbul, Southern France, and Italy. With the returning pilgrims, cholera traveled to other parts of Arabia, Mesopotomia, Syria, Palestine, and Egypt, especially Alexandria. From Alexandria, the infection traveled by sea routes to Mediterranean ports such as Istanbul, Smyrna, Ancona, and Marseilles from which it spread to the interior of Turkey and France, Cyprus, Rhodes and other Ionian islands, Bulgaria, Romania, Bukovina in Austria, and southern Italy, including Sicily. Spain and Portugal were also affected through travelers. The invasion of Luxembourg in the same period probably led to the appearance of cholera in adjacent parts of Germany.

Historians recorded one of the worst epidemics in 1866, which might have been helped by the war between Austria and Italy and between Germany and Austria. About 90,000 people are said to have perished in Russia when cholera raged from Caucasus to Leningrad. Other deaths from cholera at the time included about 4500 in Sweden, 115,000 in Germany, 80,000 in Bohemia and Moravia in Austria, 30,000 in Hungary, 20,000 in the Netherlands, and 30,000 in Belgium, but only about 15,000 in Great Britain. In 1867, although cholera was less severe in Europe in general, about 113,000 lives were lost in Italy; Switzerland recorded a limited outbreak. In 1868, cholera reappeared in only a few European localities.

Cholera ravaged Africa in 1865 when the infection probably traveled via Aden (South Yemen), to Somalia and also from Jeddah (Arabia) across the Red Sea to Ethiopia; soon the region of Kilimanjaro was reached and from there it crossed Lake Tanganyika to the upper reaches of the Congo River. Traveling southeastwards, cholera reached Zanzibar, where 70,000 people are reported to have died in 1869. From Lake Tanganyika, the disease progressed along the western shore of Lake Nyasa and reached Mozambique in May, 1870; from there it again invaded Madagascar and the Comoros islands, and the Seychelles. In North Africa, Tunisia, Algeria, and Morocco were infected and reinfected by various ways and had severe and protracted outbreaks. In 1868–1869, Senegal and the Gambia in West Africa were invaded, probably from Morocco, and suffered heavy losses of human lives.

Sanitary conditions in the United States, particularly in New York, were still deplorable and favorable[23] for the spread of cholera when it arrived again in 1865–1866. It is said that cholera arrived in New York from Le Havre in the autumn of 1865, remained suppressed during the cold weather and broke out as an epidemic in May, 1866.[23] While the spread to southern states, such as Louisiana and Texas, was by ships, the development of train services and troop movements accelerated the extension to Cincinnati, Louisville, Chicago, St Louis, and to the Midwest as far as Kansas. The outbreaks were often relatively mild and short-lived, but New Orleans suffered badly and repeatedly until 1868.[22] In New York, the threat of cholera helped in creating the Metropolitan Board of Health, which resolved to clean up the city, to use disinfectants extensively, and to identify and isolate the cases, which helped to minimize the effects of the epidemic.[22,23] In 1832, cholera was considered a consequence of sin and a chastisement by God—in other words, a "moral problem"; by 1866, the outlook had changed and cholera had come to be recognized as a social problem requiring an improved environment including better housing, clean water, and waste disposal services.[23,27] The Croton aqueduct of New York is reported to have been a direct result of the cholera epidemic of 1832. It is said that the people of New York saw for the first time that their streets were made of stones after the cleaning campaigns for cholera control.[27] Cholera reappeared in New York, New Orleans, and the Mississippi Basin in 1873–1875, but in a minor way.[22,23] Persisting rumors of its presence up until 1890 helped to keep the health agencies working to promote public health.

Canada remained free during this period, but Nicaragua and British Honduras were infected via New Orleans during 1866–1868. The disease also affected Paraguay, Brazil, Argentina, Uruguay, Bolivia, and Peru during this period.

Cholera did not cause much of a problem in Central Europe during these years, except in Russia where cases continued to occur in 1868; a severe epidemic broke out in 1869 in Kiev, and was more widespread in 1870–1872, claiming about 130,000 lives in 1871 and 1872. Fewer outbreaks were reported in 1873, but cholera was prevalent in Poland in 1873–1874. During 1871, cholera spread to Romania, Bulgaria, Istanbul, and Asia Minor; it remained active in 1872–1873 and spread to Salonica. In 1871, the disease spread westward from Russia to Finland, Sweden, Prussia (Berlin, Hamburg), and Austria. In 1873–1874, major outbreaks in many parts of Germany, including Bavaria, killed about 33,000 people; Austria had a serious outbreak in 1872, and about 190,000 died in 1872–1873 in Hungary.

Imported or indigenous sporadic cases or small outbreaks continued to occur in Great Britain, the Netherlands, Belgium, and France (Paris and Cannes), but did not cause a serious problem during this period. Cholera also recurred in Sweden and Norway in 1873.

An exacerbation of the cholera situation in Persia, in 1870, and the reappearance of cholera in Mecca, in 1872, led to the spread of infection to Turkish Kurdistan, Mesopotamia, Arabia, Egypt, Bukhara, and Russian Turkisthan, and Sudan. Syria was devastated in 1875. In India also, cholera caused a severe epidemic in 1875.

During this pandemic, the parts of Asia to the southeast or east of India suffered repeatedly. Major epidemics were recorded in China in 1862, 1864–1865, and 1877–1879, Japan in 1864–1865, and Indonesia in 1863–1864; the epidemic in Thailand and Malaysia, in 1873, also affected the people of Sumatra, Java, Madura, and Singapore, Borneo, and the Celebes seriously.

3.5. Fifth Pandemic (1881–1896)

Cholera was widespread in Europe during this period. There were serious exacerbations in India (1881) and in Mecca (1881 and 1882); returning pilgrims from Mecca and a fair in Egypt helped to disseminate the disease widely in Egypt, where it claimed more than 58,000 lives. During these epidemics, Robert Koch studied cholera in Alexandria, Egypt, and in Calcutta, India, and demonstrated conclusively, in 1883, that the disease was caused by a comma-shaped organism, which he called *Kommabazillen*.[2,21]

In Europe during 1884–1887, the pandemic was confined to France (Toulon, Marseilles, Paris), Italy (widespread, mainly Naples), and Spain (Valencia, Murcia) where case fatality was around 50%. Spain was again affected in 1890. Despite repeated invasions by imported cases, Great Britain resisted local spread thanks to the marked improvements in sanitation and water supply.[27] Disraeli's Great Public Health Act compelled all authorities to provide drainage, sewerage, and water supply, although most people in Great Britain continued to uphold the view that cholera was not contagious. The last indigenous case in the country was in 1893.[27] Cholera again came into the United States in 1887 and 1892, but did not cause any secondary cases because of general improvement in living conditions and possibly indirectly by the efforts, described by Chambers,[26] "to put bacteriology to practical use in combating an invasion by the scourge." Cholera continued to rage, however, in South America: Argentina (1886–1887 and 1894–1895), Chile (1887–1888), Brazil (1893–1895), and Uruguay (1895).

Cholera outbreaks in Afghanistan and Persia, in 1892, were followed by others in Baku, Moscow, and Leningrad (1893–1894), which claimed about 800,000 lives.[2] A large outbreak was recorded in Hamburg in 1892, (transmitted by unfiltered water from the Elbe) and in other parts of Germany in the following year. The northern part of France was affected in 1892, southern France in 1893, and sporadic cases continued to appear in 1894 in Toulon, Marseilles, and Paris.

In Africa, cholera was recorded during 1893–1896 in Libya, Tunisia, Algeria, Morocco, French West Africa, Sudan, and Egypt. Among the countries east of India, cholera was also reported during 1888–1896 in Indonesia, Sri Lanka, Thailand, Malaysia, and China (where widespread disease was found in 1881–1883, 1888, 1890, and 1895) and in Korea (1881, 1888, 1890, 1891, and 1895). Cholera epidemics in Japan in 1881, 1882, 1885, 1886, 1890, 1891, and 1895 are reported to have involved a total of about 340,000 cases. The disease was also recorded in the Philippines in 1882, 1888, and 1889.

3.6. Sixth Pandemic (1899–1923)

Pollitzer[2] felt very strongly that this pandemic was closely connected with the exacerbation of cholera in India in 1899, although Sticker (quoted by Pollitzer) had pointed out that it had not totally disappeared from Western Asia and Egypt. Cholera appeared in Afghanistan and Persia in 1900 and at a Mecca pilgrimage in 1902. Strict quarantine measures for returning pilgrims were imposed and the El Tor vibrio was discovered in 1905 from the intestines of persons who had died of diseases other than cholera in the El Tor quarantine camp in the Sinai Peninsula of Egypt.[2] Despite all efforts, cholera appeared in Asyut and elsewhere in Egypt, claiming about 34,000 victims. It then appeared in 1903 in Syria, Palestine, Asia Minor (along the Black Sea coast), Mesopotamia, Persia, and Russia.

In Western Europe, cholera was recorded as sporadic cases or restricted outbreaks like the one in Rotterdam in the Netherlands in 1909. In Central and southeastern Europe, however, there was a large outbreak in 1910–1911 in Italy, particularly in the south, reported to have been brought in by gypsies from Russia. In 1910 and 1913, cholera epidemics were recorded in Hungary. Cholera was reported in and near the camps in Hungary, Austria, and Germany where Russian war prisoners were imprisoned and in the German army camp in Turkey. According to Pollitzer, cholera was recorded in the Balkan Peninsula in Greece, Turkey, Bulgaria, Yugoslavia, Romania, and Albania during 1910–1922.

Cholera broke out at a Mecca pilgrimage again in 1907, and was rampant in Arabia in 1908–1912, after which Mecca is claimed to have remained free. Persia was badly affected in 1906 and again in 1911, 1912, 1914, 1919, and 1922–1923. During and after the First World War, cholera was present in Turkey (1916), Mesopotamia (1918–1919 and 1923), and Palestine (1918).

Inside Russia, cholera began to travel widely in 1904 and caused more than 53,000 cases; in 1910 alone there were about 230,000 cases.[2] Cholera seems to have abated after 1911, but there were about 66,000 cases in 1915 during the First World War and again about 20,000 in 1920 and 207,000 in 1921. The number of cases began to fall in 1923 and only sporadic cases were recorded in 1924–1925, after which Europe was considered free from cholera.

In 1910, infected passengers aboard a steamer from Russia on its way to South America brought the disease to Madeira, which became the westernmost limit of this pandemic. Imported cases were detected and quarantined in the US during most of these years; the last indigenous cases occurred in Massachusetts and New York in 1911.[28]

To the east of India, cholera affected Burma (Myanmar) and Malaysia in 1901, and most parts of the Far East, including China, Manchuria, Japan, Korea, and the Philippines from 1902 onwards; it continued to occur in most of these countries even after 1925.

4. CHOLERA DURING 1926–1960

Although cholera disappeared from Europe after 1925, it did not remain confined to the Indian subcontinent. It continued to occur, either regularly or intermittently, in Sri Lanka until 1953, in Nepal until 1958, in Burma (Myanmar) and Thailand until 1960, in Indonesia, Japan, Korea, Macao, and Hong Kong until 1957, in Malaysia and the Philippines until 1937, and in French Indo-China until 1958–1959. China suffered severely in 1940 and again in 1946; it reported sporadic cases until 1948, after which no information was available until 1980. In the west, cholera was present in West Pakistan until 1949; it appeared in 1930 in Afghanistan, where it caused large outbreaks during 1936–1939 and small ones in 1941 and 1946. In Iran, cholera epidemics were recorded in 1927, 1931, and 1938–1939. Iraq, particularly Basra, was also affected in 1927 and 1931.

A very significant event during this period was a large cholera outbreak in Egypt in 1947, with nearly 33,000 cases and 20,500 deaths. The origin of this epidemic remained undetermined, but it was certainly not brought by pilgrims returning from Mecca and was shown not to have been brought from India by British troops. A smaller outbreak also occurred in Syria in 1947–1948.

Two very important scientific advances in the field of cholera occurred during this period: the discovery of cholera toxin in 1953 by De,[29] and the development of an improved therapy by the team of Captain Philips.[20,21]

5. THE SEVENTH PANDEMIC (1961–?)

In 1937, a mild, choleralike disease caused by the El Tor vibrio, designated later by the taxonomists as *V. cholerae* 01, biotype El Tor, was described in Indonesia and was called "Paracholera" by de Moor[30,31] and "Enteritis choleriformis El Tor" by van Loghem.[32] Tanamal[33] later described four outbreaks of this disease in Sulawesi (Celebes), Indonesia, during 1937–1958, where it was endemic.

In 1959–1960, a small outbreak of mild, choleralike disease caused by this vibrio was detected in Ubol province of northern Thailand, but it did not spread beyond this region.[34] In May–June, 1961, however, a few cases of cholera caused by the El Tor vibrio appeared in Java and Semarang in Indonesia, and later the infection spread out to neighboring countries, and went on a pandemic rampage, defying all previous notions about its lack of epidemic potential. This seventh pandemic caught the health authorities of the region unprepared as most of the area had been free from cholera for several years. The causative agent of the first four pandemics was not isolated, but that of the fifth and sixth was the classical biotype of *V. cholerae* 01. It may therefore be safely assumed that this is the first pandemic to be caused by the El Tor vibrio and there is no doubt that it started from Sulawesi, Indonesia.*

The circumstances that helped the El Tor biotype of *V. cholerae* 01 to spread from its endemic focus in Sulawesi (Celebes), where it began to be more active than usual in January, 1961, will probably never be known. The increase in population movements as a result of political disturbances, and the availability of faster transport systems that freed small towns and villages from their isolation may both have contributed to the spread of infection. The emergence of the El Tor biotype from Celebes in 1961 strikes one as similar to that of the classical biotype from India in 1817. It is known that the El Tor vibrio, which is sturdier than the classical biotype, can cause large numbers of inapparent infections and mild cases, whose mobility remains unrestricted, and that carriers excrete the vibrio for a longer period. Today's laboratory techniques remain inadequate to detect any enhancement of the communicability or virulence of the organism that might have played a role in initiating this pandemic. It may be relevant to mention here that in 1965 both the classical and the El Tor biotype of *V. cholerae* were present in Afghanistan, but when cholera spread to neighboring Iran, all the cases there were caused by El Tor.

The number of countries affected during this pandemic has increased in two major phases: a gradual increase from 1961–1966 when there was a lull, followed by a major

---

*El Tor vibrios had been isolated earlier from surface waters unconnected with cases in several places in the Indian subcontinent, which were later found to be nontoxigenic. During this pandemic, atypical, nontoxigenic *V. cholerae* 01 of the El Tor biotype (some of them showing irregular biochemical and serological reactions) have been isolated mainly from environmental sources (clean and fecally contaminated water, sewage, oysters, etc.), having no apparent connection with cases of diarrhea. Two strains came from extraintestinal sites in two men in the US—a leg ulcer and the gall bladder. These atypical El Tor vibrios have been isolated in Asia, including Japan, the Pacific Islands, North and South America, Europe, and the Eastern Mediterranean region, suggesting that they may be free-living.

upsurge in 1970–1971 (with an extension into Africa and Europe. Since 1972, the number of countries affected in any one year has declined). A matter of continuous concern about the pandemic reaching South and Central America persisted until the end of 1990, when a dramatic flare-up had taken place (see Epilogue).

After moving out of Indonesia, the pandemic traveled from one country to its neighbors in a predictable fashion until 1966, as can be seen from Table 2 (the rumor of an extension in 1961 to Kwantung province of China could not be confirmed).[34] The etiologic agent was of the Ogawa serotype and was typical El Tor vibrio (being hemolytic by the usual test); in 1962 nonhemolytic strains began to appear in increasing numbers.[35,36] Serotype Inaba appeared later in some areas, although the Ogawa serotype nearly always remained more prevalent.

In 1962, the World Health Organization convened a Scientific Working Group meeting to review the dramatic change in the cholera situation. This group recommended inclusion of the disease caused by the El Tor vibrio in the definition of cholera under the International Health Regulations. The proposal was approved by the Fifteenth World Health Assembly in May, 1962.

In 1963, the pandemic strain reached Chittagong, East Pakistan (now Bangladesh) and Calcutta, India, in 1964. In India, the El Tor biotype almost completely replaced the classical biotype within a year of invasion, though in Bangladesh *V. cholerae* of the classical biotype remained predominant until the end of 1972. Epidemiologically, it is significant to note that in India, after the change in prevalent biotype, cholera appeared in areas of the country that never before had been affected by the disease or had been free from it for many years. While the number of infected foci increased in India, the number of reported cases continued to decline, particularly in West Bengal where there was no major outbreak after 1963 until June, 1971, when cholera broke out among refugees from East Pakistan. In 1965, the pandemic spread further westward and invaded West Pakistan, Afghanistan, Iran, and a limited area in Uzbekistan (USSR). Iraq was affected in the following year. Rigid quarantine measures to restrict the movements of people and trade, vaccination, and mass chemoprophylaxis were applied, particularly in Iran, but the spread continued. Only the provision of early treatment, along with surveillance to detect cases, reduced case–fatality and panic.

A large outbreak of the classical biotype was recorded in West Pakistan in 1968, and (despite the incompleteness of reports,) cholera was found to be more widespread in 1969. For example, Laos reported cholera for the first time. Hong Kong, Macao, and the Republic of Korea were affected again after remaining practically free from the disease since 1965. Nepal, Malaysia, and Burma (Myanmar) reported higher figures than in the preceding two or more years.

In 1970, about nine years after the beginning of this seventh pandemic, cholera invaded

TABLE 2
Extension of the Seventh Pandemic during 1961–1966 (El Tor)

1961	1962	1963	1964	1965	1966
Sarawak	Sabah	Republic of Korea	India	Brunei	Iraq
Hong Kong	Taiwan	Cambodia	Vietnam	Nepal	
Macao	West Irian	Thailand	Bahrain	Pakistan	
Philippines	North Borneo	Singapore		USSR	
		Burma		Iran	
		West Malaysia			
		East Pakistan (Bangladesh)			

Africa and Europe and dominated the world's public health problems. The first report of its westward extension beyond Iraq came from the USSR in August, 1970, when cholera appeared in Astrakhan on the coast of the Caspian Sea (serotype Inaba) and in Odessa and Kersh on the coast of the Black Sea (serotype Ogawa). Soon afterwards cholera was reported from West Asia in Lebanon, Israel, Syria, and Jordan, and from North Africa in Libya and Tunisia. There was also a strong rumor of outbreaks of "summer disease" in Egypt, in June, when mass anticholera vaccination of the whole population was undertaken.[37]

The most surprising and momentous event of this time was the report of cholera from Guinea in West Africa where the disease was most probably brought in (imported by air)[38] by students returning from a northeast African country (Egypt?)[37] (but no definite evidence of this is available). Cholera was introduced into West Africa in 1868,[8] but at that time, it failed to gain a foothold. Pollitzer[2] subsequently referred to the presence of cholera in the Sene–Gambian region in 1893–1894, without giving many details. In 1970, however, the disease caused by the Ogawa serotype invaded one West African country after another, infecting no less than 11 (Guinea, Sierra Leone, Liberia, Ghana, Ivory Coast, Mali, Togo, Dahomey, Upper Volta, Nigeria, and Niger) during the last four months of the year. Cholera spread almost systematically from west to east along the coast of West Africa,[38–40] following the routes of fishermen and traders, and set up many endemic foci in communities on the coast and around the lagoons. In November, 1970, it jumped inland and reached Mopti (Mali), an important commercial center with many road and river communications, where it caused a catastrophic situation. The spread in dry areas of Africa[38,39] continued unabated following the movements of people, large gatherings at fairs, markets, and funerals. Traditional funerary customs played a major role in transmission. Attempts to control the disease by vaccination, chemoprophylaxis, or a *cordon sanitaire* had little effect on the course of the epidemics. Case–fatality rates of more than 50% were recorded at the beginning of most new epidemics, but these came down to 7–10% when treatment procedures and facilities became organized.[38]

Cholera caused by the Inaba serotype appeared at about the same time in the Arabian peninsula, in the Trucial Sheikdoms (Dubai) and Saudi Arabia, and then, possibly after crossing the Red Sea, in Ethiopia, the French Territory of the Afars and the Issas (Djibouti) and Somalia before the end of 1970. In Europe, outside the USSR, cholera appeared in Istanbul in Turkey and in a village in Czechoslovakia. One indigenous case was detected in France.

On December 18, 1970, the US announced that cholera vaccination certificates would no longer be required from travelers entering the US from infected countries. The requirement of this certificate was abolished from the International Health Regulations later, in 1973.

During 1971, cholera spread further to Oman, Democratic Yemen, and Yemen in West Asia, to Cameroon, Chad, Mauritania, and Senegal in West Africa, to Angola, Kenya, and Uganda in East Africa, to Morocco and Algeria in North Africa, and to Spain and Portugal in Europe.

Figure 1 shows the global spread of cholera caused by the El Tor biotype from the beginning of the present pandemic until 1981. Although the number of infected territories grew considerably, the number of cholera cases reported annually to WHO did not show any remarkable increase until 1971. It is significant that cholera was reported by 10 countries in 1968, by 14 in 1969, and by 36 in 1970 as well as in 1971; 26 new countries were affected in 1970 and 14 in 1971. During 1972–1986, the number of countries reporting cholera varied from 27 to 43 with 0 to 7 new ones, but because of deficient reporting, the numbers of cases

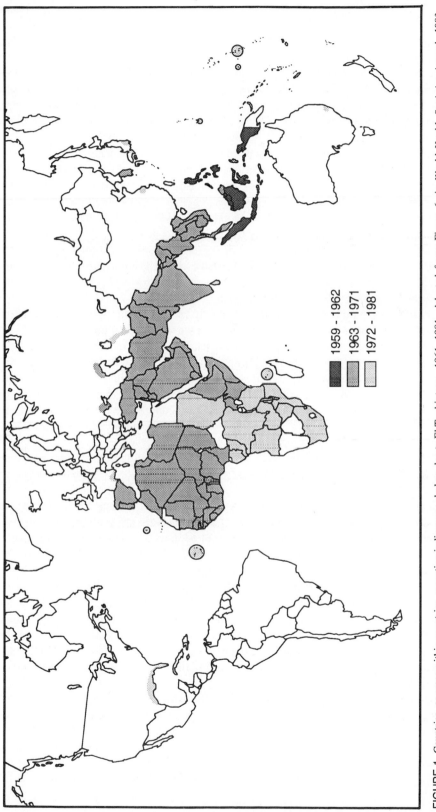

FIGURE 1. Countries, or areas within countries, reporting indigenous cholera due to El Tor biotype, 1961–1981. Adapted from: Figure 6, in *World Health Statistics Annual, 1983.* Geneva, World Health Organization (1983). Reprinted by permission.

Legend:
- 1959 - 1962
- 1963 - 1971
- 1972 - 1981

and countries notified to WHO can only indicate a trend.[38] About 155,000 cases, the largest number reported in any one year during this pandemic, were notified in 1971; about one-third of these cases were among the refugees from East Pakistan (Bangladesh) in West Bengal. Figures reported to WHO do not give a wholly accurate picture of the situation for several reasons: reports of sizeable outbreaks of cholera in some countries are not confirmed; adequate surveillance is not possible in most of the cholera-affected countries; and clinically diagnosed cholera cases represent only a fraction of the total number of cases.

There was no extension of the pandemic in 1972, but 374 passengers and 19 crew members were exposed to the infection on board a scheduled flight from London to Sidney and New Zealand with the result that 40 confirmed cases were diagnosed in Sydney and three in New Zealand, including one fatal case. A meal prepared in the flight kitchen in Bahrain and served in-flight was epidemiologically linked with this outbreak. The same meal supplied to another flight going from Sydney to London also brought on two cases of cholera.

In 1973, Italy suffered serious losses in its tourist trade when cholera broke out in August around Naples and Bari with some sporadic cases in other parts of the country. A minor outbreak, with 12 cases, was also detected in Cagliari, Sardinia. Uncooked seafood was the most important vehicle of transmission.

In Africa, the pandemic extended to Malawi, Mozambique, and Southern Rhodesia (now Zimbabwe); large numbers of cases were reported by previously infected Angola, Liberia, Nigeria, Senegal, and Upper Volta (now Burkina Faso). In Asia, Sri Lanka reported cholera for the first time since 1953; the Philippines reported 5600 cases in 1972 and 2075 in 1973, and Indonesia reported 44,300 cases in 1972 and 52,000 in 1973.

The classical biotype of *V. cholerae,* which had continued to prevail in Bangladesh despite the appearance of the El Tor biotype in Chittagong in 1963, was replaced almost entirely by the latter biotype in 1973. However, the classical biotype reappeared in small numbers in 1979 but in larger numbers in 1982, and has continued to co-exist since then with the El Tor biotype.[41] These two biotypes do, however, show different seasonal prevalences. In India, a few strains of the classical biotype were isolated in 1968,[42] but have not been seen since.

The pandemic extended still further in Africa in 1974 when Cape Verde, South Africa, and the southern part of the United Republic of Tanzania were affected; in the latter country the infection failed to spread.[43] Mozambique and Malawi again reported more than 1000 cases each. In Asia, Indonesia reported more than 41,000 cases and Sri Lanka about 4500. Guam became the first territory in Oceania to be reached by this pandemic.

A very significant event that year was the cholera outbreak at the Mecca pilgrimage— the first during this pandemic. It may be recalled[44] that this pilgrimage had been affected by 27 epidemics during 1850–1931 and had often been responsible for the wide dissemination of infection. Thirteen years after the beginning of the seventh pandemic, cholera broke out among the pilgrims there from Nigeria. Although there were more than one million people, only about 90 cases were involved. Some countries like Kuwait and France detected a few cases among returning pilgrims.

In Europe, a large outbreak affected almost the whole of Portugal. This epidemic was better investigated than many others and 42% of tested shellfish were found to harbor *V. cholerae* 01; infection was shown to be closely associated with ingestion of raw or poorly cooked cockles, water from a spring, and a brand of commercially bottled (possibly uncarbonated) water.[45]

Only one new country, Comoros (Africa), was affected in 1975, with more than 2000 cases, while Kenya continued to be troubled in this and the following year. Indonesia again reported more than 48,000 cases and Portugal about 1000 cases.

In 1976 and 1977, cholera was quiescent, but Indonesia again reported about 41,000 cases in 1976 and 17,000 in 1977. Ghana had a major epidemic again in 1976–1979, the first having occurred in 1970–1972. The third recrudescence in this country was recorded in 1983–1984. These recurrent, large and widespread epidemics occurred at a time when there were mass population movements for various reasons; there was also a severe drought in 1977 associated with food and water shortages.[46]

The United Republic of Tanzania was infected for the second time in 1977. One person developed cholera and died in a remote village of a coastal island, which had received a visitor from a country in the Middle East. The epidemic broke out after the funeral of the first case. The information did not reach the health authorities until one month later, by which time cholera cases were widespread.[43]

A second island country in Oceania, the Gilbert Islands (Kiribati), was reached by the pandemic in 1977. Japan also reported a limited outbreak in Wakayama Prefecture during that year.

An interesting report from Singapore[47] on 202 cases and 51 carriers detected during 1963–1976 indicated that 93% of the cases occurred in the ethnic group that constituted 76% of the population; also, about 91% of the houses of the cases and carriers had access to piped water and 52% were served with a water-borne sewage-disposal system. Careful epidemiological studies suggested that contaminated food sold at hawkers' stalls was an important vehicle of transmission.

In 1978, there was a marked expansion of the pandemic to 7 new countries: Burundi, Congo, Rwanda, Zaire, and Zambia in Africa, the Maldives in Asia, and Nauru in Oceania. Zaire has since been plagued by severe epidemics almost every year and had more than 10,000 cases in 1982.

The United Republic of Tanzania reported more than 6600 cases in 1978 (and continues to record large number of cases every year until now). Mass tetracycline prophylaxis had been employed in this country for cholera control in 1977 and widespread multiple drug resistance appeared within 6 months. The use of tetracycline was thereafter limited to cases and close contacts, and, in 1980, only to cases, after which the drug resistance declined significantly.[48] In Cameroon, mass chemoprophylaxis with sulfadoxine (fanasil) was employed during the large outbreak in 1983; this was followed by the isolation of a large number of strains resistant not only to sulfadoxine but also to tetracycline, chloramphenicol, and trimethoprim-sulfamethoxazole in 1984–1985.[49] Rumors of the emergence of multiple drug-resistant strains after mass chemoprophylaxis in some other countries remained unreported.

In 1979–1981, multiple drug-resistant *V. cholerae* were also prevalent in Bangladesh, but with a different pattern.[50] Easy availability to antimicrobials on the market might have led to this development as mass chemoprophylaxis was not used in this country.

In 1978, the Maldives recorded more than 11,000 cases out of its population of 200,000. In the same year Japan recorded another small outbreak, which was found to be connected with food served at several wedding receptions in a hall.

During 1979–1986 the pandemic extended to Gabon and Sudan in 1979, Swaziland in 1981, the Trust Territory of the Pacific Islands in 1982, and Equatorial Guinea in 1984, bringing the total number of countries or territories affected by the seventh pandemic to 93.

Reporting cholera accurately is difficult; reportage has seldom been complete and it has become more deficient during recent years. Bangladesh stopped reporting in 1980 and the

Philippines in 1982 mainly because of excessive trade restrictions applied by a few countries. Although such measures were often imposed on the strength of suspicion or rumors, some countries found it possible to carry on the trade by not reporting. Underreporting has become a common feature. In most cases, however, reports were received by WHO when cholera caused a public health problem or invaded a new country, though sometimes only after wide coverage in the media.

In Europe, cholera was detected again in 1979 in Cagliari (Italy) and in eight districts of Spain where many of the 267 cases appeared in sporadic fashion.

In Africa, large epidemics raged during 1979–1983 in Mozambique, Kenya, and Zaire, during 1979–1984 in South Africa, and during 1984–1986 in the drought-affected countries of Burkina Faso, Niger, Mali, Mauritania, and Senegal in addition to Ghana and the United Republic of Tanzania, mentioned earlier. Cameroon also had another epidemic in 1985. In North Africa, Algeria reported an epidemic in 1979 and sporadic cases thereafter.

Somalia reported a large number of cases in refugee camps in 1985 and 1986. Reports of similar epidemics in the camps in Ethiopia and Sudan remained officially unconfirmed.

In Asia, China reported cholera only in 1980, although the disease had been recognized as "Paracholera" in certain parts of the country before then. In 1981, for the first time, the health authorities of the Mecca Pilgrimage waived the requirement of a cholera vaccination certificate. Although a few imported cases and carriers were detected in both Medina and Mecca, no significant local transmission occurred.[51] The health authorities made ample provision for safe water supply, facilities for excreta and waste disposal, proper surveillance, and prompt action. Earlier, requirements of a stool examination report, five days' stay in a cholerafree area before arrival, and antibiotic chemoprophylaxis for pilgrims coming from infected areas had already been abolished.

During this period large numbers of cases were reported by Indonesia (1979–1985), Islamic Republic of Iran (1979, 1981), Jordan (1979, 1981), Malaysia (1979), Syrian Arab Republic (1979), and Democratic Yemen (1979, 1980). India continued to report only about 2000 to 8000 cases a year, and, in 1986, for the first time did not enforce the use of cholera vaccine during the country's largest pilgrimage at Kumbh Mela, relying instead, with success, on surveillance and sanitation measures.

The number of countries reporting cholera to WHO during 1982–1989 has varied from 30–37 each year as compared to 40 and 42 in 1980 and 1981; one new country, Guinea-Bissau was affected in 1986, and two, Sao-Tome and Principe in Africa and Yugoslavia in Europe, in 1989.

Many countries with safe water, good sanitation, and surveillance repeatedly notified imported cases during 1970–1989 and were successful in preventing local transmission or limiting it to a few indigenous cases.

There is little doubt that cholera has become endemic in most of the countries that were infected. A higher prevalence in the younger age groups and sporadic cases with seasonal and periodic exacerbations have been noted in many countries. In India alone, 56 hyperendemic districts scattered all over the country have been identified.[52] In one Asian country, an indigenous sporadic case was detected about 10 years after the last epidemic, showing that infection by *V. cholerae* 01, biotype El Tor, may remain latent or undetected for a long time, particularly in the absence of careful surveillance.

In most of the affected countries of the developing world, Africa in particular, this pattern of endemicity with occasional recrudescences to serious epidemic proportions continued during the eighties; the total number of countries annually reporting cholera to WHO decreased from 42 in 1981 to 30–37 during 1982–1990. One new country (Guinea-Bissau in

Africa) was affected in 1986, two (Sao Tome and Principe in Africa and Yugoslavia in Europe) in 1989 and three (Romania in Europe, New Zealand and Tuvalu in Oceania) in 1990. This relatively calm period, like that observed earlier during this pandemic (1966–1969), did not last, however.

For a long time cholera had refused to fulfill the predictions about transatlantic extension of the pandemic to the Western Hemisphere in the 1970s and 1980s. It finally revealed its notorious capricious propensity by appearing in early 1991 on the pacific coast of the New World in a relatively unexpected site. With this, the history of this pandemic has taken a new turn and the cholera situation has worsened considerably again, as was the case when cholera invaded Africa in the early 1970s. The Epilogue gives a separate account of this problem.

6. INDIGENOUS CHOLERA IN THE UNITED STATES AND AUSTRALIA

The first domestically acquired case of cholera in the United States after 1911 was detected in 1973 in Port Lavaca, Texas. Extensive investigation could not discover the source of this infection. Indigenous cases and carriers were again detected in 1978, 1981, and 1986 along the same Gulf Coast in Louisiana, East Texas, and Florida.[53,54] Ingestion of seafood was found to be closely associated with the infection. The organisms isolated in all three areas were similar: toxigenic and typically hemolytic *V. cholerae* 01, biotype El Tor, serotype Inaba, of a distinct but identical phage-type and having the same restriction endonuclease pattern by genetic analysis.[54] As has been mentioned earlier, by this time nearly all the pandemic strains were non- or poorly hemolytic.[35,36] These bacteriological findings strongly suggest that the Gulf Coast of the United States is a longstanding endemic focus of *V. cholerae* 01 biotype El Tor infection, like Sulawesi (Celebes) in Indonesia; therefore, these cases in the United States should not be considered as an extension of the pandemic.[21,53]

In 1977, the isolation of typically hemolytic and toxigenic *V. cholerae* 01, biotype El Tor, serotype Inaba, from an indigenous case of cholera in Queensland, Australia, led to the discovery of the presence of the same type of *V. cholerae* 01 in a section of the Albert–Logan river system with no source of contamination.[55,56] Since then, the persistence of the vibrio in a total of 13 rivers in the area and the occurrence of several sporadic cases and carriers directly or indirectly linked with some of these sources have been described.[57] These areas are probably also longstanding endemic foci of the infection, being discovered now because of better surveillance and laboratory techniques.

7. CONCLUSIONS

The history of cholera is fascinating because the disease is so elusive. Much more is known about the mechanism and treatment of cholera than about many other infectious diseases, but the reasons for its unpredictable appearances and disappearances, the emergence of *V. cholerae* 01, biotype El Tor, from obscurity to give rise to the extensive seventh pandemic, and its ability to replace the firmly established classical biotype on the Indian subcontinent (and later to reestablish coexistence with it in Bangladesh) will continue to baffle epidemiologists. The similarity in the emergence of the El Tor biotype from Celebes in 1961 and of the classical biotype from India in 1817 is also remarkable.

It is true that cholera decided the fate of several wars and caused much human suffering in the last century, but historians have commented that, at that time, cholera attracted much more attention than other infectious disease that were of equal, if not more, importance. This attitude towards cholera led to rapid sanitary reforms in many countries and to a change in their disease, which had prevented it from being looked upon purely as a technical problem. This was understandable during the previous pandemics when treatment and control measures were not known.

During the seventh pandemic, experience in many countries has shown that while the introduction of cholera into a country cannot be prevented, its spread within the country can be checked. Treatment is so successful today that no cholera patient need die if treatment can be made available. Despite these and many other developments during the last three decades (a very productive period for cholera research), attitudes towards the disease remain much the same, and there is little prospect that socioeconomic conditions in developing countries will change enough soon to bring an impact on the epidemiology of cholera.

In the closing years of the twentieth century, the global situation of cholera—with endemic areas scattered throughout Asia, Africa, and many countries of South and Central America—is far worse than it was at the end of the first quarter of the century, when the sixth pandemic ended. The quirks of cholera are therefore likely to continue to bring trouble and despair to many more people of the world for a long time to come. While the scientists remain busy unraveling the mysteries of this disease and searching for an effective vaccine, the health workers can bring much relief to the people by implementing the measures known to be effective (see Chapter 15).

ACKNOWLEDGMENT. I should like to thank Mrs. C.A. Martinez, Technical Officer, Diarrhoeal Diseases Control Programme, WHO, for her expert editorial assistance.

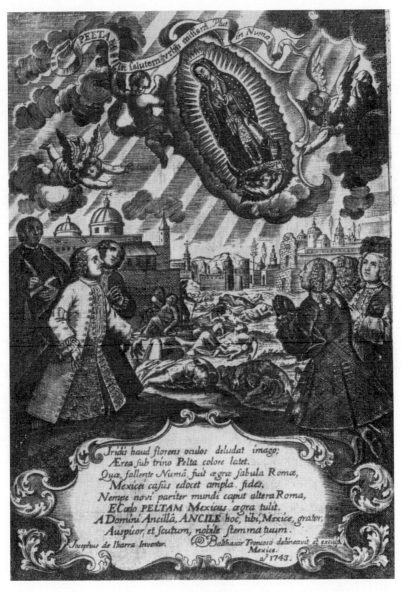

FIGURE 2.

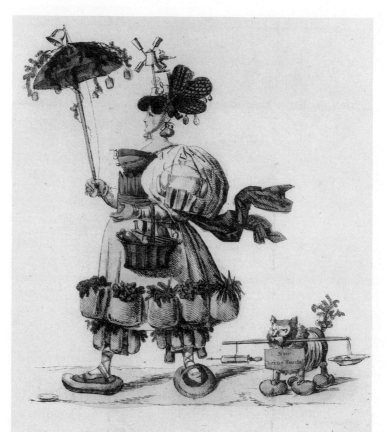

FIGURE 3.

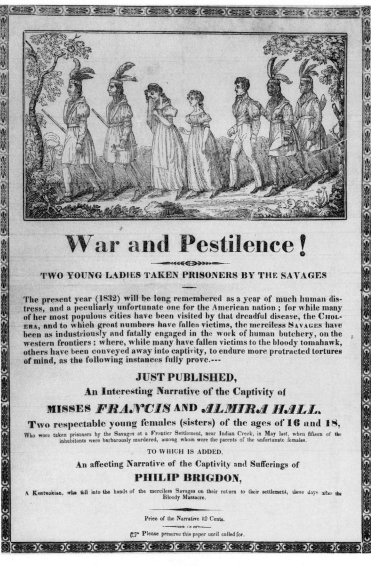

FIGURE 4.

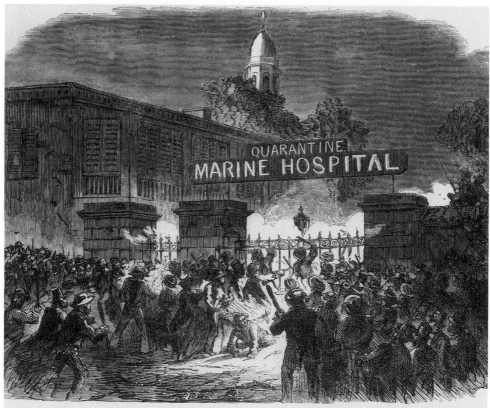

ATTACK ON THE QUARANTINE ESTABLISHMENT, ON SEPTEMBER 1, 1858.

FIGURE 5.

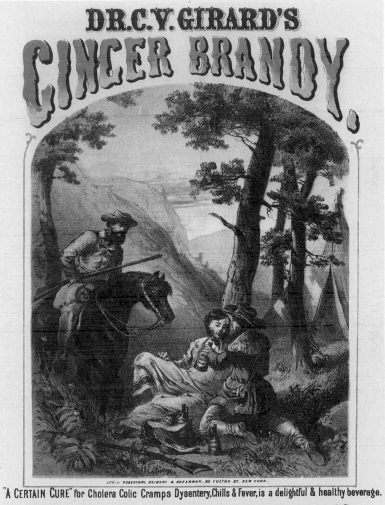

FIGURE 6.

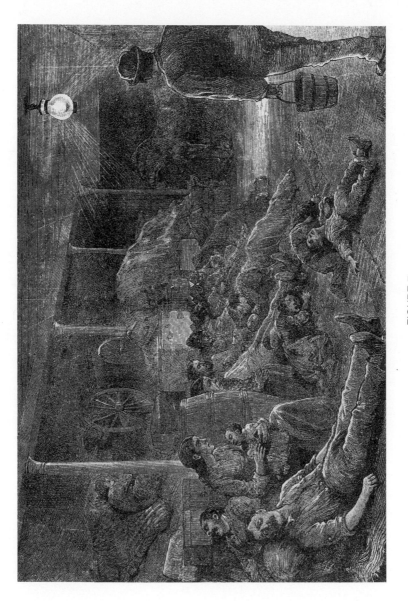

FIGURE 7.

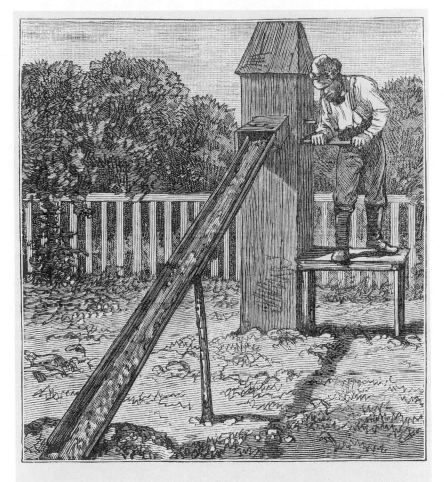

HOW TO DISPOSE OF SEWERAGE.

FIGURE 8.

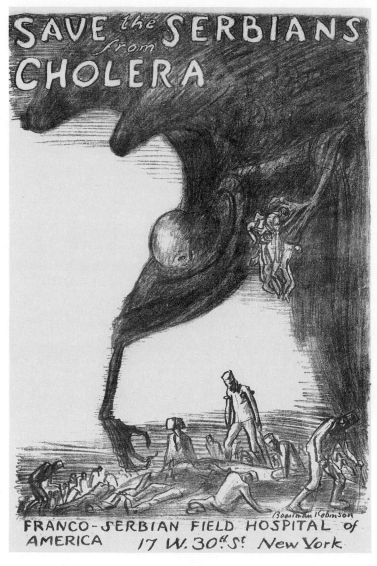

FIGURE 9.

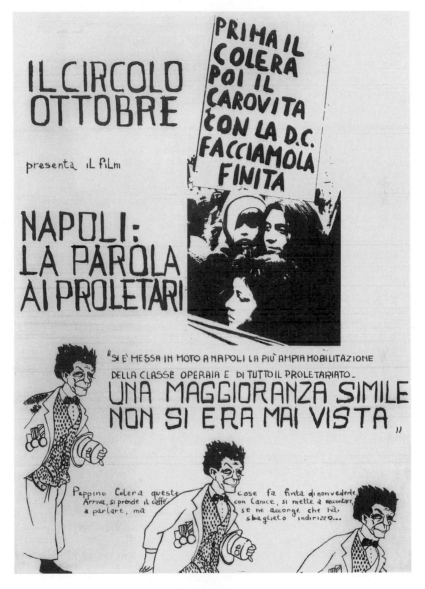

FIGURE 10.

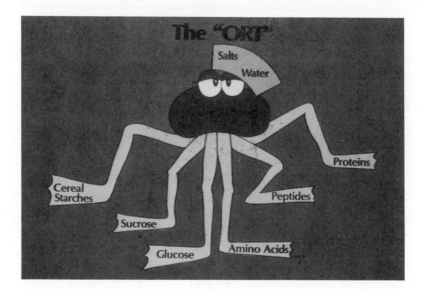

FIGURE 11.

REFERENCES

1. MacPherson J: *Annals of Cholera from the Earliest Periods to the Year 1817,* ed 2. London, HK Lewis, 1884
2. Pollitzer R: *Cholera.* Geneva, World Health Organization, 1959
3. Howard-Jones N: Cholera nomenclature and nosology: A historical note. *Bull WHO* 51:317–324, 1979
4. Littré E, Robin C: *Dictionnaire de Médecine.* Paris, JB Baillère et fils, 1878
5. MacLeod K: Cholera; history, morbid anatomy and clinical features, in Albutt TC, Rolleston HD (ed): *A System of Medicine,* Vol 2. London, 1910
6. Bhishagratna K: *An English Translation of the Sushruta Samhita,* Vol 3. Varanasi (India), The Chowkhamba Sanskrit Series Office, 1963 pp 352–356
7. Wong KC, Wu LT: *History of Chinese Medicine,* ed 2. Shanghai (China), National Quarantine Service, 1936
8. MacNamara C: *A History of Asiatic Cholera.* London, MacMillan and Co, 1876
9. De SN: *Cholera, Its Pathology and Pathogenesis.* Edinburgh, Oliver & Boyd, 1961
10. Howard-Jones N: Choleranomalies: The Unhistory of Medicine as exemplified by cholera. *Perspect Biol Med* 15:422–433, 1972
11. Creighton C: *A History of Epidemics in Britain,* ed 2, vol 2. London, Frank Cass & Co. Ltd, 1965
12. Faber K: *Nosography. The Evolution of Clinical Medicine in Modern Times.* New York, Hoeber, 1930
13. Winslow CEA: *The Conquest of Epidemic Disease. A Chapter in the History of Ideas.* Princeton, N. J., Princeton University Press, 1943
14. Dubos R: *Louis Pasteur. Free Lance of Science.* Boston, Little Brown, 1950
15. Gaskoin G: On the literature of cholera. *Medico-Chirurgical Review* 40:217–232, 1867 (English translation of work of Gaspar Correa)
16. Garcia da Orta: *Colloquies on the Simples and Drugs of India.* London, H. Southeran, 1913 (English translation by Sir Clements Markham)
17. Van Heyningen WE, Seal JR: *Cholera: The American Scientific Experience, 1947–1980.* Boulder, CO, West-view Press, 1983
18. Selwyn S: Cholera old and new. *Proc Roy Soc Med* 70:301–302, 1977
19. Wilson GS, Miles A: *Topley and Wilson's Principles of Bacteriology, Virology and Immunity,* ed 6. London, Edward Arnold, 1975
20. Carpenter CCJ: Treatment of cholera—Tradition and authority versus science, reason and humanity. *Johns Hopkins Med J* 139:153–162, 1976
21. Barua D: Cholera during the last hundred years (1884–1983), in Y. Takeda (ed): *Vibrio cholerae and Cholera.* Tokyo, KTK Scientific Publishers, 1988, pp 9–32
22. Duffy J: The history of Asiatic cholera in the United States. *Bull NY Acad Med* 47:1152–1168, 1971
23. Rosenberg CE: *The Cholera Years.* Chicago, The University of Chicago Press, 1962
24. Snow J: *On the Mode of Communication of Cholera.* London, John Churchill, 1849
25. Snow J: *On the Mode of Communication of Cholera,* ed 2. London, John Churchill, 1855
26. Chambers JS: *The Conquest of Cholera.* New York, MacMillan, 1938
27. Longmate N: *King Cholera, The Biography of a Disease.* London, Hamish Hamilton, 1966
28. *Public Health Rep* 26:2083, 1911
29. De SN, Chatterjee DN: An experimental study of the mechanism of action of *V. cholerae* on the intestinal mucous membrane. *J Path Bact* 66:559–562, 1953
30. De Moor CE: Un vibrio du type El Tor responsable dans la partie sud de l'ile de Célèbes (Indes Néerlandaises) d'une épidémie presentant les apparances complète du cholera. *Bull Off Int d'Hyg Publ* 30:1510–1519, 1938
31. De Moor CE: Paracholera (El Tor), enteritis choleriformis El Tor, Van Loghem. *Bull WHO* 2:5–19, 1949
32. Van Loghem JJ: El Tor vibrio from the Netherlands Indies. *Bull Off Int d'Hyg Publ* 30:1520–1523, 1938
33. Tanamal ST: Notes on paracholera in Sulawesi (Celebes). *Am J Trop Med Hyg* 8:72–78, 1959
34. Falsenfeld O: *The Cholera Problem.* St Louis, MO, Warren H. Green, 1967
35. Barua, D, Gomez CZ: Observations on some tests commonly employed for characterization of El Tor vibrios. *Bull WHO* 37:800–803, 1967
36. Barett J, Blake PA: Epidemiological usefulness of changes in hemolytic activity of *V. cholerae* biotype El Tor during the seventh pandemic. *J Clin Microbiol* 13:126–128, 1981
37. Kamal AM: The seventh pandemic of cholera, in Barua D, Burrows W (eds): *Cholera.* Philadelphia, WB Saunders, 1974, p 9
38. Barua D: The global epidemiology of cholera in recent years. *Proc Roy Soc Med* 65:423–428, 1972
39. Felix H: The development of the cholera epidemic in West Africa. *Bull Soc Pathol Exot Filiales* 64:561–582, 1971

40. Goodgame RW, Greenough WBG III: Cholera in Africa: A message for the West. *Ann Intern Med* 82:101–106, 1975
41. Samadi AR, Huq MI, Shahid N, et al: Classical *V. cholerae* biotype displaces El Tor in Bangladesh. *Lancet* i:805–807, 1983
42. Neogy KN, Mukherjee MK, Sanyal SN, et al: Classical cholera in West Bengal and Tripura in 1968. *Bull Calcutta Sch Trop Med* 17:39–40, 1969
43. Mahlu FS: *Cholera Problem in Central Africa.* Paper presented at the African Congress on Infectious Disease, Kigali, Rwanda, 1986
44. Dugnet MLF: Les epidémies du cholera on Hedjaz. *Rev Prat Mal Pays chauds* 11:492, 1931
45. Blake PA, Rosenberg ML, Costa JB, et al: Cholera in Portugal, 1974. 1. Modes of transmission. *Am J Epidemiol* 105:337–343, 1977
46. Arthur SA: *Cholera in Ghana.* Paper presented in the Second African Conference on Diarrhoeal Diseases, Harare, Zimbabwe, 1986
47. *WHO Wkly Epidemiol Rec* 26:311–312, 1977
48. *WHO Wkly Epidemiol Rec* 56:21, 1981
49. Garrique GP, Ndayo M, Sicard JM, et al: Resistance aux antibiotiques des souches de *Vibrio cholerae* El Tor isolées a Douala (Cameroun). *Bull Soc Pathol Exot Filiales* 79:305–312, 1986
50. *WHO Wkly Epidemiol Rec* 55:161–162, 293, 1980
51. *WHO Chron* 36:75, 1982
52. Sengupta, SK: Surveillance of cholera in India. *J Commun Dis* 7:90–94, 1975
53. Blake PA, Allegra DT, Snyder JD, et al: Cholera a possible endemic focus in the United States. *N Engl J Med* 302:305–309, 1980
54. Shandera WX, Hafkin B, Martin DL, et al: Persistence of cholera in the United States. *Am J Trop Med Hyg* 32:812–817, 1983
55. Rao A, Stockwell BA: The Queensland cholera incident of 1977. 1. The index case. *Bull WHO* 58:663–664, 1980
56. Rogers RC, Cuff RGC, Cossins YM, et al: The Queensland cholera incident of 1977. 2. The epidemiological investigation. *Bull WHO* 58:665–669, 1980
57. Bourke ATC, Cossins YN, Gray BRW, et al: Investigation of cholera acquired from the riverine environment in Queensland. *Med J Aust* 144:229–234, 1986

2

Bacteriology of *Vibrio* and Related Organisms

Riichi Sakazaki

Members of the genus *Vibrio* are natural inhabitants of the estuarine and sea environments. Until 1960, only the cholera vibrio was recognized as a human pathogen. Cholera vibrio was first found by Pacini in 1854 in the intestinal contents of patients who had died from cholera and it was given the name *Vibrio cholera* [sic]. In 1906, Gotschlich isolated organisms closely resembling but not identical to cholera vibrios in their hemolytic activity from pilgrims at El Tor in Sinai. Those hemolytic choleralike vibrios were called *V. eltor* for many years, but are now included as variants of *V. cholerae* because they do not differ sufficiently from the latter.

Vibrios found in estuarine and sea environments are generally halophilic. In recent years, interest by medical bacteriologists has been stimulated by the association of halophilic vibrios with human disease. The *Vibrio* species currently recognized to be associated with human diseases are listed in Table 1.

Other water-borne organisms that resemble vibrios in cultural and biochemical properties are *Aeromonas* and *Plesiomonas*. These two genera are included in the family *Vibrionaceae* along with the genus *Vibrio*. However, the family Aeromonadaceae has been proposed.[1] Unlike *Vibrio* species, their normal habitats are fresh-water sources and are not halophilic. Recently, they have also been associated with human diseases.

This chapter focuses on *Vibrio* species but a brief description of *Aeromonas* and *Plesiomonas* is included.

1. THE GENUS *VIBRIO*

Before the last two decades, an assortment of Gram-negative rods with polar flagellae were classified in the genus *Vibrio* of the family *Spirillaceae*. Since the International Sub-

Cholera, edited by Dhiman Barua and William B. Greenough III. Plenum Medical Book Company, New York, 1992.

TABLE 1
Vibrio Species Associated with Human Disease

Species	Diseases
V. cholerae	Cholera or cholera-like diarrhea; gastroenteritis; soft-tissue infection
V. mimicus	Cholera-like diarrhea
V. parahaemolyticus	Gastroenteritis; soft-tissue infection
V. fluvialis	Diarrhea
V. furnissii	Diarrhea (?)
V. hollisae	Diarrhea
V. alginolyticus	Soft-tissue infection
V. damsela	Soft-tissue infection
V. vulnificus	Septicemia in patient with hepatic disorder; soft-tissue infection
V. metschnikovii	Opportunistic?

committee on Taxonomy of Vibrios agreed on a definition for the genus *Vibrio* in 1966, only aerobic or facultatively anaerobic rods with fermentative metabolism have been retained in this genus. More than 30 species have been recognized as belonging to the genus *Vibrio*, although most of them are not very close to each other as measured by DNA relatedness.[1a,2]

1.1. Definition

Members of the genus *Vibrio* are Gram-negative, nonsporing, straight or curved rods. They are aerobic and facultatively anaerobic, and motile by monotrichous or lophotrichous flagella which are surrounded by a sheath in liquid media, but many species may have numerous lateral or peritrichous flagella when they grow on solid media. All species but one are oxidase positive. With few exceptions, they ferment glucose with production of acid but no gas. Sodium stimulates growth in all species and most are halophilic. They are chemoorganotrophic. They are susceptible to 2,4-diamino-6,7-diisopropylpteridine (0/129) but exceptions have been reported. The molecular % of guanine-plus-cytosine of DNA is 38–51. The exclude type species is *Vibrio cholerae* Pacini 1854.

1.2. Physiology and Biochemistry

Members of the genus *Vibrio* are brackish-water or marine organisms and many require higher concentrations of cations, particularly Na^+, K^+, Mg^{2+}, than are usual for terrestrial organisms such as *Aeromonas, Plesiomonas,* and *Enterobacteriaceae*. Most *Vibrio* species may show poor or no growth in nutrient broth which contains less than 0.5% sodium chloride. Even for *V. cholerae* and *V. mimicus,* which are the only terrestrial species of the *Vibrio,* better growth will be obtained in nutrient broth with 1% salt than in broth with lower concentrations and require Na^+ for growth.[2a] The concentration of salt for optimum growth and the range of salt tolerance differ with each species. In addition, the concentration of salt for optimum growth may be influenced by the nature of the medium used and the temperature of incubation. For example, enriched media such as blood agar or brain heart infusion agar usually support good growth of vibrios without the need for additional salt. The majority of vibrios can grow over a pH range of 5.6 to 9.6, but optimum pH for growth may be between 7.6 and 8.6. They usually grow more rapidly than other Gram-negative rods. Although some species grow poorly or not at all at 37°C, the nine *Vibrio* species associated with human diseases grow well at 30–37°C and do not at 4°C.

The biochemical characteristics of *Vibrio* species which may cause human illness are shown in Table 2.

1.2.1. *Vibrio cholerae* and *Vibrio mimicus*

These two *Vibrio* species grow well in ordinary media without additional salt but do have an absolute requirement for sodium.[2a] In the 1930s, it was recognized that the majority of vibrios found in cholera epidemics were agglutinated by a single antiserum called 01. On the other hand, organisms possessing cultural and biochemical characteristics resembling cholera vibrio but differing from it in only their somatic antigens were referred to as NCV (noncholera vibrios) or NAG (nonagglutinable) vibrios. Close DNA relatedness of these organisms with cholera vibrio has been recognized and they are now classified as *V. cholerae*.[3,4] A luminous vibrio formerly known as *V. albensis* is also included in *V. cholerae* on the basis of biochemical and nutritional characteristics and DNA homology.[4,5] Although the species *V. cholerae* should no longer be restricted to *V. cholerae* 01 and includes the "NAG" vibrios, it is accepted that these two groups of *V. cholerae* are referred to as 01 and non-01, respectively, because of the historic clinical and epidemiological importance of the former in human disease.

V. cholerae 01 is divided into two biogroups (biovars), classical and eltor. The production of dialysable, heat-labile hemolysin for sheep red cells is the main criterion for distinguishing the eltor biovar from the classical biovar, but the results obtained depend on the technique used. Hemagglutination of chicken or sheep red cells by the eltor biovar but not by the classical biovar is another distinctive feature. In addition, differences of susceptibility to polymyxin B (50 UI) and Mukerjee's phages IV and V, and a reaction on Voges–Proskauer test are seen between the two biovars, as shown in Table 3, although the differences are not always clear-cut and the results of these tests are sometimes discrepant.

Heiberg[6] described six biogroups of vibrios on the basis of fermentation reactions in sucrose, mannose, and arabinose. All strains of *V. cholerae* 01 belong to his biogroup I. Strains of *V. cholerae* non-01 belonging to the biogroup I cannot be distinguished biochemically from *V. cholerae* 01. Thus, Heiberg's biogrouping is of little use for the differentiation of 01 and non-01 strains of *V. cholerae*.

Strains of *V. mimicus* were formerly included in *V. cholerae* non-01. This species is distinguishable from *V. cholerae* only by its inability to produce acid from sucrose and acetoin from glucose, but indistinguishable by other characteristics. It is susceptible to polymyxin B.

V. cholerae and *V. mimicus* have a single polar flagellum either in liquid or on solid media. On ordinary agar medium, they usually form translucent, amorphous colonies, but wrinkled or rugous colonies may sometimes occur. In broth cultures, they show moderate turbidity and sometimes pellicle formation, especially in an alkaline broth.

1.2.2. *V. parahaemolyticus*

This organism is a typical member of the halophilic *Vibrio* species. The species is considered negative for urea decomposition, but urease positive strains have been reported recently by many investigators.[6a]

TABLE 2
Differential Characteristics of *Vibrio* Species Associated with Human Disease[a]

Test (substrate)	V. cholerae		V. mimicus		V. parahaemolyticus		V. fluvialis	
	Sign	%+	Sign	%+	Sign	%+	Sign	%+
Lateral flagella on solid media	−		−		+		d	
Growth at % NaCl								
0%	+	99	+	100	−	0	−	0
7%	−	0	−	0	+	98	d	70
10%	−	0	−	0	−	2	−	1
Indole	+	100	+	100	+	99	−	5
Voges–Proskauer	d	85	−	0	−	0	−	0
Lysine decarboxylase	+	99	+	100	+	98	−	0
Arginine dihydrolase	−	0	−	0	−	0	+	100
Ornithine decarboxylase	+	99	+	100	+	99	−	0
Urease	−	0	−	0	−	2	−	0
Gelatinase	+	100	+	100	+	100	d	75
Tween hydrolysis	+	100	d	20	+	100	+	92
Nitrate to nitrite	+	100	+	100	+	100	+	100
Fermentation								
Glucose, acid	+	100	+	100	+	100	+	100
Glucose, gas	−	0	−	0	−	0	−	0
Arabinose	−	0	−	0	d	80	d	70
Lactose	d	10	−	.5	−	0	−	0
Mannose	d	75	+	99	+	100	+	100
Sucrose	+	100	−	0	−	5	+	100
Maltose	+	100	+	100	+	100	+	100
Mannitol	+	100	+	100	+	100	+	100
Oxidase	+	100	+	100	+	100	+	100

[a] +, 90% or more positive within 48 hr; −, 90% or more negative; d, 11–89% positive reaction.

Estuarine isolates of *V. parahaemolyticus* may have to be distinguished from *V. harveyi* which is one of the indigenous estuarine vibrios. *V. harveyi* has features similar to those of *V. parahaemolyticus,* but is distinguished from the latter by some characteristics shown in Table 4.

The majority of strains of *V. parahaemolyticus* produce lateral flagella on solid medium. It grows at a range of 0.5 and 8% salt and the optimum concentration of salt is 3%. Colonies of fresh isolates on ordinary agar with 3% salt are moist, smooth, circular, and opaque in appearance, attaining a size of 2–3 mm after incubation at 35°C for 24 hr. Sometimes mucoid colonies may occur. After several subcultures, translucent or rugous colonies may dissociate from the original colonies. Some strains, especially isolates from estuarine sources yield swarming on the surface of solid media. In broth, strains of this species produce dense, homogeneous turbidity sometimes with pellicle formation on the surface.

Isolates of *V. parahaemolyticus* from patients suffering from gastroenteritis are usually hemolytic to human red cells, while the majority of isolates from marine resources do not show such activity. This reaction is possibly associated with enteropathogenicity of this vibrio and is called the Kanagawa phenomenon. Several hemolysins are found in *V. para-*

TABLE 2
(*Continued*)

V. furnissii		V. hollisae		V. alginolyticus		V. vulnificus		V. damsela		V. metschnikovii	
Sign	%+	Sign	%+	Sign	%+	Sign	%+	Sign	%+	Sign	%+
d		–		+		–		–		NT	
–	0	–	0	–	0	–	0	–	0	–	0
d	70	–	0	+	100	–	1	–	0	d	20
–	1	–	0	+	95	–	0	–	0	–	0
–	10	+	100	+	100	+	100	–	0	d	20
–	0	–	0	+	100	–	0	d	80	+	95
–	0	–	0	+	95	+	100	d	25	d	30
+	100	–	0	–	0	–	0	+	100	d	50
–	0	–	0	+	100	d	85	–	0	–	0
–	0	–	0	–	0	–	0	+	100	–	0
d	80	–	0	+	100	+	99	d	30	d	50
d	85	–	0	+	100	+	100	–	0	+	100
+	100	+	100	+	100	+	100	+	100	–	0
+	100	+	100	+	100	+	100	+	100	+	100
+	10	–	0	–	0	–	0	d	10	–	0
+	100	+	100	–	15	–	0	–	0	–	0
–	0	–	0	–	0	+	90	–	0	d	50
+	100	+	100	+	100	+	98	+	100	+	100
+	100	–	0	+	100	–	1	–	1	+	100
+	100	–	0	+	100	+	100	+	100	+	100
+	100	+	100	+	100	d	65	–	0	+	95
+	100	+	100	+	100	+	100	+	100	–	0

haemolyticus, but the thermostable extracellular hemolysin active on human red cells but inactive on horse red cells is responsible for the Kanagawa reaction.

1.2.3. *V. fluvialis* and *V. furnissii*

These halophilic vibrios grow in the presence of 6% and occasionally 8% NaCl. *V. furnissii* resembles *V. fluvialis* very closely and it was formerly known as *V. fluvialis* biovar II. *V. fluvialis* is anaerogenic, where as *V. furnissii* is aerogenic.

1.2.4. *V. hollisae*

This vibrio also belongs to the halophilic *Vibrio* species. Most of the strains are indole positive when tested in heart infusion broth with 1% salt but many strains are negative in ordinary peptone water; in a semisolid medium, none of the strains is motile after 48-hr incubation, but the majority are motile after 7 days. Unlike other enteropathogenic *Vibrio* species, *V. hollisae* may not grow on MacConkey and TCBS agars, but grows well on sheep blood agar.

TABLE 3
Differentiation of the Classical and Eltor Biovars of
Vibrio cholerae 01

Characteristics	Classical	Eltor
Hemolysis	−	+
Agglutination of chicken red cells	−	+
Susceptibility to polymyxin B (50 IU)	+	−
Voges–Proskauer	−	+
Susceptibility to bacteriophages		
IV	+	−
V	−	+

1.2.5. *V. vulnificus*

It is a halophilic organism resembling *V. parahaemolyticus*, but it fails to grow in 8% salt.

1.2.6. *V. alginolyticus*

This organism also resembles *V. parahaemolyticus*. Strains of this species grow at a range of 1 to 10% salt and grow best at 4% salt concentration. The majority of strains swarm on solid media.

1.2.7. *V. damsela*

It is a halophilic vibrio that grows in 6% salt but not in 8% salt. This species resembles *V. fluvialis* and *V. furnissii* in its amino acid reactions.

1.2.8. *V. metschnikovii*

This organism is a halophilic vibrio possessing some unusual characteristics. It is oxidase negative and fails to reduce nitrate to nitrite. Although this species requires salt for growth, some strains may grow in ordinary nutrient media without additional salt.

TABLE 4
Differentiation of *Vibrio parahaemolyticus* and *Vibrio harveyi*

Test (substrate)	*V. parahaemolyticus*	*V. harveyi*
Sucrose, acid	−	d
Cellobiose, acid (within 24 hours)	−	+
Utilization of sole C source		
Leucine	+	−
Putrescine	+	−
Ethanol	+	−
Swarming on solid media	d	−
Luminescence	−	d

1.3. Resistance and Antibiotic Susceptibility

All vibrios are killed by heat at 60°C in 10 min. Their resistance to cold is lower than that of coliform organisms, although they may survive for a few weeks at −20°C. They are easily destroyed by drying. Vibrios have a low acid tolerance and may be killed at pH 6.0 after a short period of time.

Vibrio species are usually susceptible to tetracycline, chloramphenicol, the aminoglycosides, and nalidixic acid, but susceptibility to other antibiotics may be different according to species or strains. In most strains, especially with halophilic species, resistance is likely to be intrinsic to the species rather than plasmid-mediated. Recently, however, strains of *V. cholerae* 01 with plasmid-mediated resistance to a wide range of antibiotics were reported in Tanzania and Bangladesh.[7,8] Many strains of halophilic species including *V. parahaemolyticus, V. alginolyticus, V. fluvialis, V. furnissii, V. damsela,* and *V. metschinikovii* are resistant to ampicillin, and beta-lactamase production in these species was reported.[9] On the other hand, most of all strains of *V. vulnificus* and *V. hollisae* are susceptible to ampicillin. *V. hollisae* is especially highly susceptible to most antibiotics including penicillin G.

1.4. Serology

At least two antigenic components can be recognized in strains of *Vibrio* species. The somatic (0) antigen is thermostable and is not destroyed by treatment with 50% ethanol and *n*-HCl at 37°C for 24 hrs. The flagellar (H) antigen is thermolabile; its agglutinability is inactivated by heating at 100°C for 15 min and its immunogenicity by heating at the same temperature for 2.5 hr. One characteristic of serological properties of *Vibrio* species is that all strains in a given species possess identical H antigens, although they are divided into many O-serogroups. Moreover, a common antigenic determinant is found in flagellins from the polar flagellum(a) of *Vibrio* species such as *V. cholerae, V. parahaemolyticus, V. alginolyticus, V. anguillarum, V. campbelli, V. fischeri, V. harveyi, V. metschinikovii, V. nereis,* and *V. fluvialis,* by immunodiffusion technique.[10] However, species-specific H-antiserum can be obtained by absorption with H-antigens from other species.[11] Agglutination testing with unabsorbed and absorbed H-antisera is useful to distinguish a species from other *Vibrio* species. Some species of *Vibrio* produce lateral flagella along with polar flagella, as mentioned before, when they grow on solid media. In those cultures, antigenicity of the polar flagellum is different from that of lateral flagella.

Vibrio species is subdivided into serogroups on the basis of its O-antigens. Although serovar (serotype) should be principally expressed by an assortment of O- and H-antigens, O-serogroups are referred to as serovars, because all strains of a given species share an identical H-antigen and the H-antigen determination is considered of little value for serotyping for species in the genus *Vibrio.*

There are many interspecific and extrageneric relationships of O-antigens of *Vibrio* species as summarized in Table 5.[12−14]

R-antigens of all strains of a given *Vibrio* species are serologically identical regardless of their O-serogroups.[15] The R-form is usually indistinguishable from the parent S-form in colonial morphology, but may be differentiated by agglutination with R-antiserum. So far studied, most O-antisera against strains of *Vibrio* species contain some quantity of the R-antibody, which may cause overlapping reactions in the determination of O-serogroups.

TABLE 5
Intra-, Inter-, and Extrarelationships of 0-Antigens
of *Vibrio cholerae*[a]

V. cholerae		*V. fluvialis*	*A. hydrophila*
02	09		017
06		010	
013	029		
015	025		
019			011
039		05	023
041		04	
043		02	
051			03
059			04
062			038

[a]Underlined indicates 0 identity; the other cases are cross reactions.

Some strains of a *Vibrio* species may be inagglutinable in the living state by the homologous O-antiserum because of the presence of masking antigen. This is the case particularly with *V. parahaemolyticus*. The capsular (K) antigen is one of the antigenic components for serovars of *V. parahaemolyticus*. Freshly isolated strains of this vibrio have well-developed K-antigens and may not be agglutinated by the homologous O-antiserum in the living state. In those cultures, O-agglutination may not occur unless the cultures are heated at 100°C (121°C in some cases) for 2 hr and washed with saline.

1.4.1. *V. cholerae*

More than 80 serovars (0-serogroups) have so far been recognized in *V. cholerae*[11,16]
V. cholerae 01, the caustive agent of cholera, is divided into three o-antigenic forms named Ogawa, Inaba, and Hikojima. These antigenic forms are often referred to as "serotypes" or "subtypes," but they are incorrect designations. The antigenic difference among these three forms are quantitative but not qualitative as indicated in Fig. 1. O-antigen of *V. cholerae* 01 consists of three factors designated A, B, and C.[17] The factor A is the major antigen specific for *V. cholerae* 01. Strains of the Inaba form are mutants that lost the factor B, which can be recognized as specific for the Ogawa form. Strains of Ogawa form possess a smaller quantity of the factor C, and may not be agglutinated by antiserum for the factor C. However, all agglutinins in the Inaba antiserum can be removed by repeated absorption with an excess of Ogawa cultures, while the titer of the B agglutinin in the Ogawa antiserum is not diminished when absorbed repeatedly with the Inaba cultures. The antigenic variation from the Ogawa to the Inaba may occur in patients during cholera epidemics in which the Ogawa form is the etiologic agent, and the variation is irreversible. The Hikojima form is regarded as intermediate between the Ogawa and Inaba forms, and usually unstable. Thus, the differentiation of Ogawa, Inaba, and Hikojima forms of *V. cholerae* 01 has only limited epidemiological value.

The B and C factor antigens of *V. cholerae* 01 occur not only in cholera vibrio but also in other vibrios. Shimada *et al.*[18] reported a group of halophilic vibrios possessing the B and C factors along with major antigens specific for the serogroup. An antigenic variation similar to the Ogawa to Inaba in *V. cholerae* 01 has been observed in that serogroup of halophilic

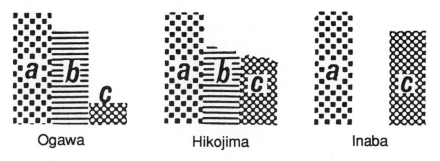

FIGURE 1. Hypothetical picture of antigenic formula of *Vibrio cholerae*.

vibrio. They have also recognized the C factor antigen in *V. cholerae* non-01 and *V. fluvialis*.[19,20]

Bhaskaran and Sinha reported that O-antigen specificity was transferable from *V. cholerae* non-01 to *V. cholerae* 01 by chromosomal hybridization.[21] Despite some dubious reports in the literature, it is difficult to believe that the change of *V. cholerae* 01 to *V. cholerae* non-01 and vice versa occurs in man or in nature because it has to be mediated by chromosomal genes.

1.4.2. *V. mimicus*

V. mimicus is indistinguishable from *V. cholerae* by serology. The H-antigen of *V. mimicus* is identical with that of *V. cholerae*. As O-serogroups of *V. mimicus* cover a wide range of O-serogroups of *V. cholerae* non-01, a single serotyping schema may be applicable for both species.

1.4.3. *V. parahaemolyticus*

V. parahaemolyticus has well-developed K-antigen. Since the H-antigens are all identical, this species is divided into serovars by a combination of the O- and K-antigens. An antigenic schema recognizing 11 O-groups and 41 K-antigens for *V. parahaemolyticus* was established by Sakazaki *et al.*[22] K-antigens 2, 4, 16, 27, and 35 were subsequently excluded because they were found to be identical to others already recognized. The antigenic schema has since been extended and is shown, as of 1986, in Table 6. The antigenic schema of this vibrio is based on strains isolated from patients. Although serovars of most strains isolated from diarrheal stools can be determined with existing, established O- and K-antisera, they may not be useful in identifying serovars of many isolates from marine sources.

1.4.4. Other Vibrios

Serotyping systems for *V. fluvialis* and *V. vulnificus* based on O-antigen determination have been developed by Shimada and Sakazaki.[15,23] The antigenic scheme for *V. fluvialis* is composed of 18 serogroups, in which *V. furnissii* is included since this species is serologically indistinguishable from the former. In *V. vulnificus*, 7 serogroups have been recognized. The majority of strains of each species mentioned above may be inagglutinable by their homologous O-antisera in the living state, although a definite capsule or a masking substance has not yet been demonstrated.

TABLE 6
Antigenic Scheme of *Vibrio parahaemolyticus*[a]

O-group	K-antigen
1	1, 25, 26, 32, 38, 41, 56, 58, 64, 69
2	3, 28
3	4, 5, 6, 7, 29, 30, 31, 33, 37, 43, 45, 48, 54, 57, 58, 59, 65
4	4, 8, 9, 10, 11, 12, 13, 34, 42, 49, 53, 55, 63, 67
5	15, 17, 30, 47, 60, 61, 68
6	18, 46
7	19
8	20, 21, 22, 39, 70
9	23, 44
10	19, 24, 52, 66, 71
11	36, 40, 50, 51, 61

[a]As of 1986.

1.5. Phage- and Bacteriocin-Typing of *V. cholerae*

A phage-typing system based on the works of Mukerjee *et al.*[24] has been used as an epidemiologic tool of cholera although not very successfully. However, Mukerjee's classical Group IV phage that lyses only classical strains and the eltor Group V phage that lyses only eltor strains have been found useful for differentiating these biovars (Table 3). For phage-typing of eltor biovar, Lee and Furniss[25] improved Mukerjee's schema by adding phages from other sources. However, it has been found that some of the phages of Lee and Furniss were contaminated and that there was no adequate set of type strains.[26] A phage-typing schema capable of typing both biovars, which also uses some of the phages of Mukerjee has been developed in the USSR.[27] Frost and Rowe[28] have evaluated the latter scheme and have found it to have a better chance of being developed into a useful scheme. (See Chapter 5 for phage-typing of *V. cholerae* 01.) For *V. cholerae* non-01, there is no phage-typing system at present, but some of these strains may react with the phages mentioned above.

Vibrio cholerae and possibly other vibrios produce different bacteriocines (vibriocines). Wahba[29] reported that susceptibility patterns of eltor strains to vibriocines are similar to those of classical strains. Mitra *et al.*[30] described a single scheme of vibriocine-typing for 01 and non-01 strains of *V. cholerae*. As reproducible results were not easily obtained, however, this method of typing has not been used much.

1.6. Isolation and Identification

1.6.1. Isolation

1.6.1.1. Clinical Specimens. Diarrheal diseases caused by *Vibrio* species are likely to be missed in clinical bacteriology laboratories because the media used for routine investigations of acute diarrhea do not support good growth of vibrios; special media for vibrios are not included unless specifically requested by the clinicians. This is particularly the case in developed countries because of cost considerations. *Vibrio* cultures usually grow on Mac-Conkey agar, but many strains may not do so or grow only with a reduced plating efficiency.

Although several media have been devised for isolating vibrios, a combination of thiosulfate–citrate–bile salt–sucrose (TCBS) agar[31] and one of the less inhibitory agar media, such as vibrio agar[32] and gelatin–taurocholate–tellurite agar (TG),[33] is recommended for use in laboratories interested in vibrio infection. TCBS agar is highly selective for *Vibrio* species, with the exception of *V. hollisae,* although lot-to-lot and brand-to-brand variation in inhibitory effect may be seen. It may be too inhibitory to cultures maintained in laboratories, but less inhibitory to freshly isolated cultures. TG agar is less selective than TCBS agar; most vibrio cultures rapidly degrade gelatin in this medium and form a turbid zone around the colony. To prepare this medium, however, caution is necessary in selecting the proper quality of gelatin and standardizing the tellurite solution. Vibrio agar is considerably less selective but supports better growth of vibrios than the former two media. TCBS and vibrio agars are the only media that are commercially available. The appearance of vibrio colonies on the three media mentioned above is shown in Table 7. Of the *Vibrio* species associated with diarrheal disease, *V. hollisae* may not grow on these media. For isolation of *V. hollisae* blood agar or marine agar (Difco and Oxoid) are the only suitable media. For isolation of *Vibrio* species from extraintestinal soft-tissue infections, special selective media may not be necessary.

Enrichment culture is not necessary in the acute stage of diarrhea, but it is useful for stool specimens from convalescent patients or asymptomatic persons. Alkaline peptone water (pH 9.0) with 1% NaCl is satisfactory for selective enrichment. Alkaline tellurite–bile salt broth of Monsur,[34] which is a more selective medium than alkaline peptone water, is also satisfactory for recovery of vibrios from feces. Tellurite–bile salt broth is prepared by adding 1% of peptone, 1% of sodium chloride, 0.5% of sodium taurocholate, and 0.1% of sodium carbonate to distilled water. The medium should be at pH 9.0–9.2. After autoclaving at 121°C for 15 min, potassium tellurite is added to give a final concentration of 1:100,000

Stool specimens should be collected in the acute stage of diarrhea, and before the patient has received any antimicrobial agents. The detection of vibrios from the stools in later stages may become difficult, because causative vibrios in the stools rapidly decrease in numbers with the recovery from the diarrhea. The specimens are taken from freshly evacuated stools using swabs tipped with calcium alginate or polyester fibers. If cotton swabs are used, treatment of cotton tips with phosphate buffer is recommended because residual fatty acids on cotton fibers may be toxic for vibrios. Cotton swabs are dipped in Sorensen buffer (7.8–

TABLE 7
Appearance of *Vibrio* Colonies on Isolation Agar Medium after 24-hr Incubation

	TCBS agar		TG agar		Vibrio agar	
Organisms	Color	Size	Cloudy zone	Size	Color	Size
V. cholerae	Yellow	1.0–1.5	+	0.5–1.0	Bluish gray	1.0–2.0
V. mimicus	Dark green	0.5–1.0	+	0.5–1.0	Pale rosy	0.5–1.0
V. parahaemolyticus	Blue green	1.5–2.0	+	1.0–2.0	Pale rosy	1.0–2.0
V. fluvialis	Yellow	0.5–1.0	Variable	0.5–1.0	Bluish gray	1.0–1.5
V. furnissii	Yellow	0.5–1.0	Variable	0.5–1.0	Bluish gray	1.0–1.5
V. hollisae	No growth		–	0.5–1.0	No growth	
V. alginolyticus	Yellow	1.5–2.5	+	1.0–2.0	Bluish gray	1.0–3.0
V. vulnificus	Blue green	0.5–1.0	+	0.5–1.0	Pale rosy	0.5–1.0
V. damsela[a]	Blue green	0.5–1.0	Variable	0.5–1.0	Pale rosy	0.5–1.0

[a]A better growth can be obtained at 25°C than at 35°C.

8.0) previously heated to boiling, drained, autoclaved, and then stored without drying at room temperature. Rectal swabs may also be used, but they are less satisfactory for convalescent and asymptomatic persons.

    If culturing must be delayed, swabs dipped in the stool specimens should be placed in Cary–Blair transport medium until examination. Cary–Blair medium is dispensed in 7-ml amounts in 9-ml screw-capped bottles. Swabs are placed in the medium and the caps tightened to prevent water loss. Otherwise, the swabs should be collected in alkaline peptone water. Specimens in the transport medium should be kept without refrigeration because low temperature may kill vibrios.

    In view of its importance in public health, the isolation procedure for *V. cholerae* 01 should always include the inoculation of stool specimens in an enrichment broth, even if the specimen is collected during the acute phase of diarrhea. The incubation period of alkaline peptone water culture is best limited to 8 hr or less to prevent overgrowth by other fecal organisms. The procedure with tellurite–bile salt broth is the same as that with alkaline peptone water, but an overnight incubation instead of 8 hr gives better results. Tellurite–bile salt broth is particularly useful for secondary enrichment from the primary culture of alkaline peptone water from convalescent patients and asymptomatic contacts when a loopful of the primary culture is transferred to tellurite–bile salt broth after 8 hr. Care should be taken to avoid shaking enrichment culture when it is taken from an incubator in order not to disturb the growth at the surface of the broth.

    For collection of extraintestinal specimens, there is no special procedure for *Vibrio* species, but specimens must not be allowed to dry because vibrios are very sensitive to desiccation. Cary–Blair medium is also useful for transport and storage of extraintestinal specimens.

    Stool specimens from diarrheal patients should be inoculated directly onto isolation agar plates as soon as possible after collection. Swabs are well washed in approximately 0.5 ml of peptone water or physiological saline to emulsify the specimens and a loopful of the emulsion is inoculated onto isolation plate. From the surface of the enrichment broth cultures, a loopful should be plated on isolation media. After overnight incubation, the plate is carefully examined for vibrio colonies.

    Extraintestinal specimens are processed with no particular attention to *Vibrio* species.

    1.6.1.2. Food and Water Samples. As a rule *Vibrio* species associated with human diseases are found in aquatic environments when the water is warmer than 15°C. The isolation of vibrios from aquatic environments and foodstuffs, especially seafish, forms an important part of special epidemiological investigations of cholera and other diarrheal diseases, of examination of seafish for exportation or when imported from areas in which cholera is epidemic, and of ecological studies of a given *Vibrio* species.

    The isolation of vibrios from food samples may be different according to the type of food and target *Vibrio* species. For food and water samples, a single enrichment culture with alkaline peptone water may hinder the isolation of target vibrio by overgrowth of other contaminants. A combination of alkaline peptone water for the primary enrichment and tellurite–bile salt broth for the secondary enrichment is recommended for the isolation of *V. cholerae*. Incubation of alkaline peptone water cultures for more than 8 hr should be avoided, otherwise overgrowth of other organisms will occur.

    The enrichment procedure is also effective for *V. parahaemolyticus,* but a more selective enrichment broth, salt–polymyxin broth,[35] may be used. This broth contains 0.3% of yeast extract, 1% of peptone, 2% of sodium chloride, and 250 IU/ml of polymyxin B (pH

8.6–9.0); the mixture is brought to a boil to dissolve completely, but is not autoclaved. It inhibits not only enteric bacteria, pseudomonads, and gram-positives, but also the main contaminants such as *V. alginolyticus*. The inoculated broth should be incubated for 8–12 hr.

There is some disagreement among investigators on the efficacy of various enrichment procedures of vibrios in seafoods, one of the reasons for which may be the type of food. When seafood is examined for the presence of a vibrio, homogenized materials are generally inoculated into enrichment broth. It is not always realized that such homogenates may contain some growth-inhibitory substances present in crustaceans like shrimp, lobster, and crabs.[36] In addition, chitin, which is contained in the carapace of these seafish, selectively adsorbs vibrios and may thus reduce the number of vibrios in the broth. Homogenate from oyster may also contain some inhibitory factors. For isolation of vibrios from seafoods, the sample should therefore be cut into small pieces, added to 10 times the volume of enrichment broth, shaken vigorously for 1–2 min or homogenized, the pieces removed, and then the broth incubated at 35°C.

For the isolation of vibrios, especially *V. cholerae,* water samples are collected in sterile 1- or 2-liter bottles containing 10–20g NaCl. At least 1 liter of the water sample is clarified by centrifugation, passed through a membrane filter, and then the filter disk is placed in 50–100 ml of enrichment broth. Since this procedure may be difficult for some laboratories, another practice in which double-strength enrichment broth is added to an equal volume of water sample is recommended. Otherwise, 1 ml of 10% FeCl may be added to approximately 1 liter of water sample, pH adjusted to 7.8–8.0 with *n*-NaOH, and then the mixture left overnight at room temperature. After discarding any supernatant, double-strength enrichment broth is added in equal volume to the resultant precipitate. The simple procedure of using Moore swab, for detection of *V. cholerae* 01 in aquatic sources has been found useful for cholera surveillance.[37,38] Spira and Ahmed have developed a simple filtration method using gauze filter.[39] A serologically specific procedure for *V. cholerae* 01 using columns of polystyrene beads coated with specific antibody has also been reported.[40]

With the exception of *V. hollisae,* TCBS agar is also commonly used for the isolation of vibrios from food and water samples. A loopful of enrichment broth culture is inoculated onto TCBS agar. However, detection of *V. cholerae* 01 in those samples is not always easy. In food and water samples containing both 01 and non-01 strains of *V. cholerae,* the growth of the latter generally far exceeds that of the former. Colonies of 01 vibrios on TCBS agar cannot be differentiated from those of non-01 strains by their appearance. A selective and differential agar medium, polymyxin–mannose–tellurite (PMT) agar (Sakazaki and Shimada, 1980, unpublished data) may be useful for detection of *V. cholerae* 01 from such samples, as all strains of *V. cholerae* 01 but only 20% of non-01 strains ferment mannose in 24 hr. PMT agar contains 5 g of Lab–Lemco powder (Oxoid), 8 g of Polypeptone (BBL), 2 g of Phytone (BBL), 10 g NaCl, 20 g of mannose, 0.1 ml of tergitol 7 (Union Carbide, Co., New York), 20 ml of 0.2% solution of cresol red, 20 ml of 0.2% solution of bromthymol blue, 180,000 IU of polymyxin B, and 15 g of agar in 1 liter of the medium. Ingredients are added to distilled water, and the mixture is boiled with gentle agitation for a minute or two, and the medium is adjusted to pH 8.4. It should not be autoclaved. After cooling to 50°C, potassium tellurite is added to give a final concentration of 1:100,000. The complete medium is then poured into petri dishes. The medium is commercially available (Nissui Seiyaku Co., Tokyo).

On PMT agar, colonies of *V. cholerae* 01 are yellow with a brown center and are easily agglutinated with 01 antiserum, while those of mannose-nonfermenting non-01 cultures are violet and rather smaller than those of the former. Moreover, many cultures of non-01 vibrios may be inhibited on PMT agar. The superiority of PMT agar to TCBS for the isolation of *V. cholerae* 01 has been demonstrated by Shimada[41] with water samples, and by Emoto[36] with shrimp.

1.6.2. Identification

When a selective plating medium such as TCBS agar is used for the isolation of vibrios from human clinical specimens, the identification of the isolates is relatively easy, because their colonial appearance provides useful information, and organisms other than those vibrios are usually inhibited. When identification of isolates from samples containing many indigenous vibrios from marine sources is very difficult, however, the following procedure may be helpful.

Testing for oxidase, glucose fermentation in Kligler iron agar, nitrate reduction to nitrite, growth in two tubes of nutrient broth of which one contains 1% NaCl and the other no salt, and lysine and ornithine decarboxylases and arginine dihydrolase in Moeller's broth are helpful as tests for first-stage identification. With the exception of *V. metschnikovii*, *Vibrio* species associated with human disease are oxidase positive and reduce nitrate to nitrite. *V. cholerae* and *V. mimicus*, and some strains of *V. metschnikovii* grow in nutrient broth containing no salt, whereas other *Vibrio* species can grow only in the broth containing 1% salt. Vibrios ferment glucose without gas production, with the exception of *V. furnissii* which produces a small quantity of gas from glucose. For the oxidase test, Kovacs' method is used, but the test should not be done with a culture on media containing a fermentable carbohydrate, otherwise a false negative reaction may be obtained. Nutrient broth used for requirement of salt for growth contains 0.5% of meat extract and 0.5% of peptone (pH 7.0–7.2), and turbidity in the broth culture is read after 24-hr incubation at 30–37°C. In addition to these tests, susceptibility to the vibriostatic agent 0/120 (2,4-diamino-6,7-diisopropylpteridine phosphate, Sigma) may be useful for the presumptive differentiation between *Vibrio* species, especially with *V. cholerae* and *V. mimicus*, and *Aeromonas*. The test is carried out by means of a diffusion method using disc containing 150 µg of the agent.

The tests for the second stage of identification may include indole, Voges–Proskauer, and acid production from L-arabinose, lactose, maltose, sucrose, mannitol, and salicin. The test procedures used to characterize cultures of *Enterobacteriaceae* work well for *Vibrio* species. However, media for characterizing vibrio cultures need to contain a concentration of NaCl. It is empirically known that 1% of sodium chloride in all media is satisfactory for the growth of *V. cholerae* as well as halophilic species. Table 2 shows some of the characteristic features.

Identification of *Vibrio* species commonly occurring in clinical specimens can also be done by commercial identification systems. However, the organisms to be tested should be suspended in saline rather than in distilled water.

1.6.2.1. Intraspecific Subdivision. Subdivision of isolates of *Vibrio* species from clinical specimens and seafoods may help outbreak investigations. Although serogrouping of *Vibrio* species associated with human diseases has been developed as mentioned before, this can only be performed in reference laboratories. One important exception is *V. cholerae* since an isolate can be easily determined to be *V. cholerae* 01 by testing the culture with 01 antiserum of the species.

For biotyping of *V. cholerae* 01, hemolysis is one of the important features. However, the conventional hemolysis testing on blood agar does not provide reliable results. A reproducible hemolysis can be obtained by incubating sheep blood agar culture at 35°C for 24 hr under anaerobic conditions without carbon dioxide.[42]

2. THE GENUS _AEROMONAS_

The genus _Aeromonas_ includes two groups of organisms having 57–63 mol% of guanine-plus-cytosine content of the DNA, a psychophilic, non-motile group and a mesophilic, usually motile group. The former group includes _A. salmonicida_ and _A. media,_ which are not found in human clinical specimens. For the latter group of aeromonads, three species, _A. hydrophila, A. sobria,_ and _A. caviae,_ are distinguished. However, the classification and nomenclature of the three mesophilic species are still in a state of flux. Although Popoff _et al._[43] reported from the results of DNA hybridization study that _A. hydrophila_ and _A. sobria_

TABLE 8
Biochemical Characteristics of Mesophilic _Aeromonas_

Test (substrate)	Sign[a]	Percent positive
Oxidase	+	100
Indole	+	92
Voges–Proskauer (25°C)	d	45
Citrate (Simmons)	d	71
H$_2$S (Kligler)	−	0
Urease (Christensen)	−	0
Gelatin (Kohn)	+	99
DNase	+	99
Tween 80 hydrolysis	+	99
Lysine decarboxylase	d	68
Arginine dihydrolase	d	85
Ornithine decarboxylase	−	0
Esculin hydrolysis	d	63
Gas from glucose	d	70
Acid from		
Arabinose	d	61
Lactose	d	55
Maltose	+	100
Melibiose	−	1
Raffinose	−	1
Rhamnose	−	1
Sucrose	+	95
Trehalose	+	100
Xylose	−	0
Adonitol	−	0
Dulcitol	−	0
Mannitol	+	99
Sorbitol	−	5
Arbutin	d	65
Salicin	d	61
Inositol	−	1
Beta-galactosidase (ONPG)	+	100

[a]For symbols, see Table 2.

are genetically heterogeneous, MacInnes *et al.*[44] suggested that these two species are not genetically distinct. *A. caviae* is genetically separate from *A. hydrophila* and *A. sobria*. Most recently, the family *Aeromonadaceae* has been proposed for membership in the genus *Aeromonas*.[1]

Members of the mesophilic *Aeromonas* are facultatively anaerobic, Gram-negative, motile rods possessing polar, monotrichous flagella. Unlike the polar flagellum of strains of the genus *Vibrio*, that of *Aeromonas* has no sheath. On solid media, young cultures of many strains may have lateral or peritrichous flagella.[45] They grow on ordinary media and on less inhibitory agar media such as MacConkey agar. Not all strains grow on TCBS agar but when they do, the colonies resemble sucrose fermenting colonies of *V. cholera*. They do not require salt for growth. The best growth is obtained at pH 7.2–7.6, but they may grow even at pH 9.0. On blood agar, many strains yield a large zone of beta-hemolysis.

Aeromonas is oxidase positive and ferments carbohydrates with or without gas formation. *A. hydrophila* and *A. sobria* are aerogenic, where as *A. caviae* is anaerogenic. They give positive reactions in tests of arginine dihydrolase but negative in ornithine decarboxylase. Different reactions may be seen with the lysine decarboxylase test, but if positive, the reaction may be weaker than that given by *Vibrio* strains. *Aeromonas* is not susceptible to the pteridine compound 0/129. The biochemical characteristics of the three species of mesophilic *Aeromonas* are shown in Table 8. Table 9 should be consulted for differentiation among these three species.

Sakazaki and Shimada[13] have distinguished 44 O-serogroups within *A. hydrophila*. They have also recognized at least 10 H-antigens in strains of the species. No difference is present between antigenicity of polar and lateral flagella. Since O- and H-antigens of *A. sobria* and *A. caviae* can be determined with antisera prepared with *A. hydrophila*, serovars of these three species could be included in a single schema.

In general, *Aeromonas* strains are susceptible to the second- and third-generation cephalosporins, the aminoglycosides, chloramphenicol, tetracycline, nalidixic acid, and trimethoprim-sulfamethoxazole, but resistant to ampicillin and carbenicillin.

TABLE 9
Differential Characteristics of Mesophilic *Aeromonas* Species

Test (substrate)	A. hydrophila		A. sobria		A. caviae	
	Sign[a]	% +	Sign[a]	% +	Sign[a]	% +
Voges–Proskauer (25°C)	d	85.5	d	37.5	−	0
Gluconate oxidation	+	95.5	+	93.5	−	0
Elastin hydrolysis	+	93.5	−	2.0	−	0
Esculin hydrolysis	+	99.0	−	5.5	+	98.5
Gas from glucose	+	99.0	+	97.5	−	0
Acid from						
Arabinose	d	85.5	d	12.5	d	87.5
Salicin	+	92.0	−	8.0	+	92.5
Arbutin	+	94.0	−	5.5	+	98.0
Citrate utilization in	+	94.5	−	5.5	+	98.0
Kauffmann–Petersen medium						

[a]For symbols, see Table 2.

3. THE GENUS *PLESIOMONAS*

In the genus *Plesiomonas,* only one species *P. shigelloides* is included. *P. shigelloides* is a facultatively anaerobic, Gram-negative motile rod with polar, lophotrichous flagella with no sheath. Occasional cells may yield lateral flagella in young cultures on solid media. *P. shigelloides* grows on MacConkey agar, SS agar, DCA agar, but not on TCBS agar; produces oxidase; and ferments glucose, inositol, and some carbohydrates without gas formation but does not with sucrose or mannitol. It gives positive reactions in tests of lysine and ornithine decarboxylases and arginine dihydrolase. *P. shigelloides* has no halophilism. Most strains are susceptible to the pteridine compound 0/129. The guanine-plus-cytosine content of the DNA is 51 mol%. Table 10 indicates biochemical characteristics of *P. shigelloides*.

TABLE 10
Biochemical Characteristics of *Plesiomonas
shigelloides*

Test (substrate)	Sign[a]	Percent positive
Oxidase	+	100
Indole	+	100
Voges–Proskauer (25°C)	−	0
Citrate (Simmons)	−	0
H$_2$ S (Kligler)	−	0
Urease (Christensen)	−	0
Gelatin (Kohn)	−	0
DNase	−	0
Tween 80 hydrolysis	−	0
Lysine decarboxylase	+	99
Arginine dihydrolase	+	99
Ornithine decarboxylase	+	95
Esculin hydrolysis	−	0
Gas from glucose	−	0
Acid from		
Arabinose	−	0
Lactose	d	40
Maltose	d	63
Melibiose	d	52
Raffinose	−	0
Rhamnose	−	0
Sucrose	−	0
Trehalose	+	100
Xylose	−	0
Adonitol	−	0
Dulcitol	−	0
Mannitol	−	0
Sorbitol	−	0
Arbutin	−	0
Salicin	d	15
Inositol	+	99
Beta-galactosidase	+	100

[a]For symbols, see Table 2.

An antigenic schema for *P. shigelloides* that included 50 O-serogroups and 17 H-antigens has been developed by Shimada and Sakazaki.[18,46,47] *P. shigelloides* was first recognized by earlier investigators because of O-antigen identity between a serogroup of this species and *Shigella sonnei*. Recently, close O-antigenic relationships between *P. shigelloides* and *Shigella* species have been demonstrated.[46,48]

Most strains of *P. shigelloides* are susceptible to the second- and third-generation cephalosporins, the aminoglycosides, chloramphenicol, polymyxin B, nalidixic acid, and trimethoprim-sulfamethoxazole, but can be resistant to ampicillin and carbenicillin.

REFERENCES

1. Colwell RR, MacDonell MT, De Ley J: Proposal to recognize the family *Aeromonadaceae* fam. nov. *Int J Syst Bacteriol* 36:473–477, 1986
1a. Baumann P, Baumann L: The marine gram-negative eubacteria: genera *Photobacterium, Beneckea, Alteromonas, Pseudomonas* and *Alcaligenes*, in Starr MP, Stolp H, Truper HG, et al (eds.): *The Prokaryotes*. Springer-Verlag, Berlin, 1981, pp. 1302–1331
2. Brenner DJ, Fanning GR, Hickman-Brenner FW, et al: DNA relatedness among *Vibrionaceae* with emphasis on the *Vibrio* species associated with human infection. *Colloq. INSERM* 114:175–184, 1983
2a. Reichelt JL, Baumann P: Effects of sodium chloride on the growth of heterotrophic marine bacteria. *Arch Microbiol,* 97:329–345, 1974
3. Sakazaki R, Gomez CZ, Sebald M: Taxonomical studies of the so-called NAG vibrios. *Japan J Med Sci Biol* 20:265–280, 1976
4. Citarella RV, Colwell RR: Polyphasic taxonomy of the genus *Vibrio:* polynucleotide sequence relationships among selected *Vibrio* species. *J Bacteriol* 104:434–442, 1970
5. Reichelt JP, Baumann P, Baumann L: Study of genetic relationships among marine species of the genera *Beneckea* and *Photobacterium* by means of in vitro DNA/DNA hybridization. *Arch Microbiol* 110:101–120, 1976
6. Heiberg C: *On the classification of Vibrio cholerae and cholera-like vibrios.* Busk, Copenhagen, 1935
6a. Kelly, MT, Stroh, EMD: Urease-positive, Kanagawa-negative *Vibrio parahaemolyticus* from patients and the environment in the Pacific Northwest. *J Clin Microbiol,* 27:2820–2822, 1989
7. Mhalu FS, Mmari PW, Ijumba J: Rapid emergence of El Tor *Vibrio cholerae* resistant to antimicrobial agents during first six months of fourth cholera epidemic in Tanzania. *Lancet* i:345–347, 1979
8. Threlfall EJ, Rowe B: *Vibrio cholerae* el tor acquires plasmied-encoded resistance to gentamicin. *Lancet* i:42, 1982
9. Joseph SW, Debell RM, Brown WP: In vitro response to chloramphenicol, tetracycline, ampicillin, gentamicin and beta-lactamase production by halophilic vibrios from human and environmental sources. *Antimicrob agents and chemother,* 13:244–248, 1978
10. Shinoda S, Kariyama R, Ogawa M, et al: Flagellar antigens of various species of the genus *Vibrio* and related genera. *Int J Syst Bacteriol* 26:97–101, 1976
11. Sakazaki R, Donovan TJ: Serology and epidemiology of *Vibrio cholerae* and *Vibrio mimicus,* in Bergan T (ed.): *Methods in Microbiology,* Vol. 16. Academic Press, London, 1984, pp. 271–289
12. Shimada T, Sakazaki R: Additional serovars and inter-O antigenic relationships of *Vibrio cholerae. Japan J Med Sci Biol* 30:275–277, 1977
13. Sakazaki R, Shimada T: O-serogrouping scheme *Aeromonas* strains. *Japan J Med Sci Biol* 37:247–255, 1984
14. Shimada T, Sakazaki R: Serological studies on *Vibrio fluvialis. Japan J Med Sci Biol* 36:315–323, 1973
15. Simada T, Sakazaki R: R antigen of *Vibrio cholerae. Japan J Med Sci Biol* 26:155–160, 1973
16. Sakazaki R, Tamura K, Gomez CA, et al: Serological studies on the cholera group of vibrios. *Japan J Med Sci Biol* 23:13–20, 1970
17. Sakazaki R, Tamuru K: Somatic antigen variation in *Vibrio cholerae. Japan J Med Sci Biol* 24:93–100, 1971
18. Shimada T, Sakazaki R, Oue M: A bioserogroup of marine vibrios possessing somatic antigen factors in common with *Vibrio cholerae* 01. *J Appl Bacteriol,* 62:453–456, 1987
19. Shimada T, Sakazaki R: A bioserogroup of *Vibrio cholerae* non-01 with Inaba antigen factor of cholera vibrio. *J Appl Bacteriol,* 64:141–144, 1988

20. Shimada T, Sakazaki R: *Vibrio fluvialis:* A new serogroup (19) possessing the Inaba factor antigen of *Vibrio cholerae* 01. *Jap J Med Sci Biol,* 40:153–157, 1987
21. Bhaskaran K, Sinha VB: Hybridization in vibrios. *Ind J Exp Biol* 9:119–120, 1971
22. Sakazaki R, Iwanami S, Tamura K: Studies on the enteropathogenic, facultatively halophilic bacteria, *Vibrio parahaemolyticus.* II. Serological characteristics. *Japan J Med Sci Biol* 21: 313–324, 1968
23. Shimada T, Sakazaki R: On the serology of *Vibrio vulnificus. Japan J Med Sci Biol* 37:241–246, 1984
24. Mukerjee S, Guha DK, Roy UK: Studies on typing of cholera by bacteriophage. Part 1. Phage-typing of *Vibrio cholerae* from Calcutta epidemics. *Ann Biochem Exp Med* 17:161–176, 1957
25. Lee JV, Furniss AL: The phage-typing of *V. cholerae* serovar O1, In Holmgren J, Holme T, Merson MH, et al (eds.): *Acute Enteric Infections of Children.* Elsevier/North Holland, Amsterdam, 1981, pp. 119–122
26. Memorandum, WHO meeting: Recent advance in cholera research. *Bull WHO* 63:841–849, 1985
27. Drozhevkina MS, Arutyunov YI: Phage typing of *Vibrio cholerae* using a new collection of phages. *J Hyg Epidem Microbiol Immunol* 23:340–347, 1979
28. Frost JA, Rowe B: Geographic variation in the distribution of phage types of *Vibrio cholerae* O1 and non-O1. *FEMS Microbiol Lett* 40:219–222, 1987
29. Wahba AH: Vibriocin production in the cholera and el tor vibrios. *Bull WHO* 33:661–664, 1965
30. Mitra S, Balganesh TS, Dastidar SG, et al: Single bacteriocin typing for the vibrio groups of organisms. *Infect Immun* 30:74–77, 1980
31. Kobayashi T, Enomoto S, Sakazaki R, et al: A new selective isolation medium for the vibrio group (modified Nakanishi medium - TCBS agar). *Japan J Bacteriol* 18:387–392, 1963, in Japanese
32. Tamura K, Shimada S, Prescott LM: *Vibrio* agar: a new plating medium for isolation of *Vibrio cholerae. Japan J Med Sci Biol* 24:125–127, 1971
33. Monsur DA: A highly selective gelatin–taurocholate–tellurite medium for the isolation of *Vibrio cholerae. Trans Roy Soc Trop Med Hyg* 55:440–442, 1961
34. Monsur KA: Bacteriological diagnosis of cholera under field conditions. *Bull WHO* 28:387–389, 1963
35. Sakazaki R, Karashima T, Yuda K, et al: Enumeration of and hygienic standard of food safety for *Vibrio parahaemolyticus. Arch Lebensmittelhyg* 30:81–84, 1979
36. Emoto M: Frozen lobster and shrimp contaminated with *Vibrio cholerae* and related vibrios, in Kurata H, Hesseltein CW (eds.): *Control of the Microbial Contamination of Foods and Feeds in International Trade: Microbial Standards and Specifications.* Saikon Publisher, Tokyo, 1982, pp 161–167
37. Isaacson M: Practical aspects of a cholera surveillance program. *S Afr Med J* 49:1699–1702, 1975
38. Barret TJ, Blake PA, Morris GK, et al: Use of Moore swabs for isolating *Vibrio cholerae* from sewage. *J Clin Microbiol* 11:385–388, 1980
39. Spira WM, Ahmed QS: Gauze filtration and enrichment procedures for recovery of *Vibrio cholerae* from contaminated waters. *Appl Environ Microbiol* 42:730–733, 1981
40. Hranitsky KW, Larson AD, Rangsdale DW, et al: Isolation of O1 serovar of *Vibrio cholerae* from water by serologically specific method. *Science* 210:1025–1026, 1980
41. Shimada T: A new selective isolation medium for *Vibrio cholerae,* eltor - PMT agar. *Media Circle* 25:6–9, 1980, in Japanese
42. Sakazaki R, Tamura K, Murase M: Determination of the hemolytic activity of *Vibrio cholerae. Japan J Med Sci Biol* 24:83–91, 1971
43. Popoff MY, Coynault C, Kiredjian M, et al: Polynucleotide sequence relatedness among motile *Aeromonas* species. *Curr Microbiol* 5:109–114, 1981
44. MacInnes JI, Trust TJ, Crosa JH: Deoxyribonucleic acid relationships among members of the genus *Aeromonas. Canad J Microbiol* 25:579–586, 1979
45. Shimada T, Sakazaki R, Suzuki K: Peritrichous flagella in mesophilic strains of *Aeromonas. Japan J Med Sci Biol* 38:141–145, 1985
46. Shimada T, Sakazaki R: On the serology of *Plesiomonas shigelloides. Japan J Med Sci Biol* 31:135–142, 1978
47. Shimada T, Sakazaki R: New O and H antigens and additional serovars of *Plesiomonas shigelloides. Japan J Med Sci Biol* 38:73–76, 1985
48. Hori M, Hayashi K, Maeshima K, et al: Food poisoning caused by *Aeromonas shigelloides* with an antigen common to *Shigella dysenteriae* 7. *J Japan Ass Infect Dis* 39:441–448, 1966, in Japanese

3

Epidemiology and Pathogenicity of Non-01 Vibrio Species and Related Organisms

S. C. Sanyal

1. INTRODUCTION

Several new species of the genus *Vibrio* have been recognized in recent years thanks to improved laboratory techniques, which have allowed the isolation and differentiation of members of the genus *Vibrio* and allied organisms. Epidemiology and pathogenesis of these new species have drawn the attention of epidemiologists and basic scientists alike. Some of these species, such as *V. vulnificus, V. alginolyticus, V. damsela*, and *V. metschnikovii*, do not cause diarrhea but cause certain extraintestinal lesions. For example, *V. vulnificus* has been implicated in fulminating septicemia and a rapidly progressing cellulitis; *V. alginolyticus* and *V. damsela*, in superficial skin and ear infections; and *V. metschnikovii* (an opportunistic pathogen), in peritonitis and bacteremia. This chapter will focus on the current status of knowledge on the epidemiology and pathogenicity of vibrios other than *V. cholerae* 01 and related organisms which cause diarrhea in humans.

2. EPIDEMIOLOGY

2.1. Natural Occurrence and Their Habitat

The natural habitats of *V. cholerae* non-01 are bodies of water such as rivers, marshes, bays, and coastal areas.[1,2] They have been found to be widely distributed in the environment

Cholera, edited by Dhiman Barua and William B. Greenough III. Plenum Medical Book Company, New York, 1992.

and have been isolated from surface and estuarine waters, sewage, seafoods (e.g., crabs and oysters), animals, poultry, cockroaches, and tadpoles.

V. mimicus appears to occur naturally in estuarine and fresh-water environments. The organism has been isolated from waters and shellfish in many parts of the world[3] including India (unpublished data).

V. parahaemolyticus is a part of the normal flora of estuarine and other coastal waters in nearly every part of the world. The organism has been isolated from sediments and fresh and sea waters and the fish in these environments.[4]

V. fluvialis and *V. furnissii* are found in coastal, estuarine, and fresh-water environments in most parts of the world.[5]

For *V. hollisae,* sea water seems to be the natural habitat[6] and seafish the most likely reservoir.

Aeromonas hydrophila is a water-borne organism appearing widely in fresh water, brackish water, sewage, and sludge in most areas of the world. In addition, it comprises a portion of the normal microbial flora of fish, as well as other aquatic animals and plants.[7]

Plesiomonas shigelloides, an inhabitant of surface water in many parts of the world,[8] is frequently isolated from stagnating as well as streaming waters, sea water, sewage, mud, the intestines of fish and other aquatic animals, and from mammals (e.g., swine, dogs, cats, goats, sheep, and monkeys).

2.2. Geographic Distribution of *V. cholerae* Non-01 Diseases

Wherever attempts have been made to isolate it, *V. cholerae* non-01 has been isolated from sporadic cases of diarrhea in all the continents. Various serotypes of *V. cholerae* non-01 have been found to cause sporadic cases of diarrhea and also limited outbreaks such as those recorded in Czechoslovakia, India, Sudan, the United States (US), in airplanes and cruise ships, and other means of transportation. However, no large epidemic, resembling those caused by *V. cholerae* 01, has been observed.

V. mimicus is a recently recognized enteropathogen, that is being isolated with increasing frequency from cases of diarrhea; so far, this infection has been reported from Bangladesh, Mexico, New Zealand, Guam, Canada, the United States, and Asia.[3,9]

V. parahaemolyticus–associated gastroenteritis has been reported in North America, Central America, Europe, Asia, and Africa. The organisms usually cause outbreaks of gastroenteritis, although sporadic cases do occur.[4]

V. fluvialis, previously kown as "Group F vibrio" or "Group EF6 vibrio," has been isolated from patients with diarrhea in Bangladesh, Bahrain, Jordan, Indonesia, India, and Thailand.[10–12] The organisms caused a large epidemic in Bangladesh during 1976–1977 affecting hundreds of adults and children.[13]

V. furnissii, formerly known as *V. fluvialis* biovar II, is an environmental organism. Its role as an etiologic agent of acute diarrhea has not yet been clearly established. It has been isolated from cases of diarrhea when other enteropathogens were also present. Careful studies are required to define its role as an enteropathogen.

V. hollisae has been isolated from feces of diarrheal patients in the US.[6]

Isolations of *Aeromonas hydrophila* from diarrheal patients have been reported from Asia, Europe, North and South Americas, Australia, and Africa.[7,14] Although *A. hydrophila* has been isolated in feces of healthy individuals, the incidence of such asymptomatic carriers is low.[14]

Plesiomonas shigelloides has been isolated from fecal specimens of diarrheal cases in Sri Lanka, India, Bangladesh, Thailand, Zaire, Cuba, Iran, Japan, Germany, Czechoslovakia, United Kingdom, Australia, and the United States, but its presence in a healthy person has been rare.[8,15] This organism has been implicated in several diarrhea outbreaks in Japan.[8]

It is said that several members of the *Vibrio* species and related organisms cause diarrheal disease worldwide but go unrecognized for lack of proper laboratory diagnosis.

2.3. Seasonal Pattern

Little is known about the seasonality of *V. cholerae* non-01 infections. Most of these infections occur in the warmer months in the United States and in Spring and Summer in Bangladesh. Although the organism is present in the water and sewage system in Varanasi, India, year-round, only a small number of cases occur during the months of May to September.[1]

Distinct seasonality of *V. parahaemolyticus*–associated gastroenteritis has been observed in at least three countries. Outbreaks of the disease occur almost exclusively during the warm summer and early fall months in the US and Japan. In Thailand, the proportion of *V. parahaemolyticus*–associated diarrhea cases varies from 3.9% in the relatively cool month of January to 2.6% in the warm month of September. This seasonal variation may reflect both enhanced opportunity of the organisms to multiply in unrefrigerated foods during the summer months and their predominance near the surface of water during warm weather; during the winter months, the organism is mostly found in the sediment.

Incidence of diarrhea associated with *A. hydrophila* and its isolation from water are noted to be higher during summer than in winter in Australia and the United States.[7] Seasonal variations with a decline in cooler months[8] have been observed in the occurrence of *P. shigelloides* in surface waters. The majority of the gastroenteritis outbreaks attributed to this organism occurred in warmer months.[16]

Very little is known about the seasonality of diseases caused by *V. fluvialis* and *V. hollisae*. Their isolation from water sources, however, also increases during warmer months.

2.4. Modes of Transmission and Incubation Period

Contaminated food and water are probably the exclusive modes of transmission of *V. cholerae* non-01 infections. Studies of three outbreaks showed that the vehicle of transmission was food (potatoes and egg and asparagus salad) in two instances, and water in one. In a case–control study, raw oysters were epidemiologically implicated in transmission of the disease.[13] In an outbreak in Sudan no secondary cases were observed and no person-to-person transmission was evident.[13] However, a study in Varanasi, India, indicated the possibility of person-to-person transmission and established the "carrier status" in humans.[17] The majority of carriers were short-term excretors for 1 to 7 days; they were detected both in association with cases and also in the absence of overt cases, in the family or in the community. The overall carrier rate was found to be 6.3%; the highest rate (8.85%) was in the 5–14 year age group, followed by children aged 1–5 years. One chronic carrier excreted the organism for 59 days. A study of sailors in the Soviet Union also indicates that carrier status could last for 60 or more days.[13] The organism has been isolated from bile, raising the possibility of the carrier state being favored by chronic biliary tract infections.

The incubation period in reported outbreaks in Czechoslovakia, in an airplane going to Australia, and to Sudan were noted to be 20–30 hour, 3–5 hour, and less than 4 days, respectively.[13]

Serotyping *V. cholerae* non-01 has been shown to be a useful epidemiologic marker, especially for studying carrier status[17,18]; however, not many carrier studies have used this procedure because the sera are not readily available.

V. parahaemolyticus is transmitted mainly through raw or partially cooked seafood; other foods, presumably cross-contaminated by raw seafoods, have also been implicated.[13] In a study in India, a third of the *V. parahaemolyticus*–associated gastroenteritis cases did not eat any type of fish or seafood during the previous seven days indicating that other modes of transmission are possible.[19]

Several factors may contribute to spread of *V. parahaemolyticus* infection.[13] It has been observed that in outbreaks involving raw seafoods, foods naturally contaminated with probably small numbers of organisms, were kept unrefrigerated long enough to allow the bacteria to proliferate to large numbers. Outbreaks involving boiled shrimp have been attributed to failure to cook the shrimp at temperatures high enough to kill the vibrios. Other outbreaks have been attributed to cooked seafood contaminated by raw seafood, followed by inadequate refrigeration. The generation time of *V. parahaemolyticus* is as short as 9 min under ideal conditions[13] enabling the organism to quickly reach the rather large infecting dose in mishandled food. The ID_{50} has been determined in volunteer studies to be about 100,000 (i.e., 10^5) organisms for persons given antacids.[20]

Asymptomatic infection has been detected although there are no reports available about hosts carrying the organisms long term; there is no evidence of infected handlers being responsible for any outbreaks.[13]

The incubation period of *V. parahaemolyticus*–associated gastroenteritis has been found to vary between 4 to 96 hr.[4] For the dysenteric illness, the incubation period may be only 2.5 hr.[13]

The usefulness of the currently available serotyping scheme for epidemiologic investigations is limited since the schema are based on strains isolated from clinical cases and may not be able to identify many strains from marine sources (see Section 1, Chapter 2).

The epidemiologic information on *V. mimicus* is scanty but the evidence of its implication in acute diarrhea linked to consumption of uncooked seafood (particularly raw oysters) is strong.[21]

V. hollisae has only recently been recognized as an etiologic agent of diarrhea, and therefore, not much is known regarding its epidemiology. The organism has been isolated from a number of patients with diarrhoea who had eaten raw seafood. It has also been isolated from the blood of a patient with hepatic cirrhosis.[22]

V. fluvialis has been isolated from cases of diarrhoea and from a number of environmental sources although the epidemiology of the disease has not yet been defined.

Analysis of various reports on *A. hydrophila*–associated diarrhea in man has brought abundant evidence of the importance of the organism as a water-borne pathogen.[14] Nosocomial spread through dialysis fluid and hospital water supplies has also been reported.[7] Nothing is known regarding the incubation period of diarrhea caused by *A. hydrophila*.

A critical analysis of the data presented in various reports of *P. shigelloides*–associated sporadic diarrhea and outbreaks indicates that contaminated water and food are the likely vehicles of transmission. The incubation period of the disease caused by *P. shigelloides* is not yet known.

3. PATHOGENICITY

3.1. Diseases Caused by *V. cholerae Non-01*

The spectrum of diarrheal disease caused by *V. cholerae* non-01 includes a choleralike disease with rice–water stools to very mild gastroenteritis; isolated cases may be clinically indistinguishable. The duration of diarrhea and the volume of fluid lost is usually less than in patients with typical cholera. With non-01 infections, fever is common and patients may have bloody stools.[1,14]

Some *V. cholerae* non-01 strains may cause wound infections, acute appendicitis, acute cholecystitis, cholangitis, cellulitis, otitis media, pneumonia, meningitis, meningoencephalitis, and septicemia.[1] These lesions indicate that some *V. cholerae* non-01 strains may possess invasive properties in addition to their enterotoxicity.

Doubts have been expressed about the pathogenicity of the free-living strains of *V. cholerae* non-01 in the environment[23]; however, cases of intestinal and extraintestinal infections due to these organisms have been reported where connection with brackish water was a common feature.[24]

V. mimicus usually causes watery diarrhea leading to varying degrees of dehydration; however, occasional mucoid and bloody stools, accompanied by abdominal cramps, have also been reported.[9] This organism has also been isolated from extraintestinal sites such as ear infections.[3]

V. parahaemolyticus causes outbreaks of gastroenteritis although sporadic cases also occur. The illness is characterized by either acute watery diarrhea or dysentery with mild fever and much abdominal pain.[4,13] *V. parahaemolyticus* has also been isolated from wounds of feet, legs, knee, infected ear, and septicemia.[13]

Gastroenteritis caused by *V. fluvialis* is usually associated with vomiting, dehydration, abdominal pain, and sometimes fever; stools often contain erythrocytes and rarely blood. Infants, children, and young adults are commonly affected.

A hydrophila has long been known as a pathogen for cold-blooded animals. In recent years the organism has attracted interest as an etiologic agent of childhood diarrhea but the relative importance of the organism as a human enteropathogen is still unknown (unpublished report of a WHO scientific group's CDD/BEI/84.4). The disease is usually characterized by watery diarrhea, but one-fifth of the sufferers may have bloody stools. The disease is often of short duration but may last for more than 2 weeks in nearly 40% of patients.[25]

A. hydrophila has also been associated with a variety of other infections such as septicemia, meningitis, endocarditis, corneal ulcers, wound infections, and peritonitis in healthy and immunocompromised humans.[7,14]

P. shigelloides has been isolated from cases with watery and dystenteric diarrhea in children and in adults; the organism has also been implicated in several outbreaks of diarrhoea.[8,26] The enteropathogenicity of the organism, however, has not been conclusively proven as yet.[27] Like most other *V. cholerae* non-01 and related organisms, *P. shigelloides* also has been associated with extraintestinal infections, such as pyometritis, cellulitis, urethritis, cholecystitis, meningitis, and bacteremia.

3.2. Virulence Factors and Probable Mechanisms of Causing Disease

The majority of the *V. cholerae* non-01 strains isolated from clinical and environmental sources produce a heat-labile, nondialysable protein enterotoxin of molecular weight ≈ 40,000 with maximum activity in the pH range 6.0–8.0 and is antigenic.[1,28] The enterotoxin causes accumulation of fluid in rabbit gut loops, increase in permeability of rabbit's skin, diarrhea in suckling rabbits, and cytotonic effect on CHO and Y1 cell monolayers. The enterotoxin of *V. cholerae* non-01 is neutralized by cholera antitoxin and anti-*Escherichia coli* LT in ileal loop and skin permeability assays; shows reaction of identity with cholera toxin in gel diffusion assay and homology with cholera toxin and *E. coli* LT at the gene level.[1] Thus, this enterotoxin is identical to cholera toxin including its pathogenic mechanism.

Quantitative differences in production of enterotoxin by certain strains of *V. cholerae* non-01 have been observed. While many of these vibrios isolated from patients in Bangladesh and in the United States have been found not to produce the toxin,[13] many of the diarrheal isolates of these vibrios produce comparable amounts of toxin like that produced by *V. cholerae* 01 as observed in rabbit loop assay.[29] Most of the environmental isolates of non-01 produce no toxin or lesser quantity of toxin.[28,30] In certain studies, the majority of the clinical and environmental isolates of these vibrios were found to be nontoxigenic. This difference in enterotoxicity may be explained by the possibility of the existence of a mechanism of repression and depression in the toxin gene, which is chromosomal in *V. cholerae*.[31] The nontoxigenic strains have been found to become toxigenic after only a couple of consecutive passages through the susceptible rabbit gut.[29,30] Further, some of these strains, especially the environmental isolates, elaborate cytotoxic substances,[32] in addition to enterotoxin, that may mask the enterotoxic activity when their culture filtrates are tested in tissue cultures. Moreover, the medium used for preparation of culture filtrates and the method of incubation—shaking or static—have profound effects on these activities.[1] It is also possible that some of these strains produce an enterotoxin not recognized previously.[33] This new toxin is a heat-labile protein, and it differs from the known cholera toxin in antigenicity, receptor site, mode of action, and genetic homology.[34] It failed to show antigenic similarity with Shiga toxin (S.C. Sanyal, unpublished data); further, some of these strains tested with Shiga toxin gene probes did not show homology (P. Echeverria, personal communication).

The *V. cholerae* non-01 strains multiply in rabbit loops by several logs, implying a capacity to colonize in the gut,[30,35] although the factors mediating mucosal adherence are not yet known.

Production of a heat-stable enterotoxin by some of the diarrheal and environmental isolates of these vibrios have been reported[1] based on the suckling mouse assay of Dean *et al.*[36] While examining 14 strains of *V. cholerae* non-01 of different serotypes for heat-stable toxin,[29] the gut/body ratio was found to be less than 0.08 which is lower than the cut-off point of 0.09 suggested to be significant by Dean *et al.*[36]

V. mimicus strains produce heat-labile protein enterotoxin, which causes accumulation of fluid in rabbit gut loops, increase in permeability of rabbits' skin, diarrhea in suckling rabbits, and cytotonic effect in CHO and Y1 cell monolayers, and can be detected by GM1 ELISA assay.[9,37] The enterotoxic activity of *V. mimicus* can be neutralized by cholera antitoxin in ileal loop and skin permeability assays.[9,37] and the toxin is identical to cholera toxin in gel-diffusion assay.[37] Further, like cholera toxin, but in contrast to *E. coli* LT, most of the toxin from *V. mimicus* is found extracellularly and is proteotypically nicked in its A subunit.[38] Colony hybridization with CT probe shows genetic homology with *V. mimicus* toxin (Sanyal, unpublished data). Thus, the toxin produced by *V. mimicus* appears to be identical to cholera toxin and it receptor site is GM1 ganglioside of the epithelial cells. Since the toxin causes cytotonic reaction in CHO and Y1 adrenal cells, its action appears to be mediated through stimulation of adenylate cyclase system simulating that of cholera toxin.

Strains of these vibrios produce a soluble hemagglutinin, which has been shown to be antigenically similar to that of *V. cholerae* 01.[38] *V. mimicus* strains multiply in rabbit ileal loops by 4–6 logs, indicating their capacity to colonize the gut mucosa[9]; however, the factors mediating mucosal adherence are not known.

The mechanism whereby *V. parahaemolyticus* causes gastroenteritis needs further investigation. Most of the strains isolated from patients with diarrhea are Kanagawa positive, i.e., they hemolyse human erythrocytes on Wagatsuma agar, but most of those strains isolated from food or other articles in the environment are Kanagawa negative.[4] *V. parahaemolyticus* produces several hemolysins, but the hemolysin responsible for the Kanagawa phenomenon is a "thermostable direct hemolysin," as it is not activated by addition of lecithin. The molecular weight of the purified and crystallized thermostable direct hemolysin is ca. 42,000 and its receptor sites are gangliosides Gt1 and Gd1a.[39] The gene encoding the direct hemolysin has been cloned and its amino acid sequence has recently been determined.[39] The thermostable direct hemolysin is cytotoxic, cardiotoxic, and lethal to small experimental animals, although its clinical significance is not clearly known. In low dose (100 μg) this toxin does not cause fluid accumulation in rabbit loop, but with very high doses (500 μg), turbid bloody fluid accumulated. On administration of 50 μg of the hemolysin by the stomach tube, all the 5- to 6-day-old mice developed diarrhea and soon died. But with a dose of 2.0–12.5 μg of the hemolysin, only some animals died while others suffered from transient diarrhea.[39] As the antiserum against the thermostable direct hemolysin could not inhibit the fluid accumulation in rabbit ileal loop by cells of Kanagawa positive strains of *V. parahaemolyticus,* enteropathogenicity of the organism could not be explained solely by the thermostable direct hemolysin.[39] The Kanagawa positive strains adhere to HeLa cells and may cause bacteremia in orally challenged infant rabbits.[39]

About 70–90% of the strains of *V. fluvialis* from patients and the environment produce a heat-labile protein enterotoxin that induces fluid accumulation in rabbit ileal loops.[10,40,41] The partially purified toxin also showed cytotonic changes in CHO cell monolayers, and its fluid outpouring activity in ileal loop was completely inhibited by chlorpromazine, indicating mediation of cyclic AMP in its mode of action.[40]

The enterotoxin produced by *V. fluvialis* strains could be neutralized by the antiserum raised against the new cholera toxin mentioned above and shows immunological identity with this toxin in gel-diffusion test.[42] No genetic homology of *V. fluvialis* enterotoxin and cholera toxin has yet been demonstrated.

V. hollisae possesses sequences that have homology with the gene encoding the thermostable direct hemolysin of *V. parahaemolyticus,*[43] produces a hemolysin which is lytic for human and rabbit erythrocytes and is antigenically similar to the thermostable direct hemolysin. Further work is needed to elucidate the virulence factors of this organism.

A. hydrophila produce an alpha and beta hemolysin which are membrane damaging. The former induces leakage of intracellular large-molecular-weight markers in human embryonic lung fibroblasts and is dermonecrotic to rabbit skin, whereas the latter induces irreversible damage with exit of small molecules, is dermonecrotic, and is lethal to small laboratory animals.[7] The beta hemolysin is a heat-labile protein of molecular weight ca. 50,000, and is toxic for a variety of cell lines.[7] It does not cause fluid accumulation in the rabbit ileal loop but is active in suckling mice.[44]

A. hydrophila strains also produce an extracellular heat-labile, protein enterotoxin.[45] Separated from hemolysin, this enterotoxin causes fluid accumulation without mucosal injury in rabbit and rat intestines.[7,44] The enterotoxin induces steroidogenesis,[46] cAMP elevation,[47] cytotonic changes in Y1 adrenal cells,[7] and elongation in CHO cells[31]; however, the cytotoxic activity of the hemolysin often masks this reaction. The molecular weight of the enterotoxin has been estimated to be ca. 15,000–20,000. A choleralike enterotoxin neutralizable by cholera antitoxin in a reverse passive latex hemagglutination assay (RPLA) has been demonstrated in culture filtrates of certain *A. hydrophila* strains; the production of choleralike toxin also has been confirmed by ELISA test.[48] However, other studies have not demonstrated any antigenic cross reaction between these two toxins.[7] The enterotoxin does not appear to bind to GM1 ganglioside or to mixtures of crude gangliosides.[7]

Hydrophobic cell-surface properties, hemagglutinating activity, and fimbriae and fimbriaelike structures are common in enterotoxigenic *A. hydrophila*.[7,49,50] Environmental isolates have been found to have different properties than those of clinical sources.[51,52] A soluble hemagglutinin unrelated to the hemolytic, enterotoxic, and proteolytic activities in cell-free extracts of diarrheal isolates of different species of *Aeromonas* has also been described recently.[53] Their role in colonization to intestinal epithelial cells has not yet been determined.

While studying 147 isolates of *A. hydrophila*, so-called *A. sobria, A. caviae,* and *A. punctata* of clinical and environmental origin in this laboratory, it has been noted that all of these isolates cause fluid accumulation in rabbit gut loop. Certain alpha-hemolytic and nonhemolytic strains required 1–2 passages through rabbit gut before becoming ileal loop positive when they also became beta-hemolytic. This indicates that these species possess the beta-hemolysin gene and are potentially enterotoxigenic (Singh and Sanyal, unpublished data).

Although *P. shigelloides* has been implicated both in sporadic cases and in outbreaks of diarrhea, its exact role as an enteropathogen is still unclear.[26,27] Live cells and culture filtrates of *P. shigelloides* strains isolated from people with diarrhea, from healthy humans, and from the environment, however, have been found to cause an accumulation of fluid in the ileal loop of rabbits. This indicates the production of enterotoxic substance(s) by this organism[15] (Table 1). A number of strains from sources other than diarrhea required 1 or 2

TABLE 1
Rabbit Ileal Loop Tests with Culture Filtrates (CF) of *Plesiomonas shigelloides*

Source	Number of CF tested	Number positive	Number of CF (range of fluid accumulated, ml/cm of gut)
Diarrheal case	48	48	14 (0.6–1.0)
			18 (1.1–1.5)
			16 (1.6–2.0)
Healthy individuals	04	04	04 (1.0–1.5)
Water			
Well water	02	02	02 (1.0–1.5)
River water	06	06	06 (0.6–1.0)
Positive control (CF of			(0.8–1.5)
V. cholerae 569B)			
Negative control (tryptic soy			0
broth with 1% inositol)			

consecutive passages through rabbit gut before causing fluid accumulation. Production of both heat-labile and heat-stable enterotoxins by *P. shigelloides* strains belonging to different serotypes have also been demonstrated[15,26] by using the techniques of time-course of fluid accumulation in ileal loops by culture filtrates with and without heat treatment and suckling mouse assay. The enterotoxins have been purified to electrophoretic homogeneity, the heat-labile toxin being active in loop and the heat-stable toxin in both loop and suckling mice assays.[54] Both toxins are stable at pH 5.0–7.0, with optimal activity observed at pH 8.0–9.0. The enterotoxins are resistant to proteolytic enzymes and organic solvents.

Certain *P. shigelloides* strains isolated from dysenterylike cases have been shown to invade the HeLa cell monolayers.[55] Very little is known regarding other virulence factors of *P. shigelloides*.

REFERENCES

1. Sanyal SC: NAG vibrio toxin, in Dorner F, Drews J (eds): *Pharmacology of Bacterial Toxins*. Oxford, Pergamon Press, 1986, pp 207–225
2. Feachem R, Miller C, Drasar B: Environmental aspects of cholera epidemiology. II. Occurrence and survival of *Vibrio cholerae* in the environment. *Trop Dis Bull* 78:865–880, 1981
3. Davis BR, Fanning GR, Madden JM, et al: Characterization of biochemically atypical *Vibrio cholerae* strains and designation of a new pathogenic species, *Vibrio mimicus*. *J Clin Microbiol* 14:631–639, 1981
4. Miwatani T, Takeda Y: *Vibrio parahaemolyticus: A Causative Bacterium for Food-Poisoning*. Tokyo, Saikon Publications, 1976, p 23
5. Baumann P, Schubert RHW: Family II. *Vibrionaceae* Veron 1965, 5245, in Krieg NR, Holt JG (eds): *Bergey's Manual of Systematic Bacteriology*, Vol. I. London, Williams and Wilkins, 1984, p 516
6. Hickman HW, Farmer JJ III, Hollis DG, et al: Identification of *Vibrio hollisae* sp. nov. from patients with diarrhoea. *J Clin Microbiol* 15:395–401, 1982
7. Ljungh A, Wadstrom T: *Aeromonas* toxins, in Dorner F, Drews J (eds): *Pharmacology of Bacterial Toxins*, Oxford, Pergamon Press, 1986, pp 289–305
8. Schubert RHW: Genus IV. *Plesiomonas* Habs and Schubert 1962, 324, in Krieg NR, Holt JG (eds): *Bergey's Manual of Systematic Bacteriology*, Vol. 1. London, Williams and Wilkins, 1984, pp 548–550
9. Sanyal SC, Huq MI, Neogi PKB, et al: *Vibrio mimicus* as an aetiological agent of diarrhoea and its pathogenesis. *Indian J Med Microbiol* 1:1–12, 1983
10. Sanyal SC, Agarwal RK, Annapurna E, et al: Enterotoxicity of group F vibrios. *Jap J Med Sci Biol* 33:217–222, 1980
11. Nishibuchi M, Roberts NC, Bradford HB, et al: Broth medium for enrichment of *Vibrio fluvialis* from the environment. *Appl Environ Microbiol* 46:425–429, 1983
12. Suthienkel O, Ohashi M, Goto S, et al: The enteropathogenicity of *Vibrio fluvialis* isolated from aquatic sources in Thailand. *J Dir Dis Res* 3:14–19, 1985
13. Blake PA, Weaver RE, Hollis DG: Diseases of humans (other than cholera) caused by vibrios. *Ann Rev Microbiol* 34:341–367, 1980
14. Kaper JB, Lockman H, Colwell RR: *Aeromonas hydrophila*: Ecology and toxigenicity of isolates from an estuary. *J Appl Bacteriol* 50:359–377, 1981
15. Sanyal SC, Saraswathi B, Sharma P: Enteropathogenicity of *Plesiomonas shigelloides*. *J Med Microbiol* 13:401–409, 1980
16. Burke V, Robinson J, Gracey M: Isolation of *Aeromonas hydrophila* from a metropolitan water supply: Seasonal correlation with clinical isolates. *Appl Environ Microbiol* 48:361–366, 1984
17. Marwah SM, Tiwari IC, Singh SJ, et al: Epidemiological studies on cholera in nonendemic regions with special reference to the problem of carrier state during epidemic and nonepidemic period. *Indian J Prev Soc Med* 6:326–337, 1975
18. Sanyal SC, Singh SJ, Tiwari IC, et al: Role of household animals in maintenance of cholera infection in a community. *J Infect Dis* 130:575–579, 1974
19. Sirkar BK, Deb BC, De SP, et al: Clinical and epidemiological studies on V. *parahaemolyticus* infection in Calcutta (1975). *Indian J Med Res* 64:1576–1580, 1976
20. Sanyal SC, Sen PC: Human volunteer study on the pathogenicity of *Vibrio parahaemolyticus*, in Fujino T,

Sakaguchi G, Sakazaki R, Takeda Y (eds): *International Symposium on Vibrio parahaemolyticus.* Tokyo, Saikon Publications, 1975, pp 227–235

21. Shandera WX, Johnson JM, Davis BR, et al: Disease from infection with *Vibrio mimicus,* a newly recognized vibrio species. *Ann Intern Med* 99:169–171, 1983

22. Morris JG, Wilson R, Hollis DG, et al: Illness caused by *Vibrio damsela* and *Vibrio hollisae. Lancet* i:1294–1297, 1982

23. WHO Scientific Working Group: Cholera and other vibrio-associated diarrhoeas. *Bull WHO* 58:353–374, 1980

24. Back E, Ljunggren, Smith H Jr: Noncholera vibrios in Sweden. *Lancet* i:723–724, 1974

25. Gracy M, Burke V, Robinson J: Aeromonas associated gastroenteritis. *Lancet* ii:1304, 1982

26. Saraswathi B, Agarwal RK, Sanyal SC: Further studies on enteropathogenicity of *Plesiomonas shigelloides. Indian J Med Res* 78:12–18, 1983

27. Sakazaki R: Serology and epidemiology of *Plesiomonas shigelloides,* in *Methods of Microbiology,* Vol. 16. London, Academic Press, 1984, p 259

28. Craig JP, Yamamoto K, Takeda Y, et al: Production of cholera-like enterotoxin by a *Vibrio cholerae* non-01 strain isolated from environment. *Infect Immun* 34:90–97, 1981

29. Shanker P, Agarwal RK, Sanyal SC: Experimental studies on enteropathogenicity of *Vibrio cholerae* serotypes other than 01. *Zantbl Bakt ParasitKde Abt I Orig A* 252:514–524, 1982

30. Singh SJ, Sanyal SC: Enterotoxicity of the so-called NAG vibrios. *Ann Soc belge Med Trop* 58:133–140, 1978

31. Vasil M, Holmes RK, Finkelstein RA: Conjugal transfer of a chromosomal gene determining production of enterotoxin in *V. cholerae. Science* 187:849–850, 1975

32. Bisgaard M, Sakazaki R, Shimada T: Prevalence of non-cholera vibrios in cavum nasi and pharynx of ducks. *Acta Path Microbiol Scand Sect B* 86:261–266, 1978

33. Sanyal SC, Alam K, Neogi PKB, et al: A new cholera toxin. *Lancet* i:1337, 1983

34. Sanyal SC, Neogi PKB, Alam K, et al: A new enterotoxin produced by *Vibrio cholerae* 01. *J Dir Dis Res* 2:3–12, 1984

35. Spira WM, Daniel RR, Ahmed QS, et al: Clinical features and pathogenicity of O group 1, non-agglutinable *Vibrio cholerae* and other vibrios isolated from cases of diarrhoea in Dacca, Bangladesh, in Takeya K, Zinnaka Y (eds): *Symposium on Cholera.* Karatsu, US–Japan Cooperative Medical Science Program, 1979, pp 137–153

36. Dean AG, Ching YC, Williams RG, et al: Test for *Escherichia coli* enterotoxin using infant mice. *J Infect Dis* 125:407–411, 1972

37. Sanyal SC, Huq MI, Neogi PKB, et al: Experimental studies on the pathogenicity of *Vibrio mimicus* strains isolated in Bangladesh. *Aust J Exp Biol Med Sci* 62:515–521, 1984

38. Dotevall H, Stromberg GJ, Sanyal SC, et al: Characterization of enterotoxin and soluble haemagglutinin from *Vibrio mimicus:* identity with *V. cholerae* 01 toxin and haemagglutinin. *FEMS Microbiol Lett* 27:17–22, 1985

39. Takeda Y: Thermostable direct haemolysin of *Vibrio parahaemolyticus,* in Dorner F, Drews J (eds): *Pharmacology of Bacterial Toxins.* Oxford, Pergamon Press, 1986, pp 183–205

40. Agarwal RK, Sanyal SC: Experimental studies on enteropathogenicity and pathogenesis of group 'F' vibrio infections. *Zbl Bakt Hyg I Abt Orig A* 249:392–399, 1981

41. Huq MI, Aziz KMS, Colwell RR: Enterotoxigenic properties of *Vibrio fluvialis* (Group F vibrio) isolated from clinical and environmental sources. *J Dir Dis Res* 3:96–99, 1985

42. Ahsan CR, Sanyal SC, Zaman A, Neogy PKB, Huq W: Immunobiological relationship between *Vibrio fluvialis* and *Vibrio cholerae* enterotoxins. *Immunol Cell Biol,* 66:251–252, 1988

43. Nishibuchi M, Ishibashi M, Takeda Y, et al: Detection of the thermostable direct haemolysin gene and related DNA sequences in *Vibrio parahaemolyticus* and other Vibrio species by the DNA colony hybridization test. *Infect Immun* 49:481–486, 1985

44. Chakraborty T, Montenegro MA, Sanyal SC, et al: Cloning of enterotoxin gene from *Aeromonas hydrophila* provides conclusive evidence that this organism produces a cytotonic enterotoxin. *Infect Immun* 46:435–441, 1984

45. Annapurna E, Sanyal SC: Enterotoxicity of *Aeromonas hydrophila. J Med Microbiol* 10:313–323, 1977

46. Dubey RS, Sanyal SC, Malhotra OP: Purification of *Aeromonas hydrophila* enterotoxin and its mode of action in experimental model, in Eaker D, Wadstrom T (eds): *Animal, Plant and Microbial Toxins.* Oxford, Permagon Press, 1980, pp 259–268

47. Dubey RS, Bhattacharya AK, Sanyal SC: Elevation of adenosine 3′5′ cyclic monophosphate level by *Aeromonas hydrophila* enterotoxin. *Indian J Med Res* 74:668–674, 1981

48. Shimada T, Sakazaki R, Harigome K, et al: Production of cholera-like enterotoxin by *Aeromonas hydrophila. Jap J Med Sci Biol* 37:141–144, 1984

49. Freer JH, Ellis A, Wadstrom T, et al: Occurrence of fimbriae among enterotoxigenic intestinal bacteria isolated from cases of human infantile diarrhoea. *FEMS Microbiol Lett* 3:277–281, 1978

50. Sanyal SC, Agarwal RK, Annapurna E: Haemagglutination properties and fimbriation of enterotoxic *Aeromonas hydroplila* strains. *Indian J Med Res* 78:324–350, 1983
51. Atkinson HM, Trust TJ: Haemagglutination properties and adherence ability of *Aeromonas hydrophila*. *Infect Immun* 27:938–946, 1980
52. Burke V, Cooper M, Robinson J, et al: Haemagglutination patterns of *Aeromonas* spp. in relation to biotype and source. *J Clin Microbiol* 19:39–43, 1984
53. Stewart GA, Bundell CS, Burke V: Partial characterization of a soluble haemagglutinin from human diarrhoeal isolates of Aeromonas. *J Med Microbiol* 21:319–324, 1986
54. Manorama, Taneja V, Agarwal RK, et al: Enterotoxins of *Plesiomonas shigelloides:* Partial purification and characterization. *Toxicon Suppl* 3:269–272, 1983
55. Mathews MA, Timmis KN, Sanyal SC: Invasive ability of *Plesiomonas shigelloides*. *Zbl Bakt Hyg A* 258:94–103, 1984

4

Genetics

James B. Kaper and Mary M. Baldini

1. INTRODUCTION

The genetic organization of *Vibrio cholerae* 01 has been investigated by a variety of classical and molecular genetic techniques. The genetic complement of this species includes plasmids, bacteriophage, and insertion sequences; however, all virulence factors so far examined are encoded on a chromosome of ca. 2.8×10^3 kb.[1] The basic features of gene structure, transcription, translation, regulation, and genetic exchange are similar to those found in common enteric bacteria, and *V. cholerae* 01 readily exchanges genetic information via conjugative plasmids with these organisms.[2,3]

2. GENE TRANSFER

2.1. Conjugation

Conjugation in *V. cholerae* 01 has been extensively studied since the discovery of the plasmid sex factor, P, by Bhaskaran in 1958.[4] P is similar to the fertility factor, F, of *E. coli;* it can encode a sex pilus seen in electron micrographs[5] and mediate transfer of chromosomal genes at a frequency of 10^{-5} to 10^{-6}.[6] Transfer of the P factor is detected by formation of "lacunae," characteristic, plaquelike clearings which are seen when P$^+$ cells are plated on a lawn of P$^-$ cells.[7] The P factor is present at one copy per cell[8] and has been isolated from several different strains, although most *V. cholerae* 01 do not carry P. It is approximately 68 kb long, based on analysis of restriction fragments and contour measurements on electron micrographs.[9] Few proteins are seen when randomly cloned fragments are examined in

Cholera, edited by Dhiman Barua and William B. Greenough III. Plenum Medical Book Company, New York, 1992.

minicells[9,10] and no readily identifiable phenotypic markers have been found on P. It has been implicated, however, in the suppression of pathogenicity in animal models.[11]

The P factor was used by Bhaskaran[12] and Parker et al.[13] to derive a linear linkage map of the V. cholerae 01 chromosome. The frequency of gene mobilization, however, is too low for efficient mapping and it appears that P and the V. cholerae 01 chromosome lack sequences that would allow homologous recombination of the sex factor into the host chromosome. Thus, unlike F in E. coli, the P factor cannot form strains capable of a high frequency of recombination (Hfr).

A novel approach was designed by Johnson and Romig[14] to generate donor strains analogous to the Hfr donors of E. coli. This transposon-facilitated recombination (Tfr) system uses transposons as "portable regions of homology" to enable P to stably integrate into the V. cholerae 01 chromosome. The ampicillin-resistance transposon, Tn1, was inserted into the chromosome and a P factor containing Tn1 was introduced into these strains. Transfer of chromosomal genes originates at the site of Tn1 insertion and proceeds in either direction depending on the orientation of the transposon in the P plasmid. The resulting Tfr donor strains transfer genes at frequencies 100- to 1000-fold higher than conventional P donors and were used to generate the first circular maps of the V. cholerae 01 chromosome.[6,15]

V. cholerae 01 bacteriophage can also provide regions of homology for stable integration of the P factor. The P derivative, pSJ15, contains the defective prophage, dVcA1, and can efficiently mobilize a variety of genes from El Tor strains lysogenized with VcA1.[16] Because all classical strains examined contained a copy of dVcA1 inserted near the his locus, pSJ15 can only mobilize transfer from this locus in the classical biotype.[17]

The efficiency of Tfr donor construction was increased by an improvement of the method by which the transposon is introduced into V. cholerae 01. Newland et al.[18] used plasmids from an incompatibility group that is unstable in V. cholerae 01 to introduce Tn5 or Tn10 into the chromosome. E. coli lambda phage has also been used to introduce transposons into V. cholerae 01.[19] First, V. cholerae 01 is made sensitive to lambda infection by the addition of a plasmid containing the gene encoding the lambda receptor, lamB,[20] then it is infected with a lambda phage carrying the transposon. Because lambda is unable to replicate in V. cholerae 01, every antibiotic-resistant cell contains the transposon inserted into the chromosome. Alternatively, a suicide plasmid vector incapable of replication in V. cholerae has been used to introduce a Tn5 derivative into the chromosome of this species.[21] Strains with chromosomal insertions of Tn5 or Tn10 can serve as Tfr donors on introduction of a P factor containing Tn5 or Tn10.[18]

Chromosomal maps derived using wild-type and Tfr donors are shown in Figure 1 and a list of genetic markers is given in Table 1. The maps of the two biotypes are quite similar except for the inversion of the regions from ilv-5 to lys-201,1 and from pro-201 to ura-201. Both maps are notable for large regions in which no markers have been identified. With the rapid progress now being made in the physical mapping of prokaryotic and eukaryotic chromosomes, a restriction endonuclease map of the entire V. cholerae chromosome should soon be achieved. Such a physical map will establish whether the clustering of genetic markers in one region of the chromosome is genuine or is merely an artifact of the conjugal mapping process.

Another fertility factor, V, was isolated from a V. cholerae non-01 strain[22] and mobilizes chromosomal genes at a very low frequency.[23] The V factor has no apparent DNA homology to the P factor,[24] but can repress the transfer of P.[22]

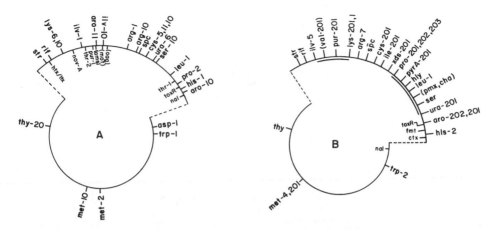

FIGURE 1. Chromosomal maps of classical strain 162 (A) and El Tor strain GN6300 (B). Although classical and El Tor strains can exchange genes, the results of such heterologous crosses must be interpreted with caution because of inverted regions found in the biotypes. Two such inversions have been confirmed (shown by inner arcs in the El Tor map) and others are suspected. Allelic designations are described in Table 1. Relative distances between genetic markers are approximate. Markers outside the circle are as originally published for these strains (taken from Sublett and Romig[6] for strain 162 and Newland et al.[18] for strain GN6300). Markers inside the circle have been mapped using non-Tfr methods (novA, thr-1, thr-2, pur-1, ams, mot, oag), or mapped in other strains with Tfr methods (htx, toxR, nal, ctx, fmt). Alleles in parenthesis have not been precisely ordered.

2.2. Transduction

Of the two types of transduction seen in *E. coli,* generalized and specialized, only generalized transduction, in which any gene is potentially capable of being transferred by bacteriophage, has been demonstrated in *V. cholerae* 01. Generalized transduction was first shown to mediate the transfer of genes encoding traits that are characteristic of the El Tor biotype.[25] A classical strain infected with a phage, CP-T1, released by an El Tor strain became resistant to polymyxin B, was Voges–Proskauer positive, and agglutinated chicken erythrocytes.

The frequency of CP-T1-mediated gene transfer, ca. 10^{-5} to 10^{-8}, corresponds to the frequency reported for the P1 transducing phage in *E. coli* and P22 in *Salmonella typhimurium*.[26] Unlike P1 and P22, however, CP-T1 has been used to study only a few genes in its host species. In a study by Ogg et al.[26] CP-T1 transferred nutritional markers, including *met, lys,* and *trp,* and genes encoding resistance to polymyxin B, streptomycin, and rifampin, from an El Tor to a classical strain. CP-T1 has been used to obtain a fine structure map of the *V. cholerae* 01 *trp* operon. The order of the structural genes for this biosynthetic pathway was determined by three factor reciprocal crosses (see below).[27] In addition, CP-T1 has been reported to mediate conversion between the Ogawa and Hikojima serotype but this has not been confirmed to be the result of transduction (see Section 4.2).[28]

By studying the mechanism of DNA packaging by CP-T1, Manning[29] and co-workers hope to devise a system for transduction of specific markers. The phage packages its DNA via a headful packaging mechanism commencing from a specific phage sequence designated *pac.* A transposon, Tn*pac,* has been constructed to introduce this site into the chromosome.

TABLE 1
Genetic Markers of *Vibrio cholerae*

Gene symbol	Phenotypic trait affected	Reference[a]
acf	Accessory colonization factor	66
ams	Mannose-sensitive adhesin biosynthesis	113
arg-1,7,10	Arginine requirement	6,14,6[b]
aro-10,11,201,202	Aromatic amino acid requirement	6,6,18,18
asp-1	Aspartic acid requirement	6
cha	Chicken erythrocyte hemagglutinin biosynthesis	93
ctx	Cholera toxin biosynthesis	58
cys-5,10,11,201	Cysteine requirement	6,6,6,18
fmt	5-Methyltryptophan resistance	61
galK,T	Galactose utilization	142
hap	Hemagglutinin/protease	117
his-1,2	Histidine requirement	6,14
hly	Hemolysin biosynthesis	93
htpG	Heat shock protein	71
htx	Increased cholera toxin biosynthesis	73
ile-201	Isoleucine requirement	18
ilv-1,5,10	Isoleucine and valine requirement	6,14,6
irgA	Iron-vibriobactin receptor	146
irgB	Positive regulation of irgA	148
leu-1	Leucine requirement	6
ltx	Decreased cholera toxin biosynthesis	73
lys-1,6,10,201	Lysine requirement	14,6,6,18
met-2,4,10,201	Methionine requirement	6,14,6,18
mot	Motility	13
mutL,S	DNA repair	139
nal	Resistance to nalidixic acid	13
nanH	Neuraminidase biosynthesis	123
nov-A	Resistance to novobiocin	13
oag (*rfb*)	O-antigen biosynthesis	13(104)
ompT,U,V,W	Outer membrane protein biosynthesis	65,65,118,121
pmx	Resistance to polymyxin B	93
pro-2,201,202,203	Proline requirement	6,18,18,18
pur-1,201	Purine requirement	13,18
pyrA-201	Pyrimidine requirement	18
recA	General recombination	135
rfb (*oag*)	O-antigen biosynthesis	104(13)
rif	Resistance to rifampin	6
ser-10	Serine requirement	6
sidA	Vibriobactin biosynthesis	101
spc	Resistance to spectinomycin	6
str	Resistance to streptomycin	6
tcp	Toxin coregulated pilus biosynthesis	65
thr-1,2	Threonine requirement	13,13
thy-20	Thymine requirement	6
toxR,S,T	Positive regulator of *ctx*	61(62),68,69a
trp-1,2	Tryptophan requirement	6,14
ura-6,201	Uracil requirement	6,18
val-201	Valine requirement	18
xds-201	Extracellular DNase biosynthesis	132

[a]Many genes have multiple references which could be cited. The references given here are those on which the chromosomal maps in Fig. 1 are based. Genes which have been cloned but not mapped on the chromosome are also included. References given are those which describe the initial cloning of these genes.

[b]Multiple mutants have been described for some genes and are designated by different numbers. The respective references are presented in the same order as the mutant numbers.

Packaging would commence at the site of the *pac* insertion, thus allowing more precise mapping of *V. cholerae* genes via transduction.

2.3. Transformation

Transformation of *V. cholerae* 01 by osmotic shock occurs at a very low frequency, mainly with small plasmids.[30] Marcus *et al.*[31] recently examined several aspects of transformation of *V. cholerae*. Using an isogenic mutant deficient in DNase production, these investigators showed that production of DNase is a significant barrier to transformation by osmotic shock. Transformation of *V. cholerae* was also affected by host restriction as transformation efficiency was greater when the plasmid DNA was from a homologous *V. cholerae* strain than when it was from *E. coli*. In contrast to the poor efficiency obtained with osmotic shock methods, transformation by electroporation is a very efficient method for the introduction of plasmids into *V. cholerae*.[31]

2.4. Mobile Genetic Elements

2.4.1. Plasmids

Nearly all classical *V. cholerae* 01 strains contain small, cryptic plasmids. Cook *et al.*[32] found that 41 of 42 classical strains contained plasmids; 80% of these strains possessed a 4.6- and a 32-kb plasmid. In contrast, El Tor strains were rarely seen to carry plasmids.[32] One-quarter of *V. cholerae* non-01 strains examined by Newland *et al.*[33] possessed small, cryptic plasmids, which could be divided into two unrelated groups based on DNA hybridization.

Although most plasmids isolated from *V. cholerae* 01 are cryptic, several have been found that encode antibiotic resistance. Generally, these R factors are large (110 to 170 kb), self-transmissible, and belong to the C incompatibility group.[34] A single resistance plasmid belonging to the J incompatibility class has also been reported.[35] The prevalence of C incompatibility group plasmids in *V. cholerae* 01 mirrors *in vitro* plasmid stability, since plasmids of the C, J, and P incompatibility groups are the most stable in this species.[36] Plasmids of the P incompatibility group have been particularly useful in constructing nontoxinogenic vaccine candidates (see Section 5.1).

V. cholerae 01 R factors can carry genes encoding resistance to ampicillin, chloramphenicol, gentamicin, kanamycin, spectinomycin, streptomycin, sulphonamides, tetracycline, and trimethoprim; up to seven different resistances have been found on a single plasmid.[37] Most of these resistance determinants are thought to have originated in the *Enterobacteriaceae*. Resistance genes from *V. cholerae* 01 show homology to three of the four classes of tetracycline resistance determinants found in gram-negative rods.[38] Other studies have shown that these R factors carry the ampicillin[34] and trimethoprim[39] resistance determinants common in enteric bacteria.

Hamood *et al.*[30] examined the effect of *V. cholerae* 01 R factors on pathogenicity in animal models. One plasmid increased fluid accumulation in the infant mouse model and a second decreased it, although both R factors increased *in vitro* production of cholera toxin. Neither R factor appeared to have an effect on colonization of the mouse gut.

2.4.2. Phage

The CP-T1 transducing phage is the best described phage for *V. cholerae* 01 but other vibriophage can act as mutagenic elements similar to the transposing phage, Mu, of *E. coli*.[40,41] These phage, designated VcA1, VcA2, and VcA3, insert randomly into the chromosome to create auxotrophic mutants, which can be used as Tfr donors for mapping studies. VcA1 and a derivative of VcA2 have also been used to generate deletions in the genes encoding cholera toxin[42]; the precise mechanism of this deletion is not known.

2.4.3. Transposons

Transposable elements other than bacteriophage have recently been isolated from *V. cholerae* 01. Resistance of an El Tor strain to trimethoprim, spectinomycin, streptomycin, and the vibriostatic agent 0/129 (2,4-diamino 6,7-diisopropropyl-pteridine) is due to a transposon inserted into the chromosome.[43] All four resistances were transferred from the *V. cholerae* 01 chromosome to a transmissible plasmid and from there onto the chromosome of *E. coli*. The 14-kb transposon mediating these resistances, Tn1527, was shown to hybridize to a probe for Tn7, which encodes resistance to trimethoprim, spectinomycin, and streptomycin.

An insertion sequence that is apparently unique to *V. cholerae* 01 is the 2.7-kb element designated RS1 (repetitive sequence 1).[44] This element is found upstream of the structural gene for cholera toxin (*ctxAB*), at the junction of tandem duplications of *ctxAB*, and, in some cases, downstream of *ctxAB*. Transposition of RS1 has been observed[45,46] and it is believed that this element is involved in the amplification of the *ctx* genetic element (see Section 3.5).

3. GENETICS OF CHOLERA TOXIN

3.1. Relationship between *elt* and *ctx*

Initial cloning[47−49] of the cholera toxin structural genes was greatly facilitated by their similarity to genes encoding the heat-labile enterotoxin (LT) of enterotoxigenic *E. coli* (*eltAB*). The *eltAB* genes hybridize under reduced stringency to sequences encoding cholera toxin[50] and DNA sequence analysis shows approximately 76% homology between the two genes.[51−53] It has been proposed that the toxin gene originated in *V. cholerae* 01 and was acquired by *E. coli* some 130 million years ago.[54] The organization of these structural genes is identical; however, the promoter and regulatory sequences are quite different. Although the *elt* promoter is very active in *V. cholerae* 01,[55] the *ctx* promoter is only weakly active in *E. coli*.[56] In addition, the *elt* genes are plasmid-borne,[57] whereas the *ctx* genes are located on the *V. cholerae* 01 chromosome, mapping between *nal* and *his*.[58]

3.2. Structure of *ctxAB*

The DNA sequence of cloned *ctxAB* genes has been determined for both El Tor[51−53] and classical[53,59] strains, allowing a detailed analysis of this operon. The sequences encoding the A subunit (*ctxA*) precede the sequences encoding the B subunit (*ctxB*) (Figure 2) and overlap by 4 nucleotides (ATGA); the first two bases of the *ctxA* translation termination signal (TGA)

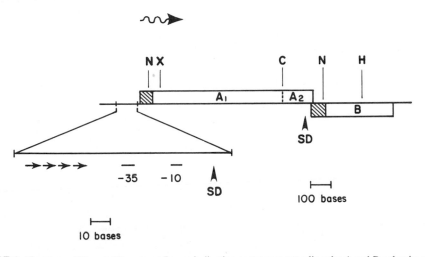

FIGURE 2. Structure of the *ctxAB* operon. Boxes indicating sequences encoding the A and B subunits are above and below the line, respectively, indicating the overlap between the termination for *ctxA* and initiation for *ctxB*. Diagonal lines indicate sequences encoding leader peptides for the A and B subunits and the arrow at the top of the figure indicates direction of transcription. Shine–Dalgarno sequences (SD) are indicated by a black triangle. The region upstream of the structural gene is expanded to show the SD sequence, the −10 and −35 regions of the *ctx* promoter and the repeated sequence, TTTTGAT. This sequence, indicated by arrows, is repeated from three to eight times, depending on the strain. Key restriction endonuclease sites (based on DNA sequence data for strains 62746[51–52] and 2125[53]) are shown: N = *Nde*I, X = *Xba*I, C = *Cla*I, H = *Hinc*II.

are the last two of the *ctxB* translation initiation codon (ATG). The *ctxA* DNA sequence predicts a translation product of 258 amino acids of which the first 18 residues are a putative signal peptide; the *ctxB* sequence predicts a protein of 124 amino acids including a putative 21-residue signal peptide.

3.3. Transcriptional and Translational Control

Immediately upstream of the structural gene sequence is the *ctx* promoter which is controlled by a positive regulatory element, *toxR* (see Section 3.4).[56] Because both subunits are transcribed from this promoter, the higher expression of the B subunit must be due to translational control. The A and B cistron possess putative ribosomal binding sites (Shine–Dalgarno sequences) immediately upstream of their start codons.[51–53] These Shine–Dalgarno (SD) sequences resemble SD sequences found in *E. coli;* however, the *ctxB* SD sequence is larger and theoretically more correct than the SD sequence for *ctxA*. Coupling of the *ctxB* structural sequences to the *ctxA* SD sequence results in a nine-fold decrease in expression of the B subunit[53] and indicates that the larger SD sequence results in more efficient translation.

3.4. Regulation

Elegant work by Mekalanos and colleagues has yielded important insights into the regulation of *ctx* and other genes of *V. cholerae* 01. Miller and Mekalanos[56] isolated the positive regulatory element, *toxR*, by examining a genomic library of *V. cholerae* 01 strain 569B for clones which increased activity of the *ctx* promoter. First, the *ctx* promoter was fused to the *lacZ* structural gene, coupling promoter activity to the level of an easily assayable product, beta-galactosidase. The genomic library of *V. cholerae* 01 569B was then introduced into an *E. coli* strain which had the *ctx–lacZ* fusion inserted into the chromosome. Clones that increased the expression of *lacZ* were selected and the gene encoding this increase was designated *toxR*. When *toxR* was introduced into *E. coli* containing cloned *ctxAB* genes, cholera toxin production increased more than 100-fold.

The *toxR* gene appears to be the same as the *tox* locus originally described by Holmes *et al.*[60] *toxR* complements the *tox* mutation in a number of hypotoxinogenic derivatives of *V. cholerae* 01 569B, increasing cholera toxin production to wild-type levels.[56] In addition, *toxR* maps near *his*,[61] on the side opposite to *ctx*, analogous to the position described for *tox*.[62]

The *toxR* gene is a *trans*-acting, positive regulator of *ctx* which activates transcription; mutants defective in this gene show greatly reduced levels of *ctxAB* mRNA.[56] The 32.5-kDa *toxR* gene product, ToxR, appears to bind to the repetitive sequence TTTTGAT in the *ctx* promoter region and activates the *ctx* promoter, possibly by changing the conformation of the promoter or interacting with RNA polymerase.[63] The number of repeats of the TTTTGAT sequence may affect binding of ToxR and thus, expression of *ctx*. *V. cholerae* 01 strains that produce low to moderate levels of cholera toxin contain 3 or 4 tandem repeats; the highly toxinogenic strain 569B contains 8 repeats.[53] The structure predicted for ToxR suggests that this protein spans the inner membrane with the amino-terminal domain mediating transcriptional control and the periplasmic carboxy-terminal domain sensing environmental stimuli.[63,64]

In addition to activating transcription of *ctx*, *toxR* can also regulate production of two outer membrane proteins encoded by the *V. cholerae ompU* and *ompT* genes and expression of a pilus colonization factor encoded by the *tcpA* (toxin coregulated pilus) locus (see Section 4.3).[65] Recent work indicates that *toxR* coordinately regulates more than 17 genes in several different operons in *V. cholerae* 01.[66] Some of these genes encode virulence factors while other genes encode functions apparently unrelated to virulence. This network of genes has been termed the *toxR* regulon.[66]

The *toxR* regulon of *V. cholerae* 01 resembles coordinate regulation systems recently described for other pathogenic bacteria such as *Bordetella pertussis, Staphylococcus aureus, Salmonella, Shigella,* and *Yersinia*.[64] Many of these systems feature a two-component system in which a sensory component perceives environmental conditions and transmits a signal to a regulatory component which in turn controls transcription of multiple genes.[64] The resulting differences in gene expression would allow a variety of responses to different environments such as the intestinal lumen, mucosal surfaces, or aquatic reservoirs. ToxR is responsive to changes in osmolarity, pH, temperature, and the levels of certain amino acids. Using a novel suicide plasmid vector to create an insertion mutation in *toxR*, Miller and Mekalanos[67] showed that not all *toxR*-regulated genes are controlled in exactly the same way. Some genes are more responsive to temperature and pH than to osmolarity and, although most genes are positively regulated, *ompT* is negatively regulated by *toxR*. Interestingly, sequences homologous to *toxR* are present in nontoxinogenic environmental strains of *V. cholerae* 01 (CT⁻)[56] as well as *V. parahaemolyticus* and the non-pathogenic *V. harveyi*,[45] suggesting that *toxR* may regulate genes in these species present in an environment other than the human intestine.

A second regulatory gene called *toxS* can significantly enhance the activity of *toxR* under some circumstances.[68,69] The *toxS* gene is located immediately downstream from *toxR* and is transcribed from the same promoter. The *toxS* gene encodes a 19-kDa transmembrane protein which is believed to interact with the periplasmic portion of ToxR. DiRita and

Mekalanos[69] propose that ToxS enhances dimerization of ToxR, thereby activating *ctx* gene expression. Various environmental signals may interact through ToxR alone or in conjunction with ToxS to influence the expression of various genes in the *toxR* regulon. Unlike other strains examined, the hypertoxinogenic strain 569B lacks *toxS* sequences,[68] raising intriguing questions about the regulation of the high toxin production seen in this strain. Perhaps a third regulatory locus, *toxT,* may be involved in the hypertoxinogenicity of 569B. *toxT* has recently been cloned from 569B and shown to activate transcription of *ctx* in *E. coli*.[69a] The *toxT* gene product can activate gene fusions that are dependent on *toxR* in *V. cholerae* but that cannot be activated in *E. coli* by cloned *toxR* alone. Transcription of *toxT* is, in turn, dependent upon *toxR* since no *toxT* mRNA was detected in a *V. cholerae toxR* mutant.[69a] DiRita *et al.*[69a] have recently provided evidence that *toxT* is a transcriptional activator of *tcpA* and other *tag* (ToxR-activated genes) genes. The picture emerging from these studies is that a "regulatory cascade" controls virulence in *V. cholerae,* whereby ToxR activates transcription of *toxT* whose gene product in turn activates several virulence genes.

Additional evidence of the complexity of the *toxR* regulon is emerging. Recently, it has been reported that expression of the *toxR* gene is regulated by the heat shock response, which is a phenomenon of organisms in both the prokaryotic and eukaryotic kingdoms. In the heat shock response, a cell responds to stressful environmental conditions, such as elevated temperature, toxic compounds, or viral infection, by inducing a set of genes that help it survive the adverse conditions. In *E. coli* these genes are induced by the production of an alternate RNA polymerase containing the sigma-32 subunit which recognizes specific promoter sequences unique to heat shock genes.[70] Parsot and Mekalanos[71] recently reported a gene in *V. cholerae* whose predicted amino acid sequence exhibits striking similarity to the heat shock proteins HtpG from *E. coli,* Hsp90 from *Saccharomyces cerevisiae,* and Hsp82 from *Drosophila melanogaster.* This gene, designated *htpG,* is located immediately upstream of *toxR* and is transcribed in the opposite direction. Because of the close proximity of the divergent promoters, only one RNA polymerase can bind to this intergenic region at any time. At low temperatures, the normal sigma-70 RNA polymerase can bind to the *toxR* promoter and transcribe the *toxR* gene. At elevated temperatures (>37°C), the increased amount of sigma-32 RNA polymerase binds to the *htpG* promoter and represses the *toxR* promoter. The decreased *in vitro* expression at 37°C of cholera toxin seems paradoxical for a virulence factor that is clearly expressed at 37°C in the intestine. Perhaps there are additional regulatory mechanisms and environmental stimuli which are involved and have not yet been elucidated.

The importance of *toxR* in the virulence of *V. cholerae* 01 was shown in a study in which volunteers were fed a derivative of Ogawa 395 mutated in the *toxR* gene.[72] Intestinal colonization of this strain was greatly reduced, thus corroborating results previously obtained in mice.[65] The reduced amounts of the *tcpA* encoded pilus produced by the *toxR* mutant may be solely responsible for the diminished colonization but reduced amounts of other *toxR*-regulated genes could also contribute.

Three other genes have been reported to affect cholera toxin production but these have not been extensively characterized. The *htx* locus[73] maps in the *str* region, distant from *ctx* and *toxR.* Mutations in *htx* result in a 3–7 fold increase in toxin production in 569B[73] when a functional *toxR* gene is present.[61] Mutations in the *ltx* locus[74] also map in the *str* region and decrease toxin production by 100-fold. *htx* and *ltx* appear to be alleles of the same gene, the product of which may interact with *ctxAB* or *toxR.* Mutations in the *tox-1000* locus also decrease cholera toxin production and map in the *his* region.[75] Given its chromosomal position, this mutation may represent an alteration in the *ctx* promoter, *toxR,* or *toxS.*

There have been reports that the presence of certain plasmids in *V. cholerae* 01 may also alter production of cholera toxin. In one case, C incompatibility group plasmids encoding multiple antibiotic resistances were reported to increase *in vitro* toxin production.[30] Introduction of the *V. cholerae* 01 sex factor P reduced cholera toxin production by 569B, according to Khan *et al.*[76] Bartowsky and colleagues,[77] however, showed that although the presence of P increased the 50% lethal dose (LD_{50}) of strain 569B more than 300-fold, the production of cholera toxin was unaltered. Rather, the attenuation was due to decreased intestinal colonization by the P^+ derivative, which appeared to produce less TCP pilus than 569B without P.

3.5. Gene Duplication

Classical strains of *V. cholerae* 01 contain two copies of the *ctxAB* operon.[44] Available DNA sequence data shows no differences between the two gene copies which both express active cholera toxin.[53] The two copies are separated on the chromosome; one copy in strain 569B maps near *nal,* as does *ctx* in El Tor strain RV79.[58] Although most El Tor strains contain only a single copy of *ctxAB,* 5 of 19 El Tor strains examined by Mekalanos[44] had two adjacent gene copies. The duplicated sequence includes an additional 6 kb of DNA upstream of *ctxAB* which is conserved in all classical and El Tor strains.

The *ctxAB* gene appears to be part of a larger genetic element which shares structural similarities to a complex transposon.[78] At the center of this element is a 4.3-kb "core region" containing the *ctx* operon. One or more copies of the transposable, 2.7-kb RS1 element flank this core region. This structure allows tandem duplication and amplification of the core element, presumably due to *recA*-dependent intramolecular recombination between RS1 copies.[78] All classical and some El Tor strains possess only an upstream copy of RS1[44,79] and this gene duplication and amplification is not seen.

Amplification of the *ctxAB* element *in vivo* was shown by Mekalanos[44] who passed El Tor strains through three sets of rabbit intestinal loops. Isolates were recovered after animal passage that produced 2- to 4-fold more toxin than the parent strain. Examination of these strains revealed that significant gene amplification had occurred with some variants acquiring as many as 6 tandem copies of the *ctxAB* region. The *in vivo* selective advantage of these variants may be due to high production of a factor other than cholera toxin; recent evidence indicates that additional potential virulence factors, including a putative enterotoxin and colonization factor, are also encoded on the 4.3-kb core region (see Section 4.6). This clustering of virulence factors suggests that this 4.3 kb region can be regarded as a "virulence cassette."

Genetic rearrangements involving the RS1 element can also lead to the deletion of *ctx* sequences.[78] Naturally occurring, nontoxinogenic *V. cholerae* 01 (CT^-) strains lack the structural genes for cholera toxin[80] and also lack sequence homology with the core region.[56] Deletion of *ctx* sequences could explain the occasional clinical isolation of nontoxinogenic *V. cholerae* 01 (CT^-) strains that are otherwise identical to toxinogenic strains.[81,82] Conversely, RS1 can mediate the acquisition of *ctx* genes by nontoxinogenic strains. The RS1 element encodes a site-specific recombination system characterized by an 18-bp sequence arranged in direct repeats at the ends of RS1.[83] An RS1 element contained on a plasmid can mediate the integration of the entire plasmid into the chromosome. This integration occurs at a site containing an 18-bp sequence nearly identical to that found at the ends of RS1. This recombination event, analogous to the establishment of lysogeny by a circular bacteriophage genome, is highly efficient and can occur even in a *V. cholerae* strain lacking a functional *recA* gene.[83]

4. GENETICS OF FACTORS OTHER THAN CHOLERA TOXIN

After the initial emphasis on the genetics of cholera toxin, increasing attention has been focused on the genetics of other determinants. A variety of genes have been cloned and characterized and, in many instances, the complete DNA sequence has been determined. Unlike *ctx* and the adjacent genes on the 4.3 kb virulence cassette, all virulence genes examined to date appear to have only a single copy on the chromosome.

Most cloned *V. cholerae* 01 genes are expressed to some extent in *E. coli*, indicating that promoter structure, translation signals, and codon usage are similar; cloned genes that are poorly expressed in *E. coli* may require positive regulatory elements present in *V. cholerae* 01. Furthermore, when genes for products that are normally secreted extracellularly from *V. cholerae* 01 are cloned into *E. coli*, the gene products are not secreted extracellularly. The nature of the extracellular secretion system of *V. cholerae* is not understood but one gene, encoding a 25-kDa protein, has been described which may play a role in this process.[84]

4.1. Hemolysin

The genetics of hemolysin production in *V. cholerae* 01 are of particular interest because of the traditional role of hemolysin in differentiating classical (hemolysin negative on sheep red blood cells) from El Tor (hemolysin positive) strains, and the number of recently isolated El Tor strains which are weakly or nonhemolytic. The possible role of this hemolysin in infection due to *V. cholerae* 01 was also of interest in light of the importance of hemolysins in other bacterial infections.

The hemolysin genes from several El Tor strains have been cloned in *E. coli* K-12.[85–88] DNA sequence analysis[88–90] of the *hlyA* gene predicts a precursor protein of 82-kDa which is processed by proteolysis to a final active form of 65 kDa.[91] The *hlyA* gene cloned from three different El Tor strains varies as much as 8% in the predicted amino acid sequence,[88–90] but is identical in two regions which show homology with the cytolysin gene of *V. vulnificus*.[92] The *hlyA* gene has been mapped to the *leu* marker by Green *et al.*[93]; genes for other characteristics that define the El Tor biotype, polymyxin B resistance (*pmx*) and chicken erythrocyte hemagglutinin (*cha*), also map near *leu*.[93] However, Goldberg and Murphy[85] positioned the cloned *hlyA* locus between *ilv* and *arg*. The reason for these discrepant results is not known.

The cloned *hlyA* gene was used by Kaper *et al.*[87] to assess the role of hemolysin in diarrheal disease. The *hlyA* gene was mutated *in vitro* and an internal deletion introduced into *V. cholerae* 01 El Tor JBK70 and *V. cholerae* classical CVD101 via site-directed mutagenesis.[87] Volunteer studies with the mutated strains did not support a role for hemolysin in the pathogenesis of cholera since no difference was seen in the ability of the isogenic *hlyA* mutant strains and the parent strains to cause diarrhea.[87,94]

Sequences homologous to *hlyA* are present in nonhemolytic classical *V. cholerae* 01 strains as well as in hemolytic *V. cholerae* non-01 and *V. mimicus* strains.[95,96] Richardson *et al.*[97] examined a gene library of classical strain 395 in *E. coli* and isolated a clone that lysed rabbit erythrocytes. The hemolysin gene contained by this clone was shown by restriction mapping and hybridization analysis to be homologous to the *hlyA* gene cloned from El Tor.

The presence of sequences homologous to the hemolysin gene in strains phenotypically nonhemolytic suggested that subtle genetic alterations were responsible for the absence of active hemolysin. For one classical strain, 569B, a specific 11-bp deletion in the *hlyA* gene leads to premature termination and production of an inactive 26.8-kDa protein.[98] A synthetic oligodeoxynucleotide probe from the region of this deletion shows promise as a diagnostic probe to distinguish El Tor from classical strains.[96] However, when the nucleotide sequences of *hlyA* genes from a nonhemolytic El Tor strain, RV79, and a hemolytic revertant of RV79 were compared, no differences were seen in the structural gene or promoter region.[89] This result suggests that additional gene products may affect hemolytic activity.

Manning *et al.*[86] described two additional genes flanking *hlyA*, *hlyB*, and *hlyC*, which affect hemolysin production. *hlyB* encodes a 60.3-kDa outer membrane protein which aids the export of hemolysin to the culture supernatant.[99] Mutagenesis of *hlyB* results in trapping of hemolysin in the *V. cholerae* periplasm. A fourth gene, *hlyR*, has been proposed as a regulatory locus for hemolysin production and maps near *his*.[100] A further level of regulation is due to iron concentration; increased levels of hemolytic activity are found in iron-starved cells compared to *V. cholerae* cells grown in iron-rich media (see Section 4.10).[101]

A second hemolysin has been cloned by Richardson *et al.*[97] from a genomic library of classical 395. This hemolysin also lysed rabbit, but not sheep, erythrocytes. A third hemolysin showing genetic similarity to the thermostable direct hemolysin (TDH) of *V. parahaemolyticus* has been found in some *V. cholerae* non-01 strains.[102] The gene encoding this hemolysin is located on a plasmid in *V. cholerae* non-01 but has not been found in *V. cholerae* 01 strains.

4.2. O-Antigen

The genetics of the O-antigen of *V. cholerae* 01 are of great interest because of the antigen's importance in identifying and typing *V. cholerae* 01 and stimulating protective immunity. The specificity of the Inaba, Ogawa, and Hikojima serotypes is believed to be due to the presence of three antigens, A, B, and C, and it appears that *V. cholerae* 01 strains possess the genetic potential to express all these antigens. Manning and colleagues[103] cloned genes (rfb) encoding the O-antigens of the Inaba serotype from 569B and of the Ogawa serotype from 017. The restriction enzyme maps for these genes show no differences and Southern blot and heteroduplex studies demonstrate the homology of these genes.[104] These results indicate that only minor changes, conceivably involving only a single nucleotide, are involved in serotype conversion. Morona *et al.*[104a] used complementation analysis to show that the Ogawa phenotype is dominant over the Inaba phenotype. These investigators identified two regions of the Ogawa *rfb* genes in which inactivating mutations would confer the Inaba phenotype. These results are consistent with previous reports that spontaneous Ogawa to Inaba variants are easier to obtain than the converse.[105]

Ogg *et al.*[28] reported the conversion of classical and El Tor Ogawa (antigens A and B) strains to the Hikojima serotype (antigens A, B, and C) after infection with phage CP-T1 grown on serotype Hikojima strain. The exact mechanism of this conversion is not clear, but it may be due to the selection of a spontaneous mutant or the effect of CP-T1 on endogenous genes rather than to a serotype-specific gene carried on the phage.

4.3. Adherence

The mechanism by which *V. cholerae* 01 adheres to the intestine is not entirely understood; however, significant progress has recently been made in elucidating this process. One factor that is essential for colonization by classical Ogawa strain 395 is a pilus colonization factor encoded by the *tcpA* gene. Taylor *et al.*[65] used the transposon Tn*phoA* to identify and clone the *tcpA* gene in *V. cholerae* 01 strain 395. In this transposon system, alkaline phosphatase activity is seen only when Tn*phoA* inserts into a target gene which encodes a secreted protein. *V. cholerae* 01 with a mutation in *tcpA* no longer produced the 20.5-kDa pilin subunit and showed a greatly reduced ability to colonize in animal models[65] and in volunteers.[72]

The *tcpA* locus is one of at least 8 genes involved in the expression and assembly of this pilus.[105] These genes are arranged in three transcriptional units which are regulated by *toxR* (hence the name toxin coregulated pilus). The number and sizes of the gene products are similar to those involved in the expression and assembly of the well-characterized PAP pilus of uropathogenic *E. coli*[106] but the protein structural features of TCP more closely resemble the *N*-methylphenylalanine (type 4) pilins of *Pseudomonas, Neisseria,* and *Moraxella* species.[107] Preliminary evidence indicates that the actual adhesive moiety is the major pilin subunit, TcpA, and not a minor pilin component as is the case in the PAP pilus.[108,109]

DNA sequences homologous to *tcpA* are present in all clinical El Tor and classical isolates of *V. cholerae* 01 examined by Taylor *et al.*[105] In contrast, *V. cholerae* non-01 strains and nontoxinogenic environmental isolates of *V. cholerae* 01 (CT$^-$) do not possess such sequences. Although *tcpA* nucleotide sequences for two classical strains are nearly identical,[107] there is greater divergence between *tcpA* genes of classical and El Tor biotypes.[105,109,110] Both El Tor and classical *V. cholerae* 01 strains produce additional pili which are morphologically, serologically, and genetically distinct from the TCP pilus.[111]

Other factors which may be involved in mucosal adhesion of *V. cholerae* have been cloned but the data supporting their role as adhesins and significant protective antigens are not as strong as are the data for TCP.[108,109,112] Mutations in a *toxR*-regulated operon called *acf* (accessory colonization factor) decrease colonization in animals, although not as severely as mutations in the *tcp* operon.[66] The *acf* operon consists of four genes designated *acfA* through *acfD* but the structural nature of this colonization factor and its importance in human colonization remain to be determined. Srivastava *et al.*[113,114] isolated a mutant of *V. cholerae* 01 defective in mannose-sensitive adhesion to rabbit intestine and cloned a gene, designated *ams,* which expresses this adhesin in *E. coli* K-12. Following the model of enterotoxigenic *E. coli* colonization, much research on colonization factors in *V. cholerae* 01 has focused on hemagglutinins. The gene (*cha*) encoding one of these hemagglutinins, the chicken erythrocyte hemagglutinin of El Tor, maps near the *leu-1* marker.[93] The *sha* gene, cloned by both Franzon and Manning[115] and Van Dongen and De Graaf,[116] encodes a factor which agglutinates erythrocytes from a variety of sources; this hemagglutination is not inhibited by D-mannose or L-fucose. The *sha* gene is poorly expressed in *E. coli* K-12, possibly due to the absence of a positive regulatory element other than *toxR*.[115] Hase and Finkelstein[117] have cloned a gene (*hap*) encoding a soluble hemagglutinin which also has proteolytic activity (HA/protease). DNA sequence analysis of the *hap* gene predicts a protein of 46.7 kda, the sequence of which shows 61.5% identity with the *Pseudomonas aeruginosa* elastase.

4.4. Outer Membrane Proteins

A number of outer membrane proteins have been described in *V. cholerae* 01 but only a few have been characterized genetically. Expression of outer membrane proteins in general appears to be highly regulated. Many outer membrane proteins are expressed only in *V. cholerae* grown *in vivo* or grown *in vitro* under iron-limited conditions (see Section 4.10). The *ompV* gene encodes a 25-kDa major outer membrane protein of *V. cholerae*.[118,119] Although OmpV is highly immunogenic in rabbits,[118] Taylor et al.[65] showed that *V. cholerae* mutated in *ompV* by insertion of Tn*phoA* were undiminished in virulence for infant mice. OmpW, a 22-kDa outer membrane protein which is a minor component of *V. cholerae* 01, is expressed in large amounts when cloned into *E. coli*.[120,121] The expression of two other outer membrane proteins is controlled by the *toxR* gene product; *ompU*, encoding a 38-kDa outer membrane protein, is positively regulated by *toxR* while *ompT*, encoding a 40-kDa outer membrane protein, is negatively regulated by *toxR*.[65,67]

4.5. Neuraminidase

The neuraminidase (sialidase) of *V. cholerae* 01 may be involved in pathogenesis by acting on enterocyte gangliosides to increase the number of G_{M1} ganglioside receptors for cholera toxin. As part of the mucinase complex,[122] neuraminidase may also aid intestinal colonization by *V. cholerae*. The gene encoding the neuraminidase, *nanH*, has been cloned and expressed in *E. coli*.[123] DNA sequence data predict a mature protein of 83.0 kDa for the *nanH* gene product[124] and the predicted protein sequence shows a repeated sequence motif that is conserved among bacterial sialidases.[125] Both insertion and deletion *nanH* mutations have been constructed in *V. cholerae*. *E. coli* lambda phage was used to introduce an insertionally inactivated *nanH* gene into *V. cholerae* 01 expressing the lambda receptor.[126] The inactivated *nanH* gene recombined into the *V. cholerae* 01 chromosome, yielding an isogenic mutant deficient in neuraminidase production. Using an isogenic *nanH* deletion mutant of strain 395, Galen and colleagues[124] concluded that neuraminidase plays a subtle but definite role in the pathogenesis of *V. cholerae* by enhancing the effect of cholera toxin.

4.6. Other Toxins

Fasano et al.[127] have recently described a putative enterotoxin of *V. cholerae* 01 which is distinct from cholera toxin. This toxin increases short circuit current in Ussing chambers by increasing tissue conductance of rabbit ileal tissue. The morphology of intercellular epithelial tight junctions (zonula occludens) is altered by this toxin which is named ZOT (zonula occludens toxin). The gene encoding ZOT (*zot*) is located immediately upstream of the *ctx* locus on the 4.3-kb virulence cassette and appears to be regulated independently of *ctx*.[128] DNA sequence data predicts a protein of 44.8 kDa for the zot gene product.[128]

Another potential enterotoxin produced by *V. cholerae* 01 has been described by Sanyal and co-workers.[129] This toxin is produced by CT$^+$ and CT$^-$ *V. cholerae* 01 strains from clinical and environmental sources but has not yet been extensively characterized nor has the gene encoding this factor been cloned. The fact that some *V. cholerae* 01 strains producing this toxin do not hybridize with the *zot* gene probe[128] demonstrates that ZOT and the toxin described by Sanyal et al. are distinctly different.

A heat-stable enterotoxin is produced by some strains of *V. cholerae* non-01 and is associated with diarrheagenicity in volunteers.[130] The gene encoding this toxin has been cloned and sequenced by Ogawa *et al.*[131] The active portion of this toxin shows considerable similarity to the ST enterotoxin of enterotoxigenic *E. coli* but *V. cholerae* 01 strains containing the gene have not been reported.

4.7. DNA Degradation, Recombination, and Repair

A structural gene for extracellular DNase, designated *xds,* was cloned by Newland *et al.*[132] *xds* was insertionally inactivated in *E. coli* by Tn5 mutagenesis, and recombined into the *V. cholerae* 01 chromosome. DNase activity of the *xds* mutant was decreased by 80% and the efficiency of transformation by osmotic shock was greatly increased.[31] This strain was used as a Tfr donor to map the chromosomal position of *xds* between *pro-1* and *ile-201*.

Focareta and Manning[133] have cloned a second gene encoding DNase activity which shows no homology to the *xds* gene. DNA sequence data predict a mature protein of 24 kDa for this DNase. The presence of this cloned DNase gene inhibited transformation in *E. coli,* suggesting that it may contribute to the low efficiency of transformation seen in *V. cholerae* 01. DNases may also be involved in the biotype-specific restriction and modification systems described by Imbesi and Manning.[134]

The gene responsible for general homologous recombination in *V. cholerae* 01, *recA,* has been cloned by complementation of a *recA* mutant of *E. coli* K-12[135−138] and encodes a protein of ca. 44 kDa in minicells.[135] An insertional mutation of *recA,* constructed *in vitro,* was recombined into the chromosome to construct a *recA* mutant of *V. cholerae* 01.[135] This mutant was used to demonstrate the important role of *recA* in duplication and amplification of the *ctx* element.[78] Another *recA* mutant constructed by Ketley *et al.*[138] showed significantly reduced colonization and immunogenicity in volunteers.

Genes involved in DNA repair in *V. cholerae* include the *mutL* and *mutS* genes which have been cloned by Bera *et al.*[139] *V. cholerae* also possesses both DNA adenine methylase (*dam*) and DNA cytosine methylase (*dcm*) activity.[139]

4.8. Motility

Only fragmentary information about the complex genetic control of motility and chemotaxis of *V. cholerae* is available. Richardson *et al.*[19] analyzed transposon-induced nonmotile mutants of *V. cholerae* and found that at least 8 different *EcoRI* chromosomal fragments were involved in motility. The relationship of these fragments to the *mot* chromosomal locus mapped by Parker *et al.*[13] is unknown. Srivastava and colleagues[140] cloned flagellar genes using RP4::mini-Mu in an *in vivo* cloning technique. The resulting clone restored motility when introduced into a nonmotile mutant of *V. cholerae* but no further characterization of these genes was reported.

Interestingly, classical strains of *V. cholerae* were found to produce spontaneous nonmotile mutants at a high frequency (ca. 10^{-4}).[141] In contrast, no spontaneous nonmotile mutants in El Tor strains were detected in the study by Mostow and Richardson.[141]

4.9. Metabolic Pathways

Although many chromosomal loci for genes encoding metabolic pathways have been mapped in *V. cholerae*, few of these genes have been characterized in detail. Genes encoding the galactose kinase (*galK*) and transferase (*galT*) in *V. cholerae* 01 were cloned on a single *EcoRI* fragment but a gene for the epimerase (*galE*) was not recovered and appears to be unlinked to *galK* and *galT*.[142] The fine structure of genes comprising the tryptophan biosynthetic pathway were mapped with the transducing phage, CP-T1.[27] The gene order determined by cotransduction, *trpE.trpD.trpC.trpB*, is identical to that for the *trp* operon from *E. coli*. The proteins encoded by the *trp* operon from *V. cholerae* 01 and *E. coli* appear to be similar as well; a plasmid-borne *E. coli trpA* gene can complement a *V. cholerae* 01 *trpA* mutant. In addition, *V. cholerae* 01 *trp* regulatory mutants were obtained that were complemented by *E. coli trpR*.[27]

4.10. Iron-Regulated Genes

When *V. cholerae* is grown under low-iron conditions, several new outer membrane proteins are expressed that are absent from cells grown in iron-rich media.[143] Many of these proteins are similar to proteins induced by *in vivo* growth of *V. cholerae* in ligated rabbit ileal loops, suggesting that the intestinal site of *V. cholerae* is a low-iron environment.[144] Conversely, expression of some outer membrane proteins appears to decrease under low-iron conditions.[143,144] Expression of hemolysin and vibriobactin, the high-affinity iron-binding compound of *V. cholerae*, are also increased under low-iron conditions.[101] In *E. coli*, coordinate regulation of iron-regulated genes involves the binding of a repressor protein, Fur, to a 21-bp operator sequence found in the promoter of these diverse genes.[145] Stoebner and Payne[101] demonstrated that a cloned *E. coli fur* gene is capable of repressing iron-regulated genes in *V. cholerae*.

Using the Tn*phoA* mutagenesis approach previously employed to identify ToxR-regulated genes, Goldberg and colleagues[146] identified at least eight distinct chromosomal loci of *V. cholerae* that were regulated by iron. Insertion into one locus, designated *irgA* (iron-regulated gene) resulted in loss of a 77-kDa outer membrane protein and reduced virulence in an infant mouse model. These investigators subsequently identified IrgA as the probable vibriobactin outer membrane receptor, based on homology of the predicted sequence of IrgA to the ferrienterochelin receptor (FepA) of *E. coli*.[147] Regulation of *irgA* by iron occurs at the transcriptional level in *V. cholerae* and requires an additional 900 bp of DNA upstream of *irgA*.[147] The upstream region contains a gene, named *irgB*, that encodes a positive transcriptional activator of *irgA*.[148] *irgA* and *irgB* are transcribed in opposite directions and the promoters for these genes overlap each other and a Fur-binding site. In the model proposed by Goldberg *et al.*,[148] transcription of both *irgA* and *irgB* is negatively regulated by the binding of a Fur-like protein in the presence of iron. Under low iron conditions, the Fur repressor does not bind and transcription of *irgB* occurs. Production of the *irgB* gene product leads to positive transcriptional activation of *irgA*. This model is an interesting example of a positive transcriptional activator that is itself negatively regulated by iron.

4.11. Antigens Expressed *in Vivo*

The observation by Sciortino and Finkelstein[143] that *V. cholerae* grown *in vivo* expresses a novel set of proteins demonstrates that studies of cells grown *in vitro* may not give an accurate and complete picture of the antigens and virulence factors that are important in infection. This observation was subsequently confirmed by both Richardson *et al.*[148a] and Jonson *et al.*,[149] although the specific novel proteins varied among the three studies. Jonson and colleagues reported a variety of proteins expressed only *in vivo* in ligated rabbit ileal loops; these proteins ranged in size from 29 to 200 kDa and most were not induced during culture in iron-depleted media. Furthermore, these investigators did not detect any increase in expression of ToxR-regulated proteins such as OmpU and TCP in the bacteria grown *in vivo*. Richardson and colleagues utilized serum and jejunal fluids from volunteers before and after experimental challenge with *V. cholerae* 01 to examine the human immune response to these proteins. Both post-challenge serum IgG and post-challenge jejunal fluid SIgA reacted to antigens unique to cells grown *in vivo,* suggesting that studies to define protective immunity should include examination of *in vivo*–grown *V. cholerae*.

These results indicate that regulation of antigens and virulence factors of *V. cholerae* is complex but elucidating the regulatory systems will lead to a fuller understanding of cholera pathogenesis and immunity. Figure 3 summarizes the major regulatory pathways of potential *V. cholerae* virulence factors described to date. The ToxR regulon is genetically the best characterized and includes important virulence factors such as cholera toxin and TCP that are up-regulated as well as factors that are down-regulated by ToxR. The heat shock regulon has only recently been described for *V. cholerae* but given the size of the heat shock regulon in other species (*E. coli* contains at least 17 heat shock genes[70]) and the fact that heat shock proteins of pathogens are often immunodominant antigens, it is anticipated that several new *V. cholerae* genes will be added to this regulon. The network of negatively iron-regulated genes includes a variety of outer membrane proteins whose expression is increased in the absence of iron. Several of these proteins are also contained in the last regulon in Figure 4, labeled "in vivo growth," due to the lack of specific information about the genes and environmental stimuli involved in this group. It is likely that antigens expressed during *in vivo* growth are not the result of a single regulon but instead involve multiple stimuli and regulatory mechanisms. In addition, there are antigens expressed *in vitro* that are down-regulated during *in vivo* growth.[148a–149]

The regulatory scheme presented in Figure 3 is an oversimplification as evidence is

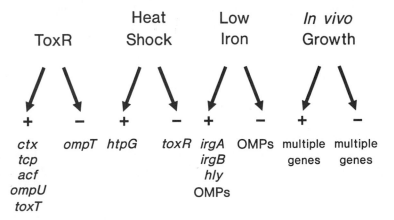

FIGURE 3. Simplified regulatory scheme of potential virulence factors of *V. cholerae*. Representative genes or proteins are listed within regulons as to whether expression is increased (+) or decreased (−) due to the modulating effect of the regulon; some of the genes listed, e.g., *tcp,* represent multiple loci. Regulatory cascades in which one regulatory factor, e.g., *toxR,* is modulated by another regulatory system, e.g., heat shock, are also present but the full extent of such cascades is not yet known.

accumulating that one regulatory factor can be positively or negatively regulated by a second factor. Examples of such regulatory "cascades" include the modulation of *toxR* by the heat shock response, the regulation of *toxT* by ToxR, and the activation of *irgA* by IrgB. Furthermore, there are undoubtedly additional regulatory systems yet to be described for *V. cholerae*. Numerous multigene regulatory systems involving environmental stimuli such as anaerobiosis, limitation of phosphate, carbon, and nitrogen, and low pH have been described in enteric bacteria. Even with the systems currently described for *V. cholerae,* little is known about interactions and hierarchies among the various regulons. It is hypothesized that the interaction of different regulatory systems and differential expression of the individual genes aids survival of *V. cholerae* in a variety of environments such as the stomach, the small bowel, or an aquatic reservoir, and prevents premature expression of virulence factors.[70] It is clear that the elucidation of the various regulatory mechanisms of *V. cholerae* 01 antigens and virulence factors will be an important area of future research in this species.

5. APPLICATIONS

5.1. Vaccine Development

The basic knowledge gained in studying the genetics of *V. cholerae* 01 provided a rationale for the construction of genetically defined vaccine strains. The first attenuated strains of *V. cholerae* 01 evaluated as live oral vaccines were chemically mutagenized using nitrosoguanidine (NTG).[150,151] NTG induces nonspecific, revertable changes that may be accompanied by secondary mutations affecting viability or immunogenicity. In contrast, precise deletion mutations can be generated *in vitro* by recombinant DNA techniques, which alter only the target genes. Recombination of these mutations into the chromosome of well-characterized *V. cholerae* 01 strains yields vaccine strains which are nonreverting and retain all other genes involved in immunogenicity.

Attenuated *V. cholerae* strains were constructed by Kaper *et al.*[152,153] and Mekalanos *et al.*[53] using similar methods. To construct the attenuated strain *V. cholerae* CVD101,[153] genes encoding cholera toxin were cloned from the parent strain, classical Ogawa 395, and digested with *Xba*I and *Cla*I to remove most of the sequence encoding the A_1 peptide (see Figure 2). The resultant plasmid, pJBK108, retains the *ctx* promoter and B subunit sequences.

The A_1-deleted *ctx* construct was recombined into the chromosome of the toxinogenic parent strain by a marker exchange procedure (Figure 4). First, an insertion mutation was constructed *in vitro,* by cloning a gene encoding tetracycline resistance (*tet*) into the *Xba*I site of the wild-type *ctxAB* operon. This construction was transferred into *V. cholerae* 01 395 by conjugation. At a low frequency, the sequences flanking the plasmid-borne, mutated genes recombine with homologous sequences flanking the chromosomal toxin genes and the *tet*-containing toxin genes displace the wild-type *ctx* in the chromosome (Figure 4B). Next, pJBK108 was mobilized into this tetracycline-resistant *V. cholerae* 01 strain. Homologous recombination of the deleted toxin gene sequences into the chromosome (Figure 4C) was detected by the loss of tetracycline resistance. The final strain, CVD101, is tetracycline sensitive, lacks the *Xba*I-*Cla*I fragment encoding the A_1 peptide, and produces the B subunit.

A different approach to vaccine development has been taken by Manning *et al.*[103] and Attridge *et al.*[154] These workers transferred the cloned genes for *V. cholerae* 01–antigen biosynthesis into the oral typhoid vaccine strain *Salmonella typhi* Ty21a. Ty21a which

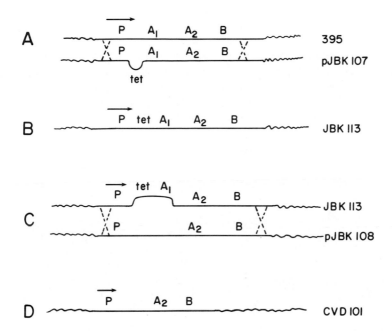

FIGURE 4. Construction of attenuated *V. cholerae* vaccine strain CVD101.[153] (A) Recombinational crossover event (indicated by dashed lines) resulting in insertion of tetracycline resistance genes (*tet*) into a chromosomal gene copy of cholera toxin A₁ subunit. The top line depicts the chromosomal toxin region of *V. cholerae* 395 and the lower line depicts the mutated, plasmid-borne toxin sequences. Plasmid pJBK107 contains cloned cholera toxin promoter (P), A₁, A₂, and B sequences with the *tet* gene cloned into the XbaI site. (B) The recombinational crossover event depicted in A results in *V. cholerae* strain JBK113 containing *tet* inserted in chromosomal A₁ sequences. (C) Recombinational crossover event resulting in displacement of *tet* gene by cholera toxin deletion mutation. Plasmid pJBK108 contains the cholera toxin promoter, A₂, and B subunit sequences with nearly all of the A₁ sequences deleted. (D) The crossover depicted in C results in *V. cholerae* CVD101 which is deleted for the A₁ sequences, produces B subunit, and is tetracycline sensitive.

expresses the *V. cholerae* 01–antigen on its surface may then stimulate intestinal immunity to *V. cholerae*. Still another approach taken by Taylor et al.[105] utilizes recent genetic information on the *tcpA* and *toxR* genes to construct strains of *V. cholerae* 01 which produce higher than normal amounts of the TCP pilus and cholera toxin B subunit. These strains could potentially be used to produce improved oral killed whole-cell vaccines.

5.2. Molecular Epidemiology

Recombinant DNA techniques provide sensitive and specific tools for studying the epidemiology of *V. cholerae* 01 and non-01. DNA hybridization analysis can detect similarities and differences in strains with greater sensitivity than serotyping or phage typing and can be used to screen thousands of strains in large-scale epidemiological surveys.[155,156]

Cloned LT genes were used as probes to assess the potential for reversion to toxinogenicity of nontoxinogenic *V. cholerae* 01 (CT⁻) strains isolated from environmental sources around the world.[80] DNA hybridization studies showed that these strains do not simply have a mutation in the toxin gene; they lack any genetic material encoding cholera toxin. Such strains, therefore, cannot revert to toxinogenicity and serve as a reservoir of cholera.

Toxin probes have been used by Kaper *et al.*[155] to study the clonal relatedness of cholera strains isolated in the U.S. All *V. cholerae* 01 strains isolated in the Gulf Coast region possessed identical probe-positive, restriction fragment patterns, indicating that a single endemic strain has persisted since 1973. Toxinogenic strains of *V. cholerae* non-01 and *V. mimicus* also hybridized to the probe but showed different patterns than the 01 strains.[157]

In addition to cloned toxin gene probes, rRNA probes[158] and *V. cholerae* 01 phage[82] have also been used as probes to assess relationships among strains. Goldberg and Murphy[82] showed that all the U.S. Gulf Coast isolates contain a VcA3 sequence in the identical chromosomal fragment, as does a nontoxinogenic strain isolated from a patient in Florida, demonstrating their clonal relatedness.

Recently isolated, classical strains from Bangladesh were probed with toxin genes and *V. cholerae* 01 phage VcA1 to assess their relationship to classical strains from previous pandemics.[32] Southern blot analysis of restricted chromosomal DNA, as well as plasmid profiles, suggests that the new classical strains are closely related to those of the sixth pandemic. These results indicate that there has been less evolutionary divergence for classical than El Tor strains.

6. CONCLUSIONS

No area of cholera research has undergone such rapid change as the genetics of *V. cholerae* 01. Prior to 1981, advances came slowly, chiefly in chromosomal gene mapping. The use of recombinant DNA techniques greatly accelerated the pace of discovery; many significant virulence factors have been characterized to the nucleotide level.

Due to its preeminent role in disease, initial research concentrated on the genetics of cholera toxin. Early workers, using classical genetic techniques, were unable to generate structural gene mutations and so, focused on regulatory mutants. The difficulty in producing structural gene mutations can now be attributed to the duplication of the *ctx* genes in all classical and some El Tor strains of *V. cholerae* 01. More recently, molecular techniques have been used to examine the structure of the genes encoding cholera toxin. These studies revealed that the genetic control of cholera toxin is considerably more complicated than first imagined. Production of cholera toxin is controlled by the number of copies of the *ctx* element and the number of repetitions of a 7-bp sequence near the *ctx* promoter, as well as regulatory elements physically removed from the *ctx* locus.

Genes encoding basic physiological functions or putative virulence factors such as hemolysin, O-antigens, and colonization factors, have also been cloned and examined. This research illuminates previously unexplained phenotypic changes in hemolysis, serology, and antibiotic resistance, as well as toxinogenicity. The cloned genes can be precisely altered, creating isogenic mutants which can be used to determine the importance of these factors for virulence.

Although molecular biological techniques have only recently been applied to *V. cholerae* 01, it is particularly satisfying that the genetic advances being made are rapidly moving out of the realm of basic research and into applications. Use of these techniques for epidemiological surveys allows the relationship of past and present *V. cholerae* 01 infections to be studied with great specificity and precision. The most significant application, however, is in vaccine development where recombinant DNA technology has been used to generate the new vaccine strains which are now being clinically evaluated. Thus, it is the contribution to the prevention of cholera that may be the most enduring legacy of this research.

REFERENCES

1. Nishibuchi M, Muroga K, Seidler RJ, Fryer JL: Pathogenic *Vibrio* isolated from cultured eels-IV. *Bull Jap Soc Sci Fish* 45:1469–1473, 1979
2. Baron LS, Falkow S: Genetic transfer of episomes from *Salmonella typhosa* to *Vibrio cholerae*. *Genetics* 46:849, 1961
3. Kuwahara S, Akiba T, Koyama K, Arai T: Transmission of multiple drug-resistance from *Shigella flexneri* to *Vibrio comma* through conjugation. *Jpn J Microbiol* 7:61–67, 1963
4. Bhaskaran K: Genetic recombination in *Vibrio cholerae*. *J Gen Microbiol* 19:71–75, 1958
5. Bhaskaran K, Dyer PY, Rogers GE: Sex pili in *Vibrio cholerae*. *Australian J Exp Biol Med Sci* 47:647–650, 1969
6. Sublett RD, Romig WR: Transposon-facilitated recombination in classical biotypes of *Vibrio cholerae*. *Infect Immun* 32:1132–1138, 1981
7. Parker C, Romig WR: Self-transfer and genetic recombination mediated by P, the sex factor of *Vibrio cholerae*. *J Bacteriol* 112:707–714, 1972
8. Datta A, Parker CD, Wohlhieter JA, Baron LS: Isolation and characterization of the fertility factor P of *Vibrio cholerae*. *J Bacteriol* 113:763–771, 1973
9. Bartowsky EJ, Morelli G, Kamke M, Manning PA: Characterization and restriction analysis of the P sex factor and the cryptic plasmid of *Vibrio cholerae* strain V58. *Plasmid* 18:1–7, 1987
10. Bartowsky EJ, Manning PA: Molecular cloning of the plasmids of *Vibrio cholerae* and the incidence of related plasmids in clinical isolates and other *Vibrio* species. *FEMS Microbiol Lett* 50:183–190, 1988
11. Sinha VB, Srivastava BS: Suppression of pathogenicity by P and V plasmids in *Vibrio cholerae*. *J Gen Microbiol* 104:251–255, 1978
12. Bhaskaran, K: Segregation of genetic factors during recombination in *Vibrio cholerae*, strain 162. *WHO Bull* 30:845–853, 1964
13. Parker C, Gauthier D, Tate A, et al: Expanded linkage map of *Vibrio cholerae*. *Genetics* 91:191–214, 1979
14. Johnson SR, Romig WR: Transposon-facilitated recombination in *Vibrio cholerae*. *Molec Gen Genet* 170:93–101, 1979
15. Johnson SR, Sublett R, Romig WR: Transposon-facilitated recombination in *Vibrio cholerae;* genetic mapping of El Tor and classical biotypes, in *Proceedings of the Fifteenth Joint Conference on Cholera*, U. S.–Japan Cooperative Medical Science Program, U.S. Dept. of Health, Education and Welfare, Bethesda, Maryland, 1979, pp 401–414
16. Johnson SR, Romig WR: *Vibrio cholerae* conjugative plasmid pSJ15 contains transposable prophage dVcA1. *J Bacteriol* 146:632–638, 1981
17. Johnson SR, Liu BCS, Schreiber D, Romig WR: Properties of the related transposable phage VcA1 and defective prophage dVcA1 in El Tor and classical biotypes of *Vibrio cholerae*, in Kuwahara S, Pierce NF (eds): *Advances in Research on Cholera and Related Diarrheas*, Vol. 1, Tokyo, KTK Scientific Publishers, 1983, pp 171–182
18. Newland JW, Green BA, Holmes RK: Transposon-mediated mutagenesis and recombination in *Vibrio cholerae*. *Infect Immun* 45:428–432, 1984
19. Richardson K, Nixon L, Mostow L, et al: Transposon-induced non-motile mutants of *Vibrio cholerae*. *J Gen Microbiol* 136:717–725, 1990
20. Harkki A, Hirst TR, Holmgren J, Palva ET: Expression of the *Escherichia coli* lamB gene in *Vibrio cholerae*. *Microbial Pathogenesis* 1:283–288, 1986
21. Taylor RK, Manoil C, Mekalanos JJ: Broad-host-range vectors for delivery of Tn*phoA:* Use in genetic analysis of secreted virulence determinants of *Vibrio cholerae*. *J Bacteriol* 171:1870–1878, 1989
22. Bhaskaran K, Sinha VB: Transmissible plasmid factors and fertility inhibition in *Vibrio cholerae*. *J Gen Microbiol* 69:89–97, 1971
23. Bhaskaran K: Recent studies on genetic recombination in *Vibrio cholerae*. *Prog Drug Res* 19:460–465, 1975
24. Smigocki AC, Voll MJ: Novel transmissible factors in a non-01 *Vibrio cholerae* and a *Vibrio* sp. *J Gen Microbiol* 132:1027–1033, 1986
25. Ogg JE, Shrestha MB, Poudayl L: Phage-induced changes in *Vibrio cholerae:* Serotype and biotype conversions. *Infect Immun* 19:231–238, 1978
26. Ogg JE, Timme TL, Alemohammad MM: General transduction in *Vibrio cholerae*. *Infect Immun* 31:737–741, 1981
27. Schreiber DB: Genetic organization in *Vibrio cholerae:* Tryptophan genes and phage VcA1. Los Angeles, University of California, Dissertation, 1984
28. Ogg JE, Ogg BJ, Shrestha MB, Poudayl L: Antigenic changes in *Vibrio cholerae* biotype *eltor* serotype Ogawa after bacteriophage infection. *Infect Immun* 24:974–978, 1979

29. Manning PA: Molecular genetic approaches to the study of *Vibrio cholerae*. *Microbiol Sci* 5:196–201, 1988
30. Hamood AN, Sublett RD, Parker CD: Plasmid-mediated changes in virulence of *Vibrio cholerae*. *Infect Immun* 52:476–483, 1986
31. Marcus H, Ketley JM, Kaper JB, Holmes RK: Effects of DNase production, plasmid size, and restriction barriers on transformation of *Vibrio cholerae* by electroporation and osmotic shock. *FEMS Microbiol Lett* 68:149–154, 1990
32. Cook WL, Wachsmuth K, Johnson SR, Birkness KA, Samadi AR: Persistence of plasmids, cholera toxin genes, and prophage DNA in classical *Vibrio cholerae* 01. *Infect Immun* 45:222–226, 1984
33. Newland JW, Voll MJ, McNicol LA: Serology and plasmid carriage in *Vibrio cholerae*. *Can J Microbiol* 30:1149–1156, 1984
34. Hedges RW, Vialard JL, Pearson NJ, O'Grady F: R plasmids from Asian strains of *Vibrio cholera*. *Antimicrob Agents Chemother* 11:585–588, 1977
35. Yokota T, Kuwahara S: Temperature-sensitive R plasmids obtained from naturally isolated drug-resistant *Vibrio cholerae* (biotype El Tor). *Antimicrob Agents Chemother* 11:13–20, 1977
36. Rahal K, Gerbaud G, Bouanchaud DH: Stability of R plasmids belonging to different incompatibility groups in *Vibrio cholerae*. *Ann Microbiol* 129A:409–414, 1978
37. Threlfall EJ, Rowe B, Huq I: Plasmid-encoded multiple antibiotic resistance in *Vibrio cholerae* El Tor from Bangladesh. *Lancet* i:1247–1248, 1980
38. Levy SB: Resistance to the tetracyclines, in Bryan LE (ed): *Antimicrobial Drug Resistance*, Orlando, Academic Press, Inc, 1978, pp 192–240
39. Young HK, Amyes SGB: Plasmid trimethoprim resistance in *Vibrio cholerae:* migration of the type I dihydrofolate reductase gene out of the Enterobacteriaceae. *J Antimicrob Chemother* 17:697–703, 1986
40. Johnson SR, Liu BCS, Romig WR: Auxotrophic mutations induced by *Vibrio cholerae* mutator phage VcA1. *FEMS Microbiol Lett* 11:13–16, 1981
41. Goldberg S, Murphy JR: Molecular epidemiological studies of United States Gulf Coast *Vibrio cholerae* strains: Integration site of mutator vibriophage VcA-3. *Infect Immun* 42:224–230, 1983
42. Mekalanos JJ, Moseley SL, Murphy JR, Falkow S: Isolation of enterotoxin structural gene deletion mutations in *Vibrio cholerae* induced by two mutagenic vibriophages. *Proc Natl Acad Sci USA* 79:151–155, 1982
43. Goldstein F, Gerbaud G, Courvalin P: Transposable resistance to trimethoprim and 0/129 in *Vibrio cholerae*. *J Antimicrob Chemother* 17:559–569, 1986
44. Mekalanos J: Duplication and amplification of toxin genes in *Vibrio cholerae*. *Cell* 35:253–263, 1983
45. Betley MJ, Miller VL, Mekalanos JJ: Genetics of bacterial enterotoxins. *Ann Rev Microbiol* 40:577–605, 1986
46. Ginzburg AL, Yanishevsky NV, Motin, VL, et al: Nature of RS1 sequences flanking the *vct* gene coding for cholera toxin synthesis in *Vibrio cholerae* El Tor. *Mol Genet Mikrobiol Virusol* (USSR) no. 2, 11–19, 1986
47. Kaper JB, Levine MM: Cloned cholera enterotoxin genes in study and prevention of cholera. *Lancet* ii:1162–1163, 1981
48. Pearson GDN, Mekalanos JJ: Molecular cloning of *Vibrio cholerae* enterotoxin genes in *Escherichia coli* K-12. *Proc Natl Acad Sci USA* 79:2976–2980, 1982
49. Gennaro ML, Greenaway PJ, Broadbent DA: The expression of biologically active cholera toxin in *Escherichia coli*. *Nucleic Acids Res* 10:4883–4890, 1982
50. Moseley SL, Falkow S: Nucleotide sequence homology between the heat-labile enterotoxin gene of *Escherichia coli* and *Vibrio cholerae*. *J Bacteriol* 144:444–446, 1980
51. Lockman HA, Galen JE, Kaper JB: *Vibrio cholerae* enterotoxin genes: Nucleotide sequence analysis of DNA encoding ADP-ribosyltransferase. *J Bacteriol* 159:1086–1089, 1984
52. Lockman H, Kaper JB: Nucleotide sequence analysis of the A2 and B subunits of *Vibrio cholerae* enterotoxin. *J Biol Chem* 258:13722–13726, 1983
53. Mekalanos JJ, Swartz DJ, Pearson GDN, et al: Cholera toxin genes: nucleotide sequence, deletion analysis and vaccine development. *Nature* 306:551–557, 1983
54. Yamamoto T, Gojobori T, Yokota T: Evolutionary origin of pathogenic determinants in enterotoxigenic *Escherichia coli* and *Vibrio cholerae* 01. *J Bacteriol* 169:1352–1357, 1987
55. Neill RJ, Ivins BE, Holmes RK: Synthesis and secretion of the plasmid-coded heat-labile enterotoxin of *Escherichia coli* in *Vibrio cholerae*. *Science* 221:289–290, 1983
56. Miller VL, Mekalanos JJ: Synthesis of cholera toxin is positively regulated at the transcriptional level by *toxR*. *Proc Natl Acad Sci USA* 81:3471–3475, 1984
57. Smith HW, Halls S: The transmissible nature of the genetic factor in *Escherichia coli* that controls enterotoxin production. *J Gen Microbiol* 52:319–334, 1968
58. Sporecke I, Castro D, Mekalanos J: Genetic mapping of *Vibrio cholerae* enterotoxin structural genes. *J Bacteriol* 157:253–261, 1984

59. Sanchez J, Holmgren J: Recombinant system for overexpression of cholera toxin B subunit in *Vibrio cholerae* as a basis for vaccine development. *Proc Natl Acad Sci USA* 86:481–485, 1989

60. Holmes RK, Vasil ML, Finkelstein RA: Studies on toxinogenesis in *Vibrio cholerae. J Clin Invest* 55:551–560, 1975

61. Miller VL, Mekalanos JJ: Genetic analysis of the cholera toxin-positive regulatory gene *toxR. J Bacteriol* 163:580–585, 1985

62. Baine WB, Vasil ML, Holmes RK: Genetic mapping of mutations in independently isolated nontoxinogenic mutants of *Vibrio cholerae. Infect Immun* 21:194–200, 1978

63. Miller VL, Taylor RK, Mekalanos JJ: Cholera toxin transcriptional activator ToxR is a transmembrane DNA binding protein. *Cell* 48:271–279, 1987

64. Miller JF, Mekalanos JJ, Falkow S: Coordinate regulation and sensory transduction in the control of bacterial virulence. *Science* 243:916–922, 1989

65. Taylor RK, Miller VL, Furlong DB, Mekalanos JJ: Use of *phoA* gene fusions to identify a pilus colonization factor coordinately regulated with cholera toxin. *Proc Natl Acad Sci USA* 84:2833–2837, 1987

66. Peterson KM, Mekalanos JJ: Characterization of the *Vibrio cholerae* ToxR regulon: identification of novel genes involved in intestinal colonization. *Infect Immun* 56:2822–2829, 1988

67. Miller VL, Mekalanos JJ: A novel suicide vector and its use in construction of insertion mutations: osmoregulation of outer membrane proteins and virulence determinants in *Vibrio cholerae* requires *toxR. J Bacteriol* 170:2575–2583, 1988

68. Miller VL, DiRita VJ, Mekalanos JJ: Identification of *toxS*, a regulatory gene whose product enhances ToxR-mediated activation of the cholera toxin promoter. *J Bacteriol* 171:1288–1293, 1989

69. DiRita VJ, Mekalanos JJ: Periplasmic interaction between two membrane regulatory proteins, ToxR and ToxS, results in signal transduction and transcriptional activation. *Cell* 64:29–37, 1991

69a. DiRita VJ, Parsot C, Jander G, Mekalanos JJ: Regulatory cascade controls virulence in *Vibrio cholerae. Proc Natl Acad Sci USA* 88:5403–5407, 1991

70. Neidhardt FC, VanBogelen RA: Heat shock response, in Neidhardt FC, Ingraham JL, Low KB, et al (eds): *Escherichia coli and Salmonella typhimurium: Cellular and Molecular Biology,* Washington DC, American Society for Microbiology, 1987, pp 1334–1345

71. Parsot C, Mekalanos JJ: Expression of ToxR, the transcriptional activator of the virulence factors in *Vibrio cholerae,* is modulated by the heat shock response. *Proc Natl Acad Sci USA* 87:9898–9902, 1990

72. Herrington DA, Hall R, Losonsky G, et al: Toxin, toxin-coregulated pili, and the *toxR* regulon are essential for *Vibrio cholerae* pathogenesis in humans. *J Exp Med* 168:1487–1492, 1988

73. Mekalanos JJ, Sublett RD, Romig WR: Genetic mapping of toxin regulatory mutations in *Vibrio cholerae. J Bacteriol* 139:859–865, 1979

74. Mekalanos JJ, Murphy JR: Regulation of cholera toxin production in *Vibrio cholerae:* genetic analysis of phenotypic instability in hypertoxinogenic mutants. *J Bacteriol* 141:570–576, 1980

75. Saunders DW, Bramucci MG: Genetic mapping of the *tox-1000* locus of *Vibrio cholerae* El Tor strain RJ1. *Infect Immun* 40:829–831, 1983

76. Khan AA, Srivastava R, Sinha VB, Srivastava BS: Regulation of toxin biosynthesis by plasmids in *Vibrio cholerae. J Gen Microbiol* 131:2653–2657, 1985

77. Bartowsky EJ, Attridge SR, Thomas CJ, et al: Role of the P plasmid in attenuation of *Vibrio cholerae* 01. *Infect Immun* 58:3129–3134, 1990

78. Goldberg I, Mekalanos JJ: Effect of a *recA* mutation on cholera toxin gene amplification and deletion events. *J Bacteriol* 165:723–731, 1986

79. Mekalanos JJ: Cholera toxin: Genetic analysis, regulation, and role in pathogenesis. *Curr Top Microbiol Immunol* 118:97–118, 1985

80. Kaper JB, Moseley SL, Falkow S: Molecular characterization of environmental and nontoxigenic strains of *Vibrio cholerae. Infect Immun* 32:661–667, 1981

81. Morris JG Jr, Picardi JL, Lieb S, et al: Isolation of nontoxigenic *Vibrio cholerae* 0 group 1 from a patient with severe gastrointestinal disease. *J Clin Micro* 19:296–297, 1984

82. Goldberg S, Murphy JR: Molecular epidemiological studies of United States Gulf Coast *Vibrio cholerae* strains: integration site of mutator vibriophage VcA-3. *Infect Immun* 42:224–230, 1983

83. Pearson GDN, Mekalanos JJ: Recombination and replication activities of RS1, a repetitive sequence associated with the cholera toxin genetic element, in: *Abstracts of the Twenty Fifth Joint Conference on Cholera,* U.S.–Japan Cooperative Medical Science Program, Grand Canyon, AZ, 1989, pp 23–24

84. Focareta T, Manning PA: Molecular cloning of a possible excretion protein of *Vibrio cholerae. FEMS Microbiol Lett* 29:161–166, 1985

85. Goldberg SL, Murphy JR: Molecular cloning of the hemolysin determinant from *Vibrio cholerae* El Tor. *J Bact* 160:239–244, 1984

86. Manning PA, Brown MH, Heuzenroeder MW: Cloning of the structural gene (*hly*) for the haemolysin of *Vibrio cholerae* El Tor strain 017. *Gene* 31:225–231, 1984

87. Kaper JB, Mobley HLT, Michalski JM, et al: Recent advances in developing a safe and effective live oral attenuated *Vibrio cholerae* vaccine, in Ohtomo N, Sack RB (eds): *Advances in Research on Cholera and Related Diarrheas*, Vol. 6, Tokyo, KTK Scientific Publishers, 1988, pp 161–167

88. Yamamoto K, Ichinose Y, Shinagawa H, et al: Two-step processing for activation of the cytolysin/hemolysin of *Vibrio cholerae* 01 biotype El Tor: Nucleotide sequence of the structural gene (*hlA*) and characterization of the processed products. *Infect Immun* 58:4106–4116, 1990

89. Rader AE, Murphy JR: Nucleotide sequences and comparison of the hemolysin determinants of *Vibrio cholerae* El Tor RV79 (Hly⁺) and RV79 (Hly⁻) and classical 569B (Hly⁻). *Infect Immun* 56:1414–1419, 1988

90. Alm RA, Stroeher UH, Manning PA: Extracellular proteins of *Vibrio cholerae:* nucleotide sequence of the structural gene (*hlyA*) for the haemolysin of the haemolytic El Tor strain 017 and characterization of the *hlyA* mutation in the non-haemolytic classical strain 569B. *Molec Microbiol* 2:481–488, 1988

91. Hall RH, Drasar BS: *Vibrio cholerae* hlyA hemolysin is processed by proteolysis. *Infect Immun* 58:3375–3379, 1990

92. Yamamoto K, Wright AC, Kaper JB, Morris JG: The cytolysin gene of *Vibrio vulnificus:* sequence and relationship to the *Vibrio cholerae* El Tor hemolysin gene. *Infect Immun* 58:2706–2709, 1990

93. Green BA, Newland JW, Holmes RK: Mapping of chromosomal genes that determine the El Tor biotype in *Vibrio cholerae. Infect Immun* 42:924–929, 1983

94. Levine MM, Kaper JB, Herrington D, et al: Volunteer studies of deletion mutants of *Vibrio cholerae* 01 prepared by recombinant techniques. *Infect Immun* 56:161–167, 1988

95. Brown MH, Manning PA: Haemolysin genes of *Vibrio cholerae:* presence of homologous DNA in non-haemolytic 01 and haemolytic non-01 strains. *FEMS Microbiol Lett* 30:197–201, 1985

96. Alm RA, Manning PA: Biotype-specific probe for *Vibrio cholerae* serogroup 01. *J Clin Microbiol* 28:823–824, 1990

97. Richardson K, Michalski J, Kaper JB: Hemolysin production and cloning of two hemolysin determinants from classical *Vibrio cholerae. Infect Immun* 54:415–420, 1986

98. Goldberg SL, Murphy JR: Cloning and characterization of the hemolysin determinants from *Vibrio Cholerae* RV79 (Hly⁺), RV79 (Hly⁻), and 569B. *J Bacteriol* 162:35–41, 1985

99. Alm RA, Manning PA: Characterization of the *hlyB* gene and its role in the production of the El Tor haemolysin of *Vibrio cholerae* 01. *Molec Microbiol* 4:413–425, 1990

100. Mechow S, Vaidya AB, Bramucci MG: Mapping of a gene that regulates hemolysin production in *Vibrio cholerae. J Bacteriol* 163:799–802, 1985

101. Stoebner JA, Payne SM: Iron-regulated hemolysin production and utilization of heme and hemoglobin by *Vibrio cholerae. Infect Immun* 56:2891–2895, 1988

102. Nishibuchi M, Khaeomanee-iam V, Honda T, et al: Comparative analysis of the hemolysin genes of *Vibrio cholerae* non-01, *V. mimicus*, and *V. hollisae* that are similar to the *tdh* gene of *V. parahaemolyticus. FEMS Microbiol Lett* 67:251–256, 1990

103. Manning PA, Heuzenroeder MW, Yeadon J, et al: Molecular cloning and expression in *Escherichia coli* K-12 of the O antigens of the Inaba and Ogawa serotypes of the *Vibrio cholerae* 01 lipopolysaccharides and their potential for vaccine development. *Infect Immun* 53:272–277, 1986

104. Morelli G, Ward HM, Kamke M, et al: A physical map of the chromosomal region determining O-antigen biosynthesis in *Vibrio cholerae* 01. *Gene* 55:197–204, 1987

104a. Morona R, Matthews MS, Morona JK, Brown MH: Regions of the cloned *Vibrio cholerae* rfb genes needed to determine the Ogawa form of the O-antigen. *Mol Gen Genet* 224:405–412, 1990.

105. Taylor R, Shaw C, Peterson K, Spears P, Mekalanos J: Safe, live *Vibrio cholerae* vaccines? *Vaccine* 6:151–154, 1988

106. Uhlin BE, Norgren M, Baga M, Normark S: Adhesion to human cells by *Escherichia coli* lacking the major subunit of a digalactoside-specific pilus-adhesin. *Proc Natl Acad Sci USA* 82:1800–1804, 1985

107. Shaw CE, Taylor RK: *Vibrio cholerae* 0395 *tcpA* pilin gene sequence and comparison of predicted protein structural features of those to type 4 pilins. *Infect Immun* 58:3042–3049, 1990

108. Sun D, Mekalanos JJ, Taylor RK: Antibodies directed against the toxin-coregulated pilus isolated from *Vibrio cholerae* provide protection in the infant mouse experimental cholera model. *J Infect Dis* 161:1231–1236, 1990

109. Sun D, Tillman DM, Marion TN, Taylor RK: Production and characterization of monoclonal antibodies to the toxin coregulated pilus (TCP) of *Vibrio cholerae* that protect against experimental cholera in infant mice. Serodiagnosis and Immunotherapy in *Infectious Diseases* 4:73–81, 1990

110. Faast R, Ogierman MA, Stroeher UH, Manning PA: Nucleotide sequence of the structural gene, *tcpA,* for a major pilin subunit of *Vibrio cholerae. Gene* 85:227–231, 1989
111. Hall RH, Vial PA, Kaper JB, Mekalanos JJ, Levine MM: Morphological studies on fimbriae expressed by *Vibrio cholerae* 01. *Microbial Pathogen* 4:257–265, 1988
112. Sharma DP, Stroeher UH, Thomas CJ, et al: The toxin-coregulated pilus (TCP) of *Vibrio cholerae:* molecular cloning of genes involved in pilus biosynthesis and evaluation of TCP as a protective antigen in the infant mouse model. *Microbial Pathogen* 7:437–448, 1989
113. Srivastava R, Srivastava BS: Isolation of a non-adhesive mutant of *Vibrio cholerae* and chromosomal localization of the gene controlling mannose-sensitive adherence. *J Gen Microbiol* 117:275–278, 1980
114. Srivastava R, Khan AA, Srivastava BS: Immunological detection of cloned antigenic genes of *Vibrio cholerae* in *Escherichia coli. Gene* 40:267–272, 1985
115. Franzon VL, Manning PA: Molecular cloning and expression in *Escherichia coli* K-12 of the gene for a hemagglutinin from *Vibrio cholerae. Infect Immun* 52:279–284, 1986
116. Van Dongen WMAM, De Graaf FK: Molecular cloning of a gene coding for a *Vibrio cholerae* haemagglutinin. *J Gen Microbiol* 132:2225–2234, 1986
117. Häse CC, Finkelstein RA: Cloning and nucleotide sequence of the *Vibrio cholerae* hemagglutinin/protease (HA/protease) gene and construction of an HA/protease-negative strain. *J Bacteriol* 173:3311–3317, 1991
118. Stevenson G, Leavesley DI, Lagnado CA, et al: Purification of the 25-kDa *Vibrio cholera* major outer-membrane protein and the molecular cloning of its gene: *ompV. Eur J Biochem* 148:385–390, 1985
119. Pohlner J, Meyer TF, Jalajakumari MB, Manning PA: Nucleotide sequence of *ompV,* the gene for a major *Vibrio cholerae* outer membrane protein. *Molec Gen Genet* 205:494–500, 1986
120. Manning PA, Bartowsky EJ, Leavesly DI, et al: Molecular cloning using immune sera of a 22-kDa minor outer membrane protein of *Vibrio cholerae. Gene* 34:95–103, 1985
121. Jalajakumari MB, Manning PA: Nucleotide sequence of the gene, *ompW,* encoding a 22 kDa immunogenic outer membrane protein of *Vibrio cholerae. Nucleic Acids Res* 18:2180, 1990
122. Stewart-Tull DES, Ollar RA, Scobie TS: Studies on the *Vibrio cholerae* mucinase complex. I. Enzymatic activities associated with the complex. *J Med Microbiol* 22:325–333, 1986
123. Vimr ER, Lawrisuk L, Galen J, Kaper JB: Cloning and expression of *Vibrio cholerae* neuraminidase gene *nanH* in *Escherichia coli. J Bacteriol* 169:1495–1504
124. Galen JE, Ketley JM, Fasano A, Richardson SH, Wasserman SS, Kaper JB: Role of *Vibrio cholerae* neuraminidase in the function of cholera toxin. *Infect Immun* 60:406–415, 1992
125. Roggentin P, Rothe B, Kaper JB, et al: Conserved sequences in bacterial and viral sialidases. *Glycoconjugate J* 6:349–353, 1989
126. Michalski J, Galen J, Kaper J: Chromosomal site directed mutagenesis in *Vibrio cholerae* using a bacterio-phage delivery system, in: *Abstracts of the 88th Annual Meeting of the American Society for Microbiology,* Miami Beach, Am. Soc. Microbio, 1988, p 106
127. Fasano A, Baudry B, Pumplin DW et al: *Vibrio cholerae* produces a second enterotoxin which affects intestinal tight junctions. *Proc Natl Acad Sci USA* 88:5242–5246, 1991
128. Baudry B, Fasano A, Ketley J, Kaper JB: Cloning of a gene (*zot*) encoding a new toxin produced by *Vibrio cholerae. Infect Immun* 60:428–434, 1992
129. Sanyal SC, Neogi PKB, Alam K, Huq MI, Al-Mahmud KA: A new enterotoxin produced by *Vibrio cholerae* 01. *J Diarrheal Disease Research* 2:3–12, 1984
130. Morris JG, Takeda T, Tall BD, et al: Experimental non-O group 1 *Vibrio cholerae* gastroenteritis in humans. *J Clin Invest* 85:697–705, 1990
131. Ogawa A, Kato J-I, Watanabe H, et al: Cloning and nucleotide sequence of a heat-stable enterotoxin gene from *Vibrio cholerae* non-01 isolated from a patient with traveler's diarrhea. *Infect Immun* 58:3325–3329, 1990
132. Newland JW, Green BA, Foulds J, Holmes RK: Cloning of extracellular DNase and construction of a DNase-negative strain of *Vibrio cholerae. Infect Immun* 47:691–696, 1985
133. Focareta T, Manning PA: Extracellular proteins of *Vibrio cholerae:* molecular cloning, nucleotide sequence and characterization of the deoxyribonuclease (DNase) together with its periplasmic location in *Escherichia coli* K-12. *Gene* 53:31–40, 1987
134. Imbesi F, Manning PA: Biotype-specific restriction and modification of DNA in *Vibrio cholerae. J Clin Microbiol* 16:552–554, 1982
135. Goldberg I, Mekalanos J: Cloning of the *Vibrio cholerae recA* gene and construction of a *Vibrio cholerae recA* mutant. *J Bacteriol* 165:715–722, 1986
136. Hamood AN, Pettis GS, Parker CD, McIntosh MA: Isolation and characterization of the *Vibrio cholerae recA* gene. *J Bacteriol* 167:375–378, 1986

137. Paul K, Ghosh SK, Das J: Cloning and expression in *Escherichia coli* of a recA-like gene from *Vibrio cholerae*. *Molec Gen Genetics* 203:58–63, 1986

138. Ketley JM, Kaper JB, Herrington D, et al: Diminished immunogenicity of a recombination-deficient derivative of *Vibrio cholerae* vaccine strain CVD103. *Infect Immun* 58:1481–1484, 1990

139. Bera TK, Ghosh SK, Das J: Cloning and characterization of *mutL* and *mutS* genes of *Vibrio cholerae*: nucleotide sequence of the *mutL* gene. *Nucleic Acids Res* 17:6241–6250, 1989

140. Srivastava R, Sinha VB, Srivastava BS: Chromosomal transfer and in vivo cloning of genes in *Vibrio cholerae* using RP4::mini-Mu. *Gene* 75:253–259, 1989

141. Mostow P, Richardson K: High-frequency spontaneous mutation of classical *Vibrio cholerae* to nonmotile phenotype. *Infect Immun* 58:3633–3639, 1990

142. Houng H-SH, Cook TM: Cloning of the galactose utilization genes of *Vibrio cholerae*. *Ann NY Acad Sci* 435:601–603, 1985

143. Sigel SP, Payne SM: Effect of iron limitation on growth, siderophore production, and expression of outer membrane proteins of *Vibrio cholerae*. *J Bacteriol* 150:148–155, 1982

144. Sciortino CV, Finkelstein RA: *Vibrio cholerae* expresses iron-regulated outer membrane proteins in vivo. *Infect Immun* 42:990–996, 1983

145. Calderwood SB, Mekalanos JJ: Confirmation of the Fur operator site by insertion of a synthetic oligonucleotide into an operon fusion plasmid. *J Bacteriol* 170:1015–1017, 1988

146. Goldberg MB, DiRita VJ, Calderwood SB: Identification of an iron-regulated virulence determinant in *Vibrio cholerae*, using Tn*phoA* mutagenesis. *Infect Immun* 58:55–60, 1990

147. Goldberg MB, Boyko SA, Calderwood SB: Transcriptional regulation by iron of a *Vibrio cholerae* virulence gene and homology of the gene to the *Escherichia coli* Fur system. *J Bacteriol* 172:6863–6870, 1990

148. Goldberg MB, Boyko SA, Calderwood SB: Positive transcriptional regulation of an iron-regulated virulence gene in *Vibrio cholerae*. *Proc Natl Acad Sci USA* 88:1125–1129, 1991

148a. Richardson K, Kaper JB, Levine MM: Human immune response to *Vibrio cholerae* 01 whole cells and isolated outer membrane antigens. *Infect Immun* 57:495–501, 1989

149. Jonson G, Svennerholm A-M, Holmgren J: *Vibrio cholerae* expresses cell surface antigens during intestinal infection which are not expressed during in vitro culture. *Infect Immun* 57:1809–1815, 1989

150. Finkelstein RA, Vasil ML, Holmes RK: Studies on toxinogenesis in *Vibrio cholerae*. I. Isolation of mutants with altered toxinogenicity. *J Infect Dis* 129:117–123, 1974

151. Honda T, Finkelstein RA: Selection and characteristics of a *Vibrio cholerae* mutant lacking the A (ADP-ribosylating) portion of the cholera enterotoxin. *Proc Natl Acad Sci USA* 76:2052–2056, 1979

152. Kaper JB, Lockman H, Baldini MM, Levine MM: Recombinant nontoxinogenic *Vibrio cholerae* strains as attenuated cholera vaccine candidates. *Nature* 308:655–658, 1984

153. Kaper JB, Lockman H, Baldini MM, Levine MM: A recombinant live oral cholera vaccine. *Bio/Technol* 2:345–349, 1984

154. Attridge SR, Daniels D, Morona JK, Morona R: Surface co-expression of *Vibrio cholerae* and *Salmonella typhi* O-antigens on Ty21a clone EX210. *Microbial Pathogenesis* 8:177–188, 1990

155. Kaper JB, Bradford HB, Roberts NC, Falkow S: Molecular epidemiology of *Vibrio cholerae* in the U.S. Gulf Coast. *J Clin Microbiol* 16:129–134, 1982

156. Roberts NC, Siebeling RJ, Kaper JB, Bradford HB Jr: Vibrios in the Louisiana Gulf Coast environment. *Microb Ecol* 8:299–312, 1982

157. Kaper JB, Nataro JP, Roberts NC, et al: Molecular epidemiology of Non-01 *Vibrio cholerae* and *Vibrio mimicus* in the U.S. Gulf Coast region. *J Clin Microbiol* 23:652–654, 1986

158. Koblavi S, Grimont F, Grimont PAD: Clonal diversity of *Vibrio cholerae* 01 evidenced by rRNA gene restriction patterns. *Res Microbiol* 141:645–657, 1990

5

Vibrio Phages and Phage-Typing

B. Rowe and J. A. Frost

1. INTRODUCTION

The first vibrio phages were identified by d'Herelle in 1926, and by the 1950s several distinct types of bacteriophage acting on *V. cholerae* had been described. These studies of cholera bacteriophages have been reviewed by Pollitzer.[1] Most early studies were directed towards the use of cholera phages for treatment or prophylaxis rather than strain discrimination. Interest in cholera phages revived with the spread of the seventh pandemic and the appearance in the 1960s of the El Tor biotype, and has proceeded along two distinct lines—the development of phage-typing schemes using lytic phages and classification using lysogeny.

2. *V. CHOLERAE* 01

2.1. Phage-Typing Schemes

Phage-typing schemes were developed by Mukerjee and his colleagues in Calcutta,[2,3] Gallut and Nicolle[4] in France, Newman and Eisenstark[5] in the United States, and Lee and Furniss[6] in the United Kingdom. The essential characteristics of these schemes are summarized in Table 1.

Studies on cholera phages and phage-typing were initiated in the Calcutta laboratory of Dr. S. Mukerjee in 1955. Their initial studies of the classical biotype screened over 600 phages which could be divided into four antigenically distinct groups. Four of these phages, isolated from the stools of cholera patients, form the phage-typing scheme for classical cholera.[2,7] Further phage adaptations enabled subdivision of type 1.[8] The replacement of the classical biotype by the El Tor biotype rendered this scheme obsolete since the classical

Cholera, edited by Dhiman Barua and William B. Greenough III. Plenum Medical Book Company, New York, 1992.

Chapter 5

TABLE 1
V. cholerae 01 Phage Typing Schemes

Author(s)	Date	Number of phages	Source of phages		Phage types		Common type	
			Previous schemes[a] (number of phages)	New	Classsical	El Tor	Classical	El Tor
Mukerjee	1957	4	—	India	5	—	>50%	
Gallut and Nicolle	1963	7	—	Egypt	5	3	50%	80%
Newman and Eisenstark	1964	8	Laboratory collections Lysogenic phages		7	—	81%	
Basu and Mukerjee	1968	5	—	India	—	6		>50%
Drozhevkina and Arutyunov	1979	7	M(4)	USSR	11	6	72%	71%
Lee and Furniss	1981	14	M(4) B&M(4) G&N(1)	Bangladesh	NT[b]	<25		41%

[a]M = Mukerjee (1957); B&M = Basu and Mukerjee (1968); G&N = Gallut and Nicolle (1963).
[b]NT = not tested.

biotype disappeared from India and neighboring countries throughout the 1960s and 1970s. There have however been recent reports of its reappearance in Bangladesh,[9,10] but not in India (National Institute of Cholera and Enteric Diseases, Calcutta, Annual Report, 1986–1987). Comparison of plasmid profiles, location of cholera toxin genes, and presence of defective VcA1 phage has suggested that the classical strains isolated in Bangladesh in 1982 are more closely related to classical strains isolated during the sixth pandemic than to El Tors or nontoxigenic 01s isolated during the seventh pandemic.[11]

The phage-typing scheme developed in Paris[4,12,13] grouped both classical and El Tor strains into eight phage types using lytic phages from various sources. The scheme was tested on 271 strains of which the majority (213) were of the classical biotype, mainly from laboratory collections. Fourteen El Tor strains were tested and 44 non-01 V. cholerae. Classical strains from the Bangkok epidemic of 1959–1960 belonged to four phage types, two of which were also identified among El Tor and non-01 isolates from the same epidemic.[13]

Newman and Eisenstark[5] investigated lysogeny in V. cholerae with the principal aim of examining the differences between the two biotypes. They concluded that phages could certainly be used to differentiate between the two biotypes and that the development of a phage-typing scheme for epidemiological studies was feasible. However, like Nicolle and his colleagues, Newman and Eisenstark used only laboratory strains and this scheme has not been tested under field conditions.

In 1965, a phage-typing scheme which distinguished nine types within the El Tor biotype was developed in Calcutta. A modification of this scheme[3] using five phages, two lytic mutants of temperate phages and three isolated from patients' stools, identifies six phage types and has been used in India for epidemiological studies. Phage-typing of 3464 strains isolated between 1937 and 1966 showed that all six phage types were present in Celebes, Indonesia, the original focus of the seventh pandemic, whereas the number of phage types isolated elsewhere declined with time and distance from Celebes so that only two phage types were isolated in Pakistan and India where the El Tor biotype first appeared in 1963/1964.[14]

Bockemühl and Meinicke[15] used the Basu and Mukerjee scheme to type 211 V. cholerae 01 El Tor strains from outbreaks of cholera in Togo between 1970 and 1973. They found that 175 strains (82.9%) belonged to type 4, 35 (16.6%) were type 1 and 1 strain (0.4%) was untypable. More recently a survey of 24,694 V. cholerae 01 isolated in India between 1975 and 1985 showed that 99.5% were El Tor and of these 47.4% belonged to type 2, 47.4% to type 4, and 0.2% to type 1.[16]

The phages of the Calcutta schemes have proved valuable in differentiating between the two biotypes of V. cholerae 01. Classical phage IV lyses all classical strains but El Tors are all resistant.[7,8] Sensitivity to phage IV together with the chicken erythrocyte agglutination test and polymixin B sensitivity have been accepted as the criteria for differentiating the two biotypes.[17]

The two biotypes can also be differentiated by their reactions with phage FK.[18] This has a similar host range to Mukerjee phage 4, that is, classical strains are sensitive and El Tors are resistant, but is morphologically distinct.

The two Calcutta schemes have been used in India to chart the progress of the seventh pandemic. Between 1955 and 1960 the classical biotype was the causative organism of cholera in India. Between 1961 and 1963 El Tor cholera spread outwards from Indonesia and, following a widespread epidemic in Burma in 1963, appeared in Bangladesh towards the end of that year and in India early in 1964. While all cholera vibrios isolated in India before March, 1964 were classical V. cholerae 01, by 1965, 89% of 2000 strains phage-typed were El Tor.[14]

In a survey of 91 *V. cholerae* 01 isolated in Bangladesh during January 1986,[19] 60 strains (65.9%) were identified as classical biotype, all of which belonged to phage type 1 of the Mukerjee scheme. The 31 El Tor vibrios identified belonged to phage types 1 (1 strain), 5 (1 strain), or 4 (19 strains) of the Basu and Mukerjee scheme, or were untypable (10 strains).

The phage-typing scheme most widely used in recent years is that developed in Maidstone, United Kingdom.[6,20] This uses 14 phages—the four classical phages of the Mukerjee scheme, four derived from the scheme of Basu and Mukerjee, Nicolle's β, and five phages isolated from sewage effluent in Bangladesh. These were used to type 1135 field strains of global origin and produced more than 25 types (Table 2). Sixty-four percent of the strains, however, gave the three most common phage reaction patterns and 11 types each accounted for less than the 1% of the strains studied. The Maidstone scheme has been used in a study of endemic cholera in a rural community in Bangladesh.[21] It was found that, in any one year,

TABLE 2
Phage Types of the Lee and Furniss Scheme[a]

Typing phages[a]

Classical				El Tor										Number of strains	Percent
Mukerjee				Basu and Mukerjee					Bangladesh						
I	II	III[b]	IV	e4	e5	β[c]	32	57	4996	13	14	16	24		
V	V	V	V	+	+	+	−	+	+	+	+	+	+	20	2
V	V	V	V	+	+	+	−	+	+	+	+	+	−	5	
−	−	−	−	+	+	+	+	−	+	+	+	+	+	4	
−	−	−	−	+	+	+	−	+	+	+	−	+	−	14	1
+	−	−	+	+	+	−	−	+	−	−	−	−	−	4	
−	−	−	−	−	+	+	+	−	+	+	+	+	+	137	12
−	−	−	−	−	+	+	+	−	−	+	+	+	+	122	11
−	−	−	−	−	+	+	+	−	−	−	+	+	+	38	3
−	−	−	−	−	+	+	+	−	−	+	−	+	+	9	
−	−	−	−	−	+	+*	+	−	+	−	+	−*	−	5	
−	−	−	−	−	+	+	−	−	+	+	+	+	+	465	41
−	−	−	−	−	+	+	−	−	+	−	+	−*	−*	49	4
−	−	−	−	−	+	+	−	−	−	+	+	+	+	13	1
−	−	−	−	−	+	+	−	−	−	−	+	−	−	6	
−	−	−	−	−	+	+	−	−	−	−	−	−	−	6	
−	−	−	−	−	+	−	−	−	+	+	+	+	+	16	1
−	−	−	−	−	+	−	−	−	+	+	−	+	+	50	4
−	−	−	−	−	+	−	−	−	+	−	−	−	−	7	
−	−	−	−	−	+	−	−	−	−	−	+	−	−	14	1
−	−	−	−	−	−	−*	−*	−	−	−	+	−	−	15	1
−	−	−	−	−*	−*	+	−	−	−	−	+	−*	−	33	3
−	−	−	−	−*	−*	+	−	+	−	−	+	−*	−	10	
−	−	−	−	−*	−	−	−	+	−	−	−	−*	−	23	2
−	−	+	+	−	−	−	−	−	−	−	−	−	−	4	
−	−	−	−	−	−	−	−	−	−	−	−	−	−	8	
													Others	58	5
													Total	1135	

[a]From Lee and Furniss, 1981.
[b]Phage III gives variable weak reactions with many El Tor strains; results not shown.
[c]β = Nicolle's β.
*, may give weak reactions of just a few plaques; +, denotes lysis; −, denotes no lysis; V = variable reactions.

TABLE 3
Phages of the USSR Scheme

Typing phage	Original designation	Source
1	I	
2	II	Mukerjee (1957)
3	IV	
4	3900	
5	455	USSR
6	7227	
7	III	Mukerjee (1957)

several phage types appeared simultaneously, suggesting multiple foci of infection. This scheme has, however, recently been evaluated by the WHO Collaborating Centre for Phage-Typing and Drug Resistance of Enterobacteria and was found to be unsatisfactory since some of the phages were contaminated, there was no suitable set of type strains available, and there were inconsistencies in the type designations between different publications.[22]

A phage-typing scheme has been developed in the USSR[23] that is designed for typing both of the biotypes of *V. cholerae* 01. It includes the four phages of Mukerjee's scheme for classical cholera and three El Tor phages isolated in the USSR (Table 3) and defines 16 phage types (Table 4). This scheme has proved useful although once again most strains fall into two phage types, types 11 and 13.[24]

TABLE 4
Current Phage Typing Chart for USSR Scheme

Type strain designation	Lysis by typing phages[a]							Phage type	Biotype
	1,	2	3	4	5	6	7		
T1	+	+	+	−	−	−	+	1	Classical
T2	−	+	+	−	−	−	+	2	
T3	+	−	+	−	−	−	+	3	
254/63 Howrah	−	−	+	−	−	−	+	4	
T5	+	+	+	−	−	−	−	5	
375	+	+	+	−	−	+	+	6	
P-4346	+	−	−	+	−	+	−	10	El Tor
806	−	−	−	+	+	−	+	11	
P-6532	−	−	+	+	−	−	−	12	
P-9263	−	−	−	+	+	+	+	13	
P-4678	−	−	−	+	−	+	−	14	
498	−	−	−	+	−	−	−	15	
10	−	−	−	−	−	+	−	16	
421	−	−	+	−	−	−	−	17	Classical
6782	+	−	+	+	−	−	−	18	El Tor
246	−	−	−	−	−	−	+	19	Classical
E26943	−	−	−	−	+	−	−	NC1[b]	El Tor
E29677	−	+	−	+	+	+	+	NC2[b]	

[a]+, denotes lysis; −, denotes no lysis (or fewer than 10 plaques).
[b]NC = non-conforming. Reacts with the typing phages but does not conform to a designated type.

Phages are prepared by the soft agar overlayer method[25] and purified by centrifugation or filtration. High-titre phage stocks are stable at 4°C–10°C for over a year but routine test dilutions (RTD) must be prepared more frequently. The RTD × 10 dilution is used for typing. Strains are phage-typed using standard techniques: phage-typing agar plates are flooded with the test strains, spotted with phage and incubated at 28°C overnight or 37°C for 6 hr.[20,22] In 1987, Frost and Rowe[24] evaluated this scheme, which at that time included the types shown in Table 4. These correspond to the phage types described by Drozhevkina and Arutyunov[23] but type strains for types 7, 8, and 9 are no longer available and types 17 and 18 have been replaced by the "new" patterns shown in the table. Table 4 is thus the currently accepted chart for this scheme and includes a further type, type 19, and two patterns provisionally identified as NC1 and NC2.

This scheme has been used to type a collection of recently isolated strains of V. cholerae 01[24] (and Frost and Rowe, unpublished results). The distribution of phage types among 360 strains of V. cholerae 01 is given in Table 5. Half of the strains tested belonged to type 13 (181 strains, 50.3%), type 11 accounted for a further 85 strains (23.6%), and type 15 for 25 strains (6.9%). Thus, three phage types represented 80.8% of the strains tested, a limitation which this scheme shares with the previous schemes described above. However the predominance of type 13 may be partially explained by the geographical bias of the sample. One hundred and forty-eight strains were from African countries and, of these, 125 (84.5%) were type 13. In contrast, of the 59 Asian strains included, only 7 (11.9%) were type 13 and the predominant phage types were types 11 (57.6%) and 15 (18.6%).

2.2. Limitations of the Above Schemes and Requirements for Future Development

The three phage-typing schemes for V. cholerae 01 which have been widely used to date, namely those of Basu and Mukerjee,[3] Lee and Furniss,[6] and Drozhevkina and Arutyunov,[23] have a number of characteristics in common. The latter two phage-typing schemes are used for both the classical and El Tor biotypes and the small number of El Tor–specific phages used, only three in the Russian scheme, means that the number of phage types defined for the El Tor biotype is necessarily limited. Furthermore, in each scheme, two or three phage types account for up to 80% of the strains examined. This variation does however appear to be epidemiologically meaningful since there are distinct geographical variations in type distribution.

Two essential requirements for a phage-typing scheme that is to be used in a number of laboratories are pure and stable phages and a well-defined set of type strains. The latter, which can be distributed with the phages, are essential for on-going quality control. The USSR scheme appears to be the only current V. cholerae 01 phage-typing scheme that meets these criteria. The extension of this scheme by the addition of new phages is a priority to improve strain discrimination within the most common types.

2.3. Lysogeny and Prophage-Typing

Before 1961, the El Tor vibrio was considered to be nonpathogenic. In 1963, Takeya and Shimodori[26] reported that strains isolated during an outbreak of El Tor cholera in the western Pacific and South East Asia were lysogenic for a phage which they designated "kappa." This phage had a very narrow host range but was easily detected in pathogenic El

Tor strains which they designated "Celebes" type. Nonpathogenic El Tor strains isolated in Ubol, Thailand in 1959 were not only nonlysogenic but also resistant to kappa. A typing scheme was proposed which appeared to correlate pathogenicity and lysogeny with this phage. Subsequent studies showed that strains sensitive to kappa could be lysogenized and could therefore be regarded as "cured" Celebes type.[27] Prophage-typing of 31 El Tor vibrios isolated in Bangladesh during January, 1986 identified 14 Ubol-type strains, 16 cured Celebes, and 1 Celebes type.[19] The fact that both the lysogenic and cured Celebes strains could cause severe disease showed that the phage was not directly involved in pathogenesis.

This phage, kappa, is widely distributed in El Tor vibrios and is synonomous with the "alpha" phage of Nicolle,[28] typing phage 3 of Basu and Mukerjee[3] and phage 32 of Lee and Furniss.[6] Thus, types that are sensitive to these phages are nonlysogenic. Nicolle[12] also demonstrated the presence of "alpha" (=kappa) in 311 of 395 (78.7%) strains tested, a further 45 strains were sensitive, i.e., "cured," Celebes type. In the same study a second lysogenic phage "beta" was identified and this has also been incorporated in the Lee and Furniss typing scheme.

Since most El Tor strains are lysogenic and the kappa phage is readily released, Takaya and others[29] developed a phage detection system for rapid and sensitive diagnosis of cholera. In untreated cases 10^3–10^6 phage particles per ml of watery stool could be detected. Phages can also be detected in the stools of carriers where isolation of the bacterium may be more difficult.

Three further phages have been described which are serologically related to kappa; VcA-1 and VcA-2 isolated from classical strain NIH41[30,31] and VcA-3 from an El Tor strain isolated in the Gulf of Mexico area of the US.[32] VcA-3 would appear to be synonomous with the phage designated T-L by Shimodori and others[33] which was present in a strain isolated in Texas in 1973 and in outbreaks in Louisiana in 1977 and 1978. VcA-1 and T-L/VcA-3 differ from kappa both in serology and host range whereas VcA-2 appears to be more closely related. "Alpha," "kappa," and VcA-2 cannot stably coexist in the same cell. VcA-1 and VcA-3 are morphologically similar and share considerable DNA homology although their restriction endonuclease digestion patterns are quite distinct, suggesting evolutionary divergence.[34] All three VcA phages can integrate randomly into the *V. cholerae* chromosome[34] and can thus be used for genetic analysis in a manner similar to that of the mutator phage Mu in *E. coli*.[11,35]

Phage CP-T1 isolated from a lysogenic El Tor strain[36,37] has been shown to mediate generalized transduction and to be capable of propagation on host cells of either biotype using the O antigen as its receptor.[38] In classical strains it appears that lysogeny with CP-T1 converts the Ogawa serotype to Hikojima.[39] All three VcA phages are able to lysogenize *V. cholerae* 01 of both the classical and El Tor biotypes and it has been shown that the phages are prevalent in both biotypes although classical strains may release only defective phage particles.[31] The role of these lysogenic phages in *V. cholerae* genetics has been recently reviewed by Guidolin and Manning.[34] This ability to transduce chromosomal genes has also been used to transmit toxin production from a hypertoxinogenic strain to one of low toxicity[40] and to mediate the transfer of the genes encoding resistance to polymixin B from an El Tor to a classical strain.[36]

3. PHAGE-TYPING OF *V. CHOLERAE* NON-01

The taxonomy and pathogenicity of *V. cholerae* belonging to serotypes other than 01 have been reviewed by Sakasaki and colleagues.[41] Recognizing their possible pathogenic

TABLE 5
Phage Type Distribution of *V. cholerae* 01 Using the USSR Scheme[a]

Country of origin	Total	Phage type													
		1	3	4	6	10	11	13	14	15	16	17	19	NC	u
Asia															
Bangladesh	10						1	3		6					
Brunei	7						7								
Japan	11						8			1					2
India	10						3	3	1	1	1			1	
Pakistan	1									1					
Philippines	10						8			2					
Taiwan	1							1							
Thailand	7						5		1				1		
Unspecified	2						2								
Total	59	—	—	—	—	—	34	7	2	11	1	—	1	1	2
Africa															
Ivory Coast	1							1							
Kenya	11						5	6							
Mali	8						1	7							
Nigeria	2							2							
Somalia	94						2	81	6	2					3

															Total
Tanzania	—	—	—	—	—	—	6	—	—	—	—	—	—	—	6
Zaire	—	—	—	—	—	2	17	1	—	—	—	—	—	—	20
Unspecified	—	—	—	—	—	—	5	1	—	—	—	—	—	—	6
Total	—	—	—	—	—	10	125	1	7	—	—	1	—	4	148
Australia	—	—	—	—	—	—	34	12	—	—	—	—	—	—	46
France	—	—	—	—	—	35	2	—	—	—	—	—	—	—	37
Infected in Algeria	—	—	—	—	—	—	—	—	—	—	—	—	—	—	—
U.K.															
Infected in Kenya	—	—	—	—	—	—	1	—	—	—	—	—	—	—	1
Infected in India	—	—	—	—	—	1	1	—	—	—	—	—	—	—	2
Infected in Pakistan	—	—	—	—	—	2	2	—	1	—	—	—	—	—	5
Prawns	—	—	—	—	—	—	—	—	1	—	—	—	—	—	1
Water	—	—	—	—	—	—	—	5	5	—	—	—	—	1	11
Unspecified	—	—	—	—	—	1	—	1	—	—	—	—	—	1	3
Total	—	—	—	—	—	4	4	6	7	—	—	—	—	2	23
Country unspecified	6	1	5	2	1	2	9	3	4	—	—	1	—	13	47
Total	6	1	5	2	1	85	181	19	25	2	1	4	2	26	360
% of total	1.7	0.3	1.4	0.6	0.3	23.6	50.3	5.3	6.9	0.6	0.3	1.1	0.6	7.2	

[a]Source: Frost and Rowe (1987) and unpublished data.

role, Sil[42] has developed a phage-typing scheme for these vibrios. The scheme uses four phages isolated from sewage and defines ten types. It was used to test 40 strains isolated in India in 1969[43] and was shown to have some epidemiological validity as a geographical variation in phage-type distribution was observed. The scheme has not been widely used to date and the relationship between phage type and 0 serotype has not been studied.

REFERENCES

1. Pollitzer R: *Cholera*. Monograph Series, No. 43. Geneva, World Health Organization, 1959
2. Mukerjee S, Guha DK, Guha Roy UK: Studies on typing of cholera by bacteriophage. I. Phage-typing of *Vibrio cholerae* from Calcutta epidemics. *Ann Biochem Exp Med* 17:161–176, 1957
3. Basu S, Mukerjee S: Bacteriophage typing of *Vibrio eltor*. *Experientia* 24:299–300, 1968
4. Gallut J, Nicolle P: Lysogenie et lysotypie de *V.cholerae* et *V. El Tor* d'origines géographiques diverses. *Bull WHO* 28:389–393, 1963
5. Newman FS, Eisenstark, A: Phage–host relationships in *Vibrio cholerae*. *J Infect Dis* 114:217–225, 1964
6. Lee JV, Furniss AL: The phage typing of *Vibrio cholerae* serovar 01, in Holme T, Holmgren J, Merson MH, Molby R (eds): *Acute Enteric Infections in Children: New Prospects for Treatment and Prevention*. Amsterdam, Elsevier/North Holland Biomedical Press, 1981, pp 119–122
7. Mukerjee S: Bacteriophage-typing of cholera. *Bull WHO* 28:337–345, 1963
8. Mukerjee S, Guha Roy UK, Rudra BC: Studies on typing of *Vibrio cholerae* by bacteriophage. III. Phage-typing of strains of Calcutta epidemics of 1959. *Ann Biochem Exp Med* 20:181–188, 1960
9. Samedi AR, Huq MI, Shahid N, et al: Classical *Vibrio cholerae* biotype displaces El Tor in Bangladesh. *Lancet* i:805–807, 1983
10. Khan MU, Samedi A-R, Huq MI, et al: Simultaneous classical and El Tor cholera in Bangladesh. *J Diar Dis Res* 2:13–18, 1984
11. Cook WL, Wachsmuth K, Johnson SR, et al: Persistence of plasmids, cholera toxin genes, and prophage DNA in Classical *Vibrio cholerae* 01. *Infect Immun* 45:222–226, 1984
12. Nicolle P, Gallut J, LeMinor L: Étude lysogenique, lysotypique, serologique et biochimique (choléra-roth et récherche de la lysine decarboxylase) d'une collection de vibrions cholériques El-Tor. *Ann Inst Pasteur* 99:664–671, 1960
13. Nicolle P, Gallut J, Ducrest P, et al: Research with a view to establishment of a lysotype for *Vibrio cholerae* and *Vibrio eltor*. *Rev Hyg Med Soc* 10:91–126, 1962
14. Mukerjee S: Vibrio phages and phage-typing of cholera vibrios, in Barua D, Burrows W (eds.): *Cholera*, Philadelphia, W.B. Saunders Co., 1974, pp 61–74
15. Bockemühl J, Meinicke D: Value of phage typing of *V.cholerae* biotype eltor in West Africa. *Bull WHO* 54:187–192, 1976
16. Niyogi SK, De SP: Prevalence of biotypes, serotypes and phage-types of *Vibrio cholerae* 01 in India (1975–1985). *Ind J Med Res* 85:1–4, 1987
17. Barua D, Burrows W, Gallut J: *Principles and Practice of Cholera Control*. Public Health Paper No. 40, Geneva, World Health Organization, 1970, pp 128–129
18. Takeya K, Otohuja T, Tokiwa H: FK phage for differentiating the classical and El Tor groups of *Vibrio cholerae*. *J Clin Microbiol* 14:222–224, 1981
19. Nakasone N, Iwanaga M, Eeckels R: Characterization of *Vibrio cholerae* 01 recently isolated in Bangladesh. *Trans Roy Soc Trop Med Hygiene* 81:876–878, 1987
20. Furniss AL, Lee JV, Donovan TJ: *The Vibrios*. Monograph No. 11 Public Health Laboratory Service, 1978
21. Glass RI, Becker S, Huq I, et al: Endemic cholera in rural Bangladesh 1966–1980. *Am J Epidemiol* 116:959–967, 1982
22. Recent advances in cholera research: Memorandum from a WHO meeting. *Bull WHO* 13:841–849, 1985
23. Drozhevkina MS, Arutyunov YI: Phage-typing of *Vibrio cholerae* using a new collection of phages. *J Hyg Epidem Microbiol Immunol* 23:340–347, 1971
24. Frost JA, Rowe B: Geographical variations in the distribution of phage types of *V.cholerae* 01 and non-01. *FEMS Microbiol Lett* 40:210–222, 1987
25. Adams MH: *Bacteriophages*. New York, Interscience Publishers, Inc, 1959
26. Takeya K, Shimodori S: "Prophage-typing" of El Tor vibrios. *J Bacteriol* 85:957–958, 1963

27. Takeya K: El Tor cholera, with special reference to Kappa-type cholera phage. *Jap J Trop Med* 8:5–9, 1967

28. Nicolle P, Gallut J, Schraen MF, et al: Diversité des états lysogenes parmi les vibrions cholériques El Tor de provenances variés. *Bull Soc Path Exot* 604:603–612, 1971

29. Takeya K, Shimodori S, Zinnaka Y: New method for early diagnosis of Celebes type El Tor vibrio carriers. *J Bacteriol* 90:824–825, 1965

30. Weston L, Drexler H, Richardson SH: Characterization of vibrio phage VA-1. *J Gen Virol* 21:155–158, 1973

31. Gerdes JC, Romig WR: Complete and defective bacteriophages of classical *Vibrio cholerae:* relationship to the Kappa type bacteriophage. *J Virol* 15:1231–1238, 1975

32. Goldberg S, Murphy JR: Molecular epidemiological studies of United States Gulf Coast *Vibrio cholerae* strains: integration site for mutator vibriophage VcA-3. *Infect Immun* 42:224–230, 1983

33. Shimodori S, Takeya K, Takade A: Lysogenicity and prophage type of the strains of *Vibrio cholerae* 0-1 isolated mainly from the natural environment. *Am J Epidemiol* 120:759–768, 1984

34. Guidolin A, Manning PA: Genetics of *Vibrio cholerae* and its bacteriophages. *Microbiol Rev* 51:285–298, 1987

35. Johnson SR, Romig WR: *Vibrio cholerae* conjugative plasmid pSJ15 contains transposable prophage dVcA1. *J Bacteriol* 146:632–638, 1981

36. Ogg JE, Strestha MB, Poudayl L: Phage induced changes in *Vibrio cholerae* serotype and biotype conversions. *Infect Immun* 19:231–238, 1978

37. Ogg JE, Timme JL, Alemohammad MM: General transduction in *Vibrio cholerae. Infect Immun* 31:737–741, 1981

38. Guidolin A, Manning PA: *Vibrio cholerae* bacteriophage CP-T1: Characterization of the receptor. *Eur J Biochem* 153:89–94, 1985

39. Ogg JE, Ogg BJ, Shretstha MB, et al: Antigenic changes in *Vibrio cholerae* biotype eltor serotype Ogawa after bacteriophage infection. *Infect Immun* 24:974–978, 1979

40. Siddiqui KAI, Bhattacharyya FK: Phage-induced change of toxigenesis in *Vibrio cholerae. J Med Microbiol* 23:331–334, 1987

41. Sakasaki R, Gomez CZ, Sebald M: Taxonomical studies of the so-called NAG vibrios. *Jap J Med Sci Biol* 20:265–280, 1967

42. Sil J: Studies on NAG vibrios and NAG bacteriophages. Doctoral thesis. Calcutta, India, Calcutta University, 1970

43. Sil J, Dutta NK, Sanyal SC, et al: Phage-typing of *Vibrio cholerae* strains other than 0 serotype 1 isolated in different states of India in 1969. *Indian J Microbiol* 12:110–113, 1972

6

The Ecology of *Vibrio cholerae*

Rita R. Colwell and William M. Spira

1. INTRODUCTION

Until the late 1970s and early 1980s, *Vibrio cholerae* was believed to be highly host-adapted and incapable of surviving longer than a few hours or days outside the human intestine. This view, enunciated by Felsenfeld,[1] was that "some authors claimed that cholera vibrios may survive in water, particularly seawater, for as long as 2 months. This is, however, scarcely possible under natural conditions if reinfection of the water does not take place." This perspective of cholera ecology had dominated the literature since the organism was first identified by Robert Koch. Interestingly, Koch himself held a rather less stringent opinion:

> There remains still the important question to be answered, whether the infectious material can reproduce or multiply itself outside the human body. I believe it can. . . . I would not certainly assume that multiplication . . . takes place in . . . river water without any assistance, for these fluids do not possess the concentration of nutritious substances which is necessary for the growth of the bacilli. But I can easily imagine that . . . some spots may contain sufficient concentrations of nutritive substances [for bacilli to flourish].[2]

The speculations of Koch have proven to be prescient, since the most recent data show that toxigenic *V. cholerae* 01 exist outside the human intestine and the autochthonous nature of *V. cholerae* 01 is an important factor in the epidemiology of cholera, significantly so in endemic areas.

V. cholerae historically has been divided into subgroups, but both environmental and clinical isolates have been shown to be identical by 5S rRNA sequencing.[3] Interestingly, both the 5S rRNA and 16S rRNA data indicate a deep branching of *V. cholerae* from other vibrios, reported by Colwell and MacDonell[4] and E. Stackebrandt (personal communication).

Thus, the common wisdom for about 100 years was that the only reservoir of toxigenic

Cholera, edited by Dhiman Barua and William B. Greenough III. Plenum Medical Book Company, New York, 1992.

V. cholerae 01 and, hence, endemic cholera, was the human intestinal tract and that *V. cholerae* 01 was taxonomically separate from *V. cholerae* non-01, the "non-agglutinable vibrios," found in aquatic, predominantly estuarine, environments. An important advance was made when it was shown by Citarella and Colwell in 1970, using DNA/DNA hybridization, that both 01 and non-01 *V. cholerae* comprise a single species.[5] The distinction between "cholera vibrios" and other *V. cholerae* was vigorously championed at that time[6] and, even today, some investigators continue to maintain this position, despite the overwhelming evidence to the contrary. The evidence, including numerical taxonomy,[7] DNA/DNA hybridization,[5] and nucleic acid sequence data,[3,4] supports the conclusion that *V. cholerae,* both 01 and non-01, represents a single species.

For purposes of discussion, toxigenic *V. cholerae* 01, i.e., the "cholera vibrio," is defined as possessing the 01 antigen and being capable of producing enterotoxin and, therefore, causing cholera in susceptible hosts. Both classical and El Tor *V. cholerae* are included in *V. cholerae* 01 (CT[+]). Nontoxinogenic *V. cholerae* 01 comprise those isolates which agglutinate in 01 antiserum but do not possess the cholera toxin gene. Nevertheless, these strains may produce diarrheal disease and are designated *V. cholerae* 01 (CT[-]).

Vibrio cholerae non-01, both environmental and clinical isolates, do not agglutinate in 01 antiserum, although some cultures may contain 01 cells when examined by direct epifluorescent microscopy.[8] These strains have been implicated in many, well-documented cases of diarrheal disease and outbreaks, but, in general, not with major cholera epidemics. Some non-01 *V. cholerae* isolates produce an enterotoxin indistinguishable from cholera toxin and, as recently shown for *V. cholerae* 01,[9] are capable of a free-living existence in the aquatic environment.

The following is a review of *V. cholerae* 01 (CT[+]) ecology, a subject which, until recently, was in a state of transition and engendered a great deal of controversy amongst some clinical investigators. A brief presentation of the earlier literature (pre-1970) on survival of bacteria in the natural environment is provided. The term "survival" had been viewed as highly host-adapted "cholera vibrios" being able to exist for only very short periods of time outside the human intestine, when, in fact, the evidence that has accumulated over the past decade shows that *V. cholerae* is an autochthonous inhabitant of brackish water and estuarine systems.[10] Thus, the very early studies of *V. cholerae,* prior to 1970, were aimed at identifying environmental conditions associated with unusual delays in the inevitable "death" of the "cholera vibrios," in order to establish the length of time after which an environment could be considered cholera-free, if it were not recontaminated with infected stool.

The discoveries of the past decade have revealed the existence of a dormant state entered into by *V. cholerae* 01 (CT[+]) and other *V. cholerae* in response to nutrient deprivation and other environmental parameters.[9] This phenomenon presents a new perspective and imparts a dynamic meaning to "survival," with the evidence showing *V. cholerae* cells do not die when discharged into aquatic environments and are capable of transforming into a dormant state when environmental conditions are not favorable.[11] The implications of dormancy of *V. cholerae* 01 are both significant and relevant, considering that the dormant forms are not recoverable on bacteriological media routinely employed in cholera microbiology laboratories.

Thus, there is a growing body of evidence, based primarily on physiological studies of *V. cholerae* in aquatic environments, that transcends mere survival and addresses the more fundamental questions of adaptation and response of microorganisms to environmental conditions.[12] The first of these studies is based on observations using microcosms simulating saline, estuarine, and brackish- and fresh-water environments. Important new information gained from the studies of *V. cholerae* physiology has shed light on: (1) temperature and salinity relationships, (2) adherence, and (3) colonization of chitinaceous macrobiota.

With the foregoing supplying a brief overview of the new information on the ecology of *V. cholerae* 01, the balance of this chapter presents the model of *V. cholerae* 01 (CT$^+$) as a free-living species of estuarine vibrios, the salient parameters of its optimum environment, and the relationship between its adaptation to the human intestinal tract and its primordial adaptation to the aquatic environment and, consequently, implications for the epidemiology of cholera.

2. HISTORICAL PERSPECTIVE ON SURVIVAL

An exhaustive historical review of the many published studies on the occurrence of *V. cholerae* 01 (CT$^+$) in stool, night soil, sewage, water, and other environments has been provided by Pollitzer[13] and updated in a recent review by Feacham *et al.*[14]

Virtually all earlier studies, i.e., prior to 1970, were based on methods for isolation and characterization of *V. cholerae* originally developed for clinical diagnosis of cholera in hospital laboratories.[15] The many difficulties associated with isolation of *V. cholerae* 01 (CT$^+$) from the aquatic environment can be related to the simple fact that methods employed to isolate *V. cholerae* were developed for clinical specimens containing large numbers of actively growing cells, whereas environmental samples are likely to contain cells exposed to and, thereby, adapted to, a variety of environmental conditions, most commonly, low nutrient concentration, pH in the range of 7–8 (seawater), fluctuating temperatures, variations in oxygen tension, and exposure to UV via sunlight.[16]

The finding by Colwell *et al.*[9] that *V. cholerae* 01 (CT$^+$) present in environmental samples may not grow on laboratory media routinely used for isolation was pivotal in the debate concerning the ecology of *V. cholerae*, i.e., that viable but "non-culturable" cells may go undetected unless direct methods of detection, e.g., microscopy, are employed. Given that virtually all studies of *V. cholerae* 01 (CT$^+$) in the environment were based solely on culturing cells, historical information in the literature on the ecology of *V. cholerae* must be interpreted with caution, since it is possible that large populations of viable but non-culturable cells may have been present in the environments sampled. The range of reported survival times in the literature prior to 1980 can, however, be usefully reexamined, both to provide a historical perspective and to estimate how long *V. cholerae* 01 (CT$^+$) continue in a fully active, culturable state in the environment before going nonculturable, i.e., unable to be detected by standard culture methods.

2.1. Survival in Nonaquatic Environments

V. cholerae 01 (CT$^+$) is reported to be recoverable from nonaquatic environments for limited periods of time following introduction. For example, in feces, *per se,* culturable organisms are rarely found after 5–7 days[17] under any conditions of storage. On the other hand, there is ample evidence that *V. cholerae* 01 (CT$^+$) can be isolated from nightsoil in cholera endemic areas,[18,19] even when active cholera cases are not reported. Survival on dry surfaces is relatively short (e.g., a matter of hours) and *V. cholerae* 01 (CT$^+$) is reported to be extremely sensitive to desiccation.[20]

In a study by Gerichter et al.,[21] V. cholerae 01 (CT+) inoculated at a concentration of $10^7/g$ in soil and stored at ambient temperature (<28°C) could be recovered only up to four days later if the soil were dry, but could be isolated up to ten days later if the soil were kept moist by adding uncontaminated sewage. The same authors found that V. cholerae 01 (CT+) could be recovered from sewage-contaminated vegetables for several days. These results are typical of the many studies of sewage-irrigated or sewage-freshened fruits and vegetables as potential vehicles of cholera.[22,23] In general, most authors concluded that the El Tor biotype survives for a relatively longer time under these conditions, compared with the classical biotype. However, only a few studies have been reported which compare El Tor and classical biotypes directly.[22]

It should be noted that foodstuffs most often incriminated in cholera outbreaks have been fish and shellfish. In these animals, V. cholerae 01 (CT+) may not simply be surface contaminants but may also be present in the intestinal tract, or gut, either as transient or colonizing flora. Such nutrient-rich, moist, and nonacidic environments permit multiplication, as well as maintenance of active populations of the organism for long periods of time.[24] Unfortunately, in light of reported cholera outbreaks associated with fish in Peru and neighboring countries in 1991, this aspect of V. cholerae ecology has been sadly neglected.

2.2. Survival in Aquatic Environments

Since it is by water that cholera transmission has traditionally occurred, survival of V. cholerae 01 (CT+) in water and wastewater has been the subject of many published studies. A consistent theme of this aspect of the literature on V. cholerae 01 (CT+), is that, when suspended in fresh or saline water, V. cholerae shows a steady decrease in number of cells enumerated over time by plate counts. However, many of these reports are difficult to interpret since the data reported are not quantitative.

Feacham et al.[14] collected data from studies in which the initial concentrations of vibrios were reported and estimated the average time of a 1-log decline in cell number (t_{90}) as a function of the type of water to which the organism was exposed, as well as biotype. The t_{90} for classical V. cholerae strains in fresh surface water (nonsterile) and sea water (nonsterile) was, respectively, 18 hr (range: 0.16–36 h) and 95 h (range: 0.36–161 h). For the El Tor biotype, the parallel values were 53 h (range: 1–230 h) and 56 h (range: 3–235 h). These results are remarkably similar to those of laboratory microcosms showing the conversion of V. cholerae from the culturable to the viable but nonculturable state.[25,26]

The conclusion drawn from these studies was that survival is enhanced in saline waters and that the organism maintains itself less well in potable water, consistent with the finding by Singleton and Colwell[27] that V. cholerae has an absolute requirement for Na+ for growth. Comparison between types of environmental waters has additional significance, since many of the studies were designed to compare different types of water using the same strain of V. cholerae. However, comparisons between biotypes are less rigorous since different strains and different experimental techniques were used in most of the pre-1980 studies. Nevertheless, the corroboration of earlier studies in the field with laboratory microcosm data is significant.

Another argument that had been employed to support the view that V. cholerae 01 (CT+) does not survive in environmental waters is the failure to isolate the organism from environmental water sources unless existing cases of cholera were in close proximity. For example, epidemiologic surveillance in the intensively monitored Matlab area in

Bangladesh, published in 1969, failed to isolate *V. cholerae* 01 (CT$^+$) from water sources between cholera seasons or from water not subject to contamination by active cholera cases.[24] In contrast, Huq *et al.*,[11] in 1990, showed that, if direct immunofluorescent microscopy were used, *V. cholerae* 01 could be detected in these waters when the organism could not be isolated, i.e., cultured, from water except when cases of cholera were nearby.

Thus, in light of recent findings that demonstrate the existence of a viable but non-culturable state in which *V. cholerae* 01 (CT$^+$) can maintain itself in the aquatic environment, i.e., in a form that would have been missed by surveillance methodologies other than direct detection by fluorescent antibody or gene probes, it is useful to examine the concept of dormancy and to identify physico–chemical conditions positively correlated with the presence of culturable *V. cholerae* 01 (CT$^+$) in the natural environment.

3. DORMANCY AS A RESPONSE TO NUTRIENT DEPRIVATION

Probably the most profound challenge to prior dogma concerning *V. cholerae* 01 (CT$^+$) ecology derives from studies by Colwell *et al.*[9] suggesting that *V. cholerae* 01 (CT$^+$) possesses the ability to enter a state of, or one approximating, dormancy in response to nutrient deprivation, elevated salinity, and/or reduced temperature. The response to nutrient deprivation of bacteria, in general, has only recently been recognized and appears to be one of many examples of a common strategy for survival among bacteria in nutrient-poor environments.[12] Novitsky and Morita[28–30] demonstrated that cultures of the marine psychrophilic *Vibrio* sp. ANT-300 responded to starvation in either natural or artificial seawater by increasing cell numbers and producing cells which were significantly decreased in volume and altered in morphology from the typical bacillus, i.e., rod-shape, to coccoid cells. The coccoid cells exhibited an endogenous respiration less than 1% of original, as well as a 40% decrease in cellular DNA, but remained culturable. Novitsky and Morita did not postulate a viable but nonculturable state, but, rather, presented excellent evidence of adaptation of cells to a low-nutrient environment.

These and other studies,[31–33] including those employing *Vibrio* ANT-300,[34,35] suggested that certain gram-negative bacteria, under conditions of nutrient deprivation, respond by: (1) continuing cell division and increasing cell numbers while the total biomass remains constant, (2) forming small (0.2 to 0.4 μm) coccoid cells, and (3) reducing overall metabolic rate. These changes are associated with long-term survival and maintenance of culturability under conditions of virtually complete nutrient deprivation.

The process by which cell numbers increase without increasing biomass (reductive division) appears to be the result of the ability of an organism to continue reproducing with energy derived from endogenous sources, while simultaneously employing previously initiated multiple replication forks to continue DNA synthesis in the absence of exogenous nutrients.[36] The resulting small cells reduce their maintenance requirements and metabolic turnover rates, and ultimately achieve a state in which they remain culturable but in which they are highly resistant to starvation. These dwarfed cells, produced by starvation under laboratory conditions, resemble the "ultramicrobacteria" (size <0.3 μm) that occur naturally in estuarine and marine waters and demonstrate low metabolic rates.[32,37,38] Many of these ultramicrobacteria appear to be *Vibrio* sp.[39] and a subgroup of the more widely recognized class of "filterable" marine bacteria (i.e., < 0.45 μm).[40]

Cells much reduced in size are not an anomaly in the aquatic environment. Indeed, such microorganisms may represent the "true" autochthonous microflora of the marine environment, or, at the least, the more common state of many bacterial species in the deep-sea environment. The putative adaptive mechanism described above is not limited to aquatic organisms, but has also been reported for soil bacteria such as *Agromyces*[41] and *Arthrobacter*,[42] and for gram-negative enteropathogens such as *Salmonella enteritidis*[43] and *Campylobacter jejuni*,[44] as well as *Escherichia coli*.[45]

Because the standard plate count is not successful in enumerating such organisms, alternative methods were developed to enumerate viable bacteria based on direct counting, the most common of which is epifluorescence microscopy of preparations stained with acridine orange.[46–49] The acridine orange direct count (AODC) is taken as a presumptive count of viable organisms since, in general, intact, double-stranded DNA binds monomers of the dye which fluoresce with a green color but broken, single-stranded DNA binds dye as dimers which fluoresce red-orange. At the very least, the AODC permits enumeration of unlysed cells containing intact DNA. However, the color shift cannot be used to measure viable versus nonviable cells.

A more convincing assay for viability is the direct viable count (DVC) of Kogure *et al.*,[50] in which active cells are identified by growth, after incubation for 6 hr at 25°C, in response to the addition of yeast extract in the presence of nalidixic acid. Under these conditions, active cells carry out protein synthesis in the absence of DNA replication or cell division and, hence, produce elongated cells that are easily identified. In general, the AODC count is higher than DVC enumeration for a given bacterial suspension, suggesting that non–substrate responsive cells may not be viable. However, this observation requires further study because the substrate employed for the direct viable count can influence the result.

In many studies, the discrepancy between the number of organisms identified by these direct methods in environmental samples or in laboratory microcosms (designed to mimic relevant environmental conditions; see Kosinski *et al.*[51]), and the number identified by direct plating has suggested that a significant population of nonculturable cells is present. Torrella and Morita,[32] for example, observed marine ultramicrobacteria which were characterized by reduced growth rate and many cells which formed microcolonies not visible on nutrient-rich plating media. In early studies of bacterial growth and death, Postgate[52] suggested that small aquatic bacteria may be susceptible to "substrate-accelerated death," if they are exposed to high levels of nutrient directly upon isolation. Chan,[53] Stevenson,[54] and MacDonell and Hood[39] also suggested that many filterable bacteria or ultramicrobacteria may be in an almost dormant state and may not be recoverable with nutrient-rich standard media but may be resuscitated under other conditions.

Colwell and colleagues[9,11,12,25,26] demonstrated, by both field and laboratory studies, that *V. cholerae,* indeed, undergoes conversion to a viable but nonculturable state, whereby the cells are reduced in size, become ovoid, but, in contrast to starved cells, do not grow at all on standard laboratory media, but remain responsive to nalidixic acid and continue to take up radiolabeled substrate.[12,55] Thus, there is now overwhelming evidence: (1) that *V. cholerae* responds to nutrient deprivation by altered morphology, i.e., "round body" formation (first described by Felter *et al.* in 1969[56]), eventually entering dormancy, i.e., the viable but nonculturable state; (2) that this state comes about through a definable physiological process, with several important aspects in common with that of other marine, estuarine, and brackish-water vibrios; and (3) that viable cells in this state may not be culturable by routine methods. These small cells of *V. cholerae* 01 (CT$^+$) can return to an active state of growth and multiplication under appropriate environmental conditions and must be assumed to have both clinical and epidemiological virulence potential.

The first report that a nonculturable state could be induced in *V. cholerae* 01 (CT$^+$)

under laboratory conditions was made by Xu et al.,[25] who reported that V. cholerae ATCC 14035 (classical) suspended in cold, sterile Chesapeake Bay water (1.1‰ salinity and 4–6°C) had a t_{90} of approximately 41 h, based on recovery on Trypticase Soy Agar (Difco Labs, Detroit, MI) and 29 h, based on recovery on Thiosulfate Citrate Bile Sucrose Agar[57] (Oxoid Ltd, Columbia, MD). Cells were not recoverable after nine days by either direct plating or alkaline peptone enrichment: a decrease of more than five logs in culturable count during this period. Concomitant evidence obtained from AODC and a fluorescent antibody (FA) direct counting procedure indicated the continued presence of intact cells at the same concentration as when the experiment was initiated.[25]

Another set of experiments was carried out with V. cholerae strain CA401 (classical) inoculated into microcosms of chemically defined sea-salts solution adjusted to 0.5% or 2.5% salinity and incubated at 10°C or 25°C for 24 or 96 h. In contrast to experiments employing V. cholerae ATCC 14035, these microcosms showed increases in cell number by AODC, DVC, and culturable counts between 24 and 96 h. Also, there was no more than a 0.5 log difference between results of the three counting methods, in all cases. The DVC represented, in all cases, ca. 98% of the AODC, while the percentage of culturable cells compared with AODC counts, ranged from 13% (10°C, 2.5% salinity) to 87% (25°C, 0.5% salinity).

The DVC was also employed in survival experiments with E. coli in Chesapeake Bay water (1.1‰ salinity and 4–6°C). DVC decreased significantly over time and was, at 13 days, close to the culturable count obtained on tryptic soy agar, ca. 1 $\log_{10}$ lower than AODC and FA counts (which remained constant from the start of the trial).

Hood and Ness[58] reported results similar to those obtained by Xu et al.,[25] but using a nontoxigenic VC-01 (oyster isolate) and five nontoxigenic V. cholerae non-01 (environmental isolates), as well as a clinical isolate of V. cholerae 01 (CT$^+$). They monitored survival in estuarine waters and sediments (both sterile and nonsterile) at 20°C with AODC and plate counts on trypticase soy–1.5% NaCl agar. All strains showed the same pattern. In sterile estuarine water, the culturable counts remained relatively constant for the duration of monitoring (up to 15 days) and were consistently 0.5 to 1 $\log_{10}$ less than the AODC counts.

A subsequent publication by the same group[59] provided evidence for the formation of small coccoid cells by both an environmental (WF110 from shellfish) and a clinical (CA401) strain of V. cholerae exposed to nutrient-free artificial seawater and filter-sterilized natural seawater microcosms. Total counts (TC) were determined by direct epifluorescence microscopy on preparations stained with 4′,6-diamino-2-phenylinodole (DPAI). Viability was determined by DVC and plate counts on a seawater-based, complete medium insulated and incubated for 72 h at 30°C. Microcosms were maintained at 21°C for up to 330 days following inoculation with approximately 5×10^3 cells (by culturable count).

The results showed no significant difference between the two seawater solutions or between the two strains of V. cholerae with respect to starvation survival. Upon exposure to starvation conditions, the clinical as well as the environmental isolate underwent reductive cell division, increased cell numbers, and formed coccoid cells while greatly reducing individual cell volume. By two days after inoculation, the culturable counts increased approximately 2.5 $\log_{10}$. From that peak, all counts decreased steadily and gradually (<0.5 $\log_{10}$ overall) until the experiment was terminated at 55 or 75 days. At the time of inoculation, the total (AODC) count was approximately 0.5 $\log_{10}$ greater than the DVC and 1 $\log_{10}$ greater than the culturable count. By 20 days and thereafter, this difference increased to 1 $\log_{10}$ and 2 $\log_{10}$, respectively. The relationship between the slopes for TC, DVC, and culturable counts remained essentially constant throughout; there was no sudden or rapid decrease in viability or increase in viable but nonrecoverable cells in any of the time periods monitored. Since incubation was at 21°C, in contrast to the much lower temperature employed by Xu *et al.*,[25] these data indicate the importance of temperature in inducing the viable but nonculturable state in *V. cholerae*.

The morphological response to starvation, monitored by electron microscopy, appeared to be uniform for the two strains studied.

At 24 h, cells of both strains were uniformly electron dense, vibroid, and of normal size (1.5 μm × 0.38 μm). At 48 h, small regions of electron transparency appeared at the periphery of cells which were unchanged in size or shape, as observed in 1970 by Felter *et al.*[56] and Kennedy *et al.*[60] who reported "round body" formation by marine vibrios.

At day 18, cells were spherical, with an electron-dense region in the center (0.56 μm diameter), surrounded by a remnant cell wall, again, as observed by Felter *et al.*[56] for marine and estuarine vibrios.

The coccoid-shaped cells studied by Hood and Ness[58] regained normal size and vibroid shape within 2 h after nutrient supplementation with a dilute solution of peptone and yeast extract. The beginning of the reversion process was observed within 10 min after nutrient addition and initiation of cell division occurred within 4–5 h. Thus, Hood and Ness[58] did not induce the viable but nonculturable state in *V. cholerae* but, instead, provided some useful information concerning nutrient depletion in this species, showing that generation times during exponential growth were significantly longer than control, nutrient-conditioned cells, suggesting nutrient depletion induces a starvation response, as opposed to complete dormancy in *V. cholerae*.

The overall response to nutrient deprivation of *V. cholerae* is similar to that of other estuarine and marine gram-negative bacteria. The pattern (e.g., initial increase in viable cells followed by a decrease to a constant level), noted by Amy and Morita[61] in their study of freshly isolated open-ocean bacteria (the other two patterns reported were "immediate decrease to constant level" and "increase to constant level with no decrease"), is but one aspect of adaptation to environmental conditions. The small coccoid cells associated with starvation survival, survive for long periods of time with little or no loss in viability, at least 5 years at ambient temperature in solutions of carbon-free, 1.5–2.0% basal salts.[61]

The starvation response of *V. cholerae* CA401 at the macromolecular level was further characterized by Hood *et al.*[62] and Guckert *et al.*[63] Nutrient deprivation included rapid decline in total lipids and carbohydrates within the first seven days and a constant decline over 30 days (the time period of monitoring) in protein and DNA. After 7 days, 88.7% of carbohydrates and 99.8% of total lipids were noted, with little change thereafter. After 30 days, a reduction of 70% in protein and 75% in the DNA content was noted. RNA concentrations, on the other hand, remained relatively constant. Profiles of lipids and carbohydrates changed during the time of maximum loss, i.e., neutral lipids declined much more slowly than did phospholipids, poly-*b*-hydroxybutyrate disappeared completely, and a relative decline in ribose and *N*-acetylglucosamine and a relative increase in six-carbon sugars, especially glucose, were noted.

The morphological response of *V. cholerae* CA401 to starvation shared some, but not all, characteristics of that of the marine vibrio ANT-300.[28,61] Important common features included conservation of ribosomal structure, disappearance of granules, and compression of the nuclear region into the center of the cell surrounded by a denser cytoplasm. On the other hand, ANT-300 showed little distortion of the cell wall while *V. cholerae* CA401 exhibited a great deal of convolution.[56,60]

The ancillary characterization of fatty acids carried out by Guckert *et al.*[63] demonstrated that lipid utilization by strain *V. cholerae* CA401 was preferential for fatty acids most easily and rapidly metabolized (*cis*-monoenoic fatty acids), but conservative of cyclopropyl and *trans*-monoenoic fatty acids, believed to be important in the maintenance of membrane integrity and fluidity. The strikingly reproducible pattern of lipid degradation during starvation in the clinical isolate *V. cholerae* CA401 paralleled, in several respects, the pattern of starvation survival of other organisms studied, including the psychrophilic marine *Vibrio*,[37] and demonstrates clearly that *V. cholerae* 01 (CT$^+$) possesses a well-regulated set of starvation responses.

As suggested by Colwell *et al.*,[9] however, taking into account annual distribution, *V. cholerae* demonstrates seasonality, observable using fluorescent antibody for detection and enumeration, as reported by Huq *et al.*[11] Seasonality, coupled with the starvation response and dormancy phenomena, reflects the origin of *V. cholerae* as an autochthonous estuary dweller.

The capacity of *V. cholerae* to undergo starvation response makes it clear that long-term survival of this organism in the culturable state in the environment as viable cells, perhaps for years, must be considered a source of the organism in cholera epidemics. But if, in addition to nutrient depletion, the cells are subjected to reduction in temperature and/or elevation in salinity, the cells rapidly go nonculturable, but remain viable and potentially pathogenic, as demonstrated by Colwell *et al.*,[64] who employed rabbit loop assays to recover viable but not culturable *V. cholerae* exposed to cold, full-strength seawater.

Thus, viable but nonculturable cells are not detected by standard plating methods currently employed in bacteriological laboratories. In fact, viable but nonculturable cells will not form colonies on agar media or grow in broth culture, a response to nutritional deprivation similar to that reported for *E. coli*,[25] *C. jejuni*,[44] *S. enteritidis*,[43] and other gram-negative and gram-positive bacteria.[45] The starvation response, leading to formation of small coccoid cells may be a preliminary step in the induction of the viable but nonculturable state in *V. cholerae*. The latter requires reconsideration of the role of the environment, with respect to transmission of disease in the future, not just for cholera, but for many bacterial enteric pathogens.

4. PHYSIOLOGY OF *V. CHOLERAE* IN THE AQUATIC ENVIRONMENT

Colwell and associates[9,65–69] first hypothesized that *V. cholerae* 01 (CT$^+$) is an estuarine and brackish water bacterium, demonstrating characteristics primarily of environmental advantage but, possibly, also accidentally causing diarrheal disease in humans.

Physiological characteristics studied, which are significant determinants in the ecology of *V. cholerae*, were: salinity and temperature relationships; adherence to surfaces; chitinolytic capability; and colonization of macrobiota possessing structures composed of chitin, e.g., crustacea. More important is the fact that the life cycle of free-living *V. cholerae* in natural estuarine waters and in laboratory microcosms simulating the environment show both *V. cholerae* 01 (CT$^+$) and *V. cholerae* non-01 to behave similarly under these ecological conditions.

4.1. Temperature and Salinity Relationships

The isolation of both *V. cholerae* 01 and non-01 from natural water sources and the suggestion that this species may be autochthonous to the brackish and estuarine aquatic ecosystems was noted in very early studies reported from the Indian subcontinent (see

Pollitzer[13]). However, the close relationship of *V. cholerae* non-01, which is easily isolated from environmental sources, and *V. cholerae* 01 (CT$^+$) was not appreciated until the 1970s when Citarella and Colwell[5] showed that by numerical taxonomy and by DNA/DNA hybridization,[65] *V. cholerae* non-01 were the same species. Later, Craig *et al.*[70] demonstrated that strains of *V. cholerae* non-01 isolated from the environment can also produce toxin which is biologically and immunologically indistinguishable from choleragen produced by *V. cholerae* 01 serovar. Subsequent analyses of 5SrRNA sequencing by MacDonell and Colwell[3] confirmed species relationships of 01 and non-01 *V. cholerae*. In fact, the conclusion was drawn in pre-1970 studies that the ecology of *V. cholerae* non-01 had no significant implication for the epidemiology of cholera, an unfortunate perspective of studies on the ecology of *V. cholerae* since it was tenaciously adopted by clinical personnel with no experience in microbial ecology but influential in shaping the dogma of the time.

Following demonstration of the taxonomic relatedness of *V. cholerae* 01 and non-01 strains[5,65] at the species level, Colwell and colleagues reported the isolation of *V. cholerae* 01 and non-01 from the Chesapeake Bay and other natural environments.[66] They described the ecology of *V. cholerae* 01 in Chesapeake Bay on the north–central Atlantic coast of the United States.[66] They later added information from a major study on the ecology of *V. cholerae*[67] and reported the isolation of nontoxigenic *V. cholerae* 01 (Inaba) from Chesapeake Bay[67] and bayous in the Gulf state of Louisiana.[69] In results of analyses of water samples collected along transects in Chesapeake Bay, salinity and fecal pollution gradients were studied, with the conclusion that there was no correlation between *V. cholerae* counts and counts of total heterotrophic bacteria, coliforms, or fecal coliforms. This finding was in contrast to a clear, positive correlation of *Salmonellae* counts with pollution indicators.

Isolation of *V. cholerae* from the natural aquatic environment, however, was patchy and the concentration of cells, determined by culture methods for detection, was low (the highest count being 46/liter), with more frequent isolations occurring in the summer months. A linear correlation with salinity was observed, with greater frequency of isolations at sites of salinities between 0.2–2.0 0/00. The effect of temperature was more strongly correlated; isolations were more frequent and readily obtained when the water temperature was greater than 17°C. From these data, Colwell *et al.*[69] concluded that *V. cholerae* is autochthonous in brackish water and estuarine environments.

This finding was subsequently confirmed by Hood and co-workers[71] who reported strong linear correlations between *V. cholerae* non-01 and temperature and salinity in two estuaries in Florida. *V. cholerae* non-01 was detected in highest numbers in water samples with salinities between 1.0–2.5 0/00, with a calculated optimum at 1.8% and temperatures between 20°C–35°C. In addition to being able to isolate *V. cholerae* non-01 from 50% of water samples examined, they detected the organism in 45% of oyster, 30% of sediment, and 75% of blue crab samples collected at the same sites as the water samples. Nontoxigenic *V. cholerae* 01 was isolated only once during these studies. It is important to point out that only cultural methods were employed until 1982 when the fluorescent antibody method was developed by Xu *et al.*[25] and subsequently employed for enumeration of *V. cholerae* in the environment by Brayton and Colwell[26] and Huq *et al.*[11]

A significant number of reports of the isolation of *V. cholerae* non-01 and nontoxigenic *V. cholerae* 01 from fresh and saline waters,[67–69,71–76] as well as an extensive computer-assisted statistical analysis of data on the isolation of *V. cholerae* from four U.S. coastal areas,[77] supported the conclusion that environmental parameters heavily influence the distribution of *V. cholerae* in brackish and estuarine waters.

The constantly changing conditions in tidal estuaries suggest an association of the ability of *V. cholerae* to adapt to a wide range of saline and temperature conditions and its natural ecological habitat.

To refine the understanding of salinity and temperature relationships for *V. cholerae*, laboratory microcosms, which simulate environmental conditions and can be controlled and replicated, were employed. This approach also provided the advantage of being able to measure quantitatively the effects of temperature and salinity on *V. cholerae* 01 (CT[+]), as well as effects of other environmental parameters on pathogenic properties. *V. cholerae* 01 (CT[+]), in uncontaminated natural waters, are not consistently detectable by culture methods, as described above. In fact, detection, enumeration, and monitoring *V. cholerae* in the environment is of little value except at times of cholera outbreak and when done in tandem with fluorescent antibody direct staining. This approach has proven more effective for samples collected from the natural environment.[11]

The first extensive studies of salinity and temperature relationships using microcosms were reported by Singleton *et al.*,[27,78] using *V. cholerae* 01 (CT[+]) strain LA4808, isolated from the 1978 El Tor cholera outbreak in Louisiana, and nine other clinical or environmental strains, including both non-01 and non-*V. cholerae* 01 (CT[+]). The number of bacterial cells in the microcosms, over time, were calculated from viable plate and AODC microscopic counts using samples taken from microcosms prepared with a chemically defined sea salts solution in which the salinity, organic nutrient concentration, or temperature was varied.

An optimum salinity of 2.5% for growth of *V. cholerae* was observed in all microcosms in which the organic nutrient concentration was less than 1.0 mg/liter, but salinity was less of a controlling factor when the nutrient concentration was greater than 1.0 mg/liter, a finding significant in that highly eutrophic waters can mask salinity effects, including requirement for NaCl for growth. At 10°C, counts declined at all salinities above 0.5% to 3.5%. At 15°C, growth occurred at salinities of 1.5% and 2.5%, but not outside that range. Comparative trials between strains showed no significant difference between clinical and environmental isolates in salinity/temperature relationships.

Specific uptake (per culturable cell) of [^{14}C] amino acids by *V. cholerae* grown in media of different salinities was greater at the extremes, compared to 1.5%–2.5%, suggesting that cells were metabolically more active at lower or higher salinity concentrations. The saline optimum, midway between fresh water and full-strength sea water provides additional evidence that *V. cholerae* is, in fact, an estuarine bacterium, as concluded by Singleton *et al.*[27,78] The salt-sparing effect of organic nutrients suggests at least one mechanism whereby the organism can survive in fresh water, including drinking water, namely by colonizing a niche sufficiently rich in nutrients or by attaching to surfaces and concentrating nutrients at the surface.

Following the initial studies by Singleton *et al.*,[27,78] survival and growth of *V. cholerae* under various conditions of salinity, pH, temperature, and presence of cations was reported by Miller *et al.*[79] A total of 59 strains, representing a variety of biotypes, were examined, using viable plate counts on trypticase soy agar. Six *V. cholerae* 01 (CT[+]) isolates were extensively studied. The results were similar to those of Singleton *et al.*,[27,78] presenting, again, a definitive picture of the importance of salinity as a factor in the distribution of *V. cholerae* in the environment. Survival of *V. cholerae* in sea salt solutions, without nutrient and incubated at 25°C, was at least 70 days. The optimal salt concentration for survival was 2.0%, but initial growth and long-term survival (72 days) occurred in microcosms of the salinity range 0.25%–3.0% NaCl.

Strains of *V. cholerae* varied greatly in survival in the culturable state under conditions of low salinity (0.05%), a result that was unrelated to serotype, i.e., whether 01 or non-01, source (clinical or environmental), or country of origin (Tanzania or Bangladesh). Variation among strains was less at optimal salinity and 18 of the 20 strains tested remained viable for more than 40 months at 25°C.

An elegant differentiation between a specific requirement for Na^+ and osmotic effect of Na^+ was shown by Singleton et al.[27,78] Results of a series of cation substitution experiments showed very clearly that at low salinities, osmolarity, rather than $[Na^+]$, is the dominant factor influencing growth and survival. However, the response of V. cholerae to different sodium concentrations, in a modified M9 minimal medium with NH_4Cl as the sole nitrogen source and 800 mg glucose/liter, pH 8.0), showed that the salinity-sparing effect of nutrients, reported by Singleton et al.,[27,78] has a lower limit, even at very high levels of organic nutrient. Growth was linearly correlated with Na^+ concentration at levels below 0.5% and an absolute requirement for Na^+ growth, i.e., more than 0.0001% but less than 0.0005%, was demonstrated.

Results of in situ studies have demonstrated that V. cholerae comprises the normal flora in many aquatic environments, with presence of V. cholerae strongly influenced by salinity and temperature. Parallel laboratory microcosm studies showed that the strict requirement for Na^+ is not limiting in natural waters, but that salinity, as the key determinant of osmolarity, normally would restrict the distribution of V. cholerae to water of more than potable salinity. Results provided by Colwell et al. and her associates[64-68] also suggest that actual growth of V. cholerae in the environment will be limited to waters with temperatures greater than 10°C. Survival through cold seasons, however, depends on the capacity of the organism to enter a dormant state, as discussed above.

Results of studies accomplished to date demonstrate the close similarity of salinity/temperature relationships between clinical V. cholerae 01 (CT$^+$) and environmental V. cholerae non-01 or 01 both (CT$^+$) and (CT$^-$). The data suggest that V. cholerae 01 (CT$^+$) is, indeed, part of the normal flora of many, if not all, aquatic environments. It is useful, as a corollary, to consider the effect of salinity and related physico-chemical parameters on production of enterotoxin by V. cholerae 01 (CT$^+$).

Tamplin and Colwell[81] demonstrated that toxin production in microcosm cultures was related to salinity, demonstrating a salinity optimum between 2.0%–2.5% for toxin production that was independent of cell concentration and toxin stability. Results of a study reported by Miller et al.[80] showed that cells do not lose enterotoxigenicity after long-term exposure (64 days) in microcosms under a variety of conditions, nor did a selection for either hyper- or hypotoxigenic mutants occur. Clearly, CT$^+$ strains do not dramatically alter their toxigenic character in the aquatic environment.

4.2. Adherence to Surfaces

For an individual microbial cell, survival is often not so much a function of macrohabitat, that is, whether the intestine or an estuary, as of microhabitat, namely, the immediate vicinity of cells, often measurable in square micrometers, of one or a cluster of cells. Interfaces are significant physical features in most macrohabitats and can have a profound effect on the ecology of indigenous microorganisms.[82] The ecology of V. cholerae in aquatic environments can be influenced significantly by ability of the cells to associate with specific surfaces and to create, thereby, a more favorable microenvironment.

Of great interest is the adherence of V. cholerae to chitin,[83] a semitransparent material, predominantly mucopolysaccharide, which is the principal component of crustacean shells.

Nalin *et al.*,[84] following on findings reported by Kaneko and Colwell[85–87] for *V. parahaemolyticus*, found that *V. cholerae* suspended in a 4.2% salt solution at pH 6.2 and 20°C adhered strongly to particles of powdered crabshell added to the suspension. After 6 h in an incubator–shaker, sedimentation of the chitinous particles was found to remove approximately 70% of the platable cells. The chitin-absorbed *V. cholerae* were subsequently able to survive immersion for 13 min in a dilute HCl solution at pH 1.6–1.8, suggesting that such adherent organisms might be able to pass the gastric acid barrier in humans ingesting *V. cholerae* adhered to crustacean shell. All biotypes of *V. cholerae* had been shown by Colwell in taxonomic studies done in 1970 to produce chitinase[65] and both Colwell[65] and Nalin *et al.*[84] were able to demonstrate growth of *V. cholerae* 01 (CT+) in media with chitin as the sole carbon source.

These findings suggest that *V. cholerae*, indeed, resembles *V. parahaemolyticus*,[85–87] with a life cycle alternatively involving colonization of chitinaceous planktonic crustacea during times of plankton blooms and survival in sediment between blooms, such as the winter in temperate climates or the monsoon season in Bangladesh. Evidence for a life cycle of this type for *V. cholerae* 01 was provided by Huq *et al.*,[11] using the direct detection method employing monoclonal antibody.

Adherence of *V. cholerae* to chitin appears to be specific and, to some extent, the polar flagellum may play a role in mediating adherence. Belas and Colwell[88] showed that adsorption of polarly flagellated vibrios, such as *V. cholerae*, tended to follow proportional saturation kinetics, rather than the Langmuir adsorption kinetics evidenced by *V. parahaemolyticus* when cells were grown under conditions favoring production of lateral flagella by *V. parahaemolyticus*. The binding index (product of number of binding sites and bacterial affinity to the surface) was also significantly different between the two groups, suggesting that they bind to chitin by different mechanisms.

MacDonell and Hood[39] reported an effect of nutrient deprivation on adherence of *V. cholerae*, depending on whether the surface involved was inert material, such as $CaCO_3$ and glass, or if it was chitinaceous. Nutrient-enriched cells of the *V. cholerae* strain adhered at high rates to both $CaCO_3$ (50% of culturable cells) and chitin (42%). However, there was virtually no adherence when chitin was added to nutrient-deprived cells (produced by maintaining cells for 35 days in an unsupplemented marine salts solution, e.g., 2.0% salinity), while 53% of a parallel suspension of nutrient-deprived cells adhered to $CaCO_3$.

When nutrient-deprived cells not adhering to chitin were subsequently exposed to $CaCO_3$ particles, 55% adhered. When the sequence was reversed, however, 62% of cells adhered to the $CaCO_3$ added initially and none of the residual nonadherent cells adhered to the chitin added subsequently. It appears that changes in physiological state and morphology associated with nutrient deprivation and dormancy include alterations in the bacterial surface characteristics of the *V. cholerae* cells.

This phenomenon may be common to survival of bacteria in natural, low-nutrient aquatic environments. Starvation-induced changes in bacterial surface topography and hydrophobicity, electrostatic interaction, and irreversible binding to glass surfaces have been reported for several strains of marine bacteria by Kjelleberg and Hermansson.[89] In *V. cholerae*, there appears to be a predilection for association with inert particles over chitinaceous surfaces, which might be interpreted as an ecological advantage. For example, enhanced attachment to inert suspended matter can provide a mechanism for transport of the bacteria to sediment during periods of nutrient-depletion in the overlying water column. In the sediment, cells would be in close contact with more nutrient than in the water column, hence better able to survive and reproduce for extended periods of time.[58]

A few examples of adherence to nonchitinaceous surfaces described for *V. cholerae* include adherence to roots of water hyacinth by *V. cholerae* 01 (CT[+]) in fresh water in cholera-endemic areas, an association that appears to confer some measure of protection to *V. cholerae*.[90] A report by Daniel and Lloyd[91] showed that trickling filters installed to treat sewage effluent from Oxfam Sanitation Units became colonized by *V. cholerae* non-01 in very high numbers. The vibrios appeared to compete successfully for a niche on the solid matrix of the filters and to grow rapidly by more efficient access to nutrients in the constant flow of sewage through the system.

4.3. Colonization of Macrobiota with Chitinaceous Exoskeletons

The role of zooplankton, specifically copepods, in the survival and multiplication of *V. cholerae* in the aquatic environment is significant in the natural history of this species. Efforts to study this phenomenon clearly have as a model the life cycle elucidated for *V. parahaemolyticus* in Chesapeake Bay,[85–87] for which there is unambiguous evidence that the life cycle of the microorganisms is intimately linked with that of zooplankton blooms. *V. parahaemolyticus* associates with zooplankton during the summer months and is involved in mineralization and degradation of plankton following blooms of the latter, which occur in spring and fall months in Chesapeake Bay.

In situ evidence has been obtained showing association of *V. cholerae* with copepods in Chesapeake Bay, which demonstrates that *V. cholerae* non-01 can be isolated from plankton samples when water temperatures are greater than 17°C.[67,68] Comparable studies of viable but nonculturable *V. cholerae* 01, employing the fluorescent antibody method, need to be done. FA studies have shown that *V. cholerae* 01 can be observed in Chesapeake Bay water (Xu and Colwell, unpublished data), but a seasonal study employing several transects for sampling in Chesapeake Bay has not yet been done.

Data from laboratory microcosm studies by Huq *et al.*,[92] however, suggest strongly that *V. cholerae* of all types are capable of colonizing surfaces of copepods. The specific sites of attachment appear to be the oral region and the egg sac: the former probably being a reflection of the normal ingestion of bacteria as a food source and the latter suggesting a selective advantage for the *Vibrio*, since spawning of fertilized eggs thus affords an excellent vehicle for dissemination. It also has been hypothesized that *V. cholerae*, being proteolytic, may play a role in the life cycle of the copepod, since the eggs are dispersed into the water upon rupture of the egg sack.

Association with copepods appears to be a property associated with *V. cholerae*, *V. parahaemolyticus*, and other vibrios, but not necessarily a generalized characteristic of all aquatic bacteria. Kaneko and Colwell[85] suggested that the electrostatic charge of the epicuticle covering the copepod may be a factor limiting attachment. Huq *et al.*[93] found attachment and growth of copepod-associated *V. cholerae* 01 (CT[+]) to be optimum in microcosms with salinity (1.5%), pH (8.5), and temperatures (30°C), similar to conditions optimum for growth and survival of planktonic *V. cholerae* observed in earlier microcosm studies.

Huq *et al.*[94] have also reported attachment of *V. cholerae* 01 (CT[+]) to the hindgut of the blue crab (*Callinectes sapidus*). The hindgut in crustacea is an extension of the exoskeleton and is chitin-lined. The midgut, which does not contain a chitinaceous lining, did not support attachment of the vibrios. Hindgut-specific attachment was observed both in feeding experiments with live crabs and in experiments using excised guts suspended in saline and inoculated with bacterial cells, i.e., ligated crab loops.

The observation that there is specific attachment by vibrios in crabs has important implications for the epidemiology and transmission of cholera in the aquatic environment, since ingestion of shellfish is well established as a major risk factor for cholera in endemic areas. The hypothesis, first raised by Colwell et al.,[68] that V. cholerae in the crab may play a role in osmoregulation and, therefore, in the migration of crabs or other crustacea from the open ocean to the uppermost reaches of the Chesapeake Bay and vice versa, is based on the premise that V. cholerae produces cholera toxin or related toxins, such as tetrodotoxin, which act on the gut mucosa to increase Cl^- secretion and reduce Na^+ absorption. The production of tetrodotoxin by V. cholerae was shown by Tamplin et al.[95] Another hypothesis that has been proposed is that V. cholerae 01 (CT^+) is not as robust or prolific in the aquatic environment, since it has evolved in a different niche than other biotypes or serotypes of the species V. cholerae. In Bengal, the putative home of cholera, there has been massive, intimate human contact with water sources containing V. cholerae (as an autochthonous species) for many centuries. It seems obvious that such conditions are not unfavorable for selecting a mutant capable of utilizing the human intestinal tract as part of its life cycle without necessarily losing its ability to exist in the aquatic environment. This may be much less an intellectually attractive hypothesis than that of association with blooms of other components of the aquatic ecosystem. That is, blooms of zooplankton and/or phytoplankton, for example, may exert significant effects on the bacterial species composition. This hypothesis is under study by Huq, Colwell, and Russek-Cohen (unpublished data), who have gathered multi-year data on V. cholerae culturable, AODC, FA, and DVC counts, along with counts and taxonomic identification of plankton for several sites in Bangladesh. Seroconversion of 01 to non-01 and vice-versa also is not totally improbable, based on results obtained by Brayton and Colwell[8] (Proc. Proceedings of the International Union of Microbiological Societies Congress, Manchester, UK) and may occur in the environment. The most successfully adapted strain over time obviously can dominate a niche to the exclusion of other V. cholerae. At least two strain lines successfully compete for niches today: the classical and El Tor biotypes of V. cholerae 01 (CT^+).

A model, suggested by Miller et al.,[96] suggests marginal survival capabilities of V. cholerae in aquatic environments and an ability to maintain itself at very low levels in the autochthonous estuarine microbial population and is invoked to explain occurrences of cholera in both Bangladesh and the southeastern U.S. However, this suggestion does not take into account viable but nonculturable V. cholerae in the environment.

In Bangladesh, thousands of water samples can be analyzed without a single isolation of V. cholerae 01 (CT^+) in culture.[97] At the same time, millions of people, several times daily, ingest water directly from these water sources, creating a much greater "sampling" intensity that leads to a finite number of primary cases [i.e., arising from ingestion of autochthonous V. cholerae 01 (CT^+)]. From each of these derives a "burst" of numerous secondary cases, arising from the standard fecal–oral route of transmission, most of which appear to involve ingestion of fecally contaminated water.[97] The result is thousands of cases of cholera each year.

In Louisiana, on the other hand, where secondary transmission is unlikely, millions of meals of fresh shellfish are consumed each year, many of them not cooked well enough to kill vibrios, leading to one or two isolated cases of cholera. These have been of the same epitype of V. cholerae 01 (CT^+) biotype El Tor that has existed, apparently autochthonously, in the Gulf region since it was first isolated in 1978.[98,99]

The seasonality of cholera in Bengal may also be explained by the model in that primary transmission would be controlled by environmental factors such as temperature, salinity, nutrient concentration, and zooplankton blooms; as well as by seasonal variations in seafood harvesting and consumption, and in direct water contact.[101]

Using this as the context, Miller et al.[102] reviewed historical data to produce graphs showing a coincidence between cholera seasons in Calcutta (1956–1958) and London (1893–1894) and seasonal increases in the salinity of the Hooghly (premonsoon season) and Thames rivers, respectively. They also pointed out that since V. cholerae 01 (CT[+]) is best maintained in water too saline to be potable, based on the work of Singleton et al.[27,78] and Miller et al.,[102] ingestion of contaminated shellfish and other seafood may be the most important mode of transmission.

On the other hand, Colwell et al.[103] and Tamplin et al.[104] have demonstrated a significant role of plankton, based on the work of Huq et al.,[11] who showed that culturability of V. cholerae was associated with living copepods, one component of the plankton population, i.e., an active, dynamic association of V. cholerae with components of the plankton community. At least 10^4–10^5 V. cholerae may attach to a single copepod. If there is, in fact, a bloom of copepods, for example, the total number of V. cholerae in a given volume of water can rise by several orders of magnitude, well within the number for an infective dose.

Tamplin et al.[104] showed attachment of V. cholerae to components of plankton, other than copepods, e.g., Volvox. Work in progress (Huq, Colwell, and Russek-Cohen, unpublished data) is examining the linkage(s) between V. cholerae and members of the plankton community.

Association of V. cholerae with shellfish, notably crustaceans, has been well documented. Association with vertebrate fish should prove interesting, as well, in light of cholera outbreaks in Peru and Ecuador in 1991, which have been traced to seafood.

In rural Bangladesh, the peak cholera season is after the summer monsoon, varying from September to December. This is not the season of peak salinity (which is premonsoon), but is a period associated with a heavy bloom of zooplankton,[101] maximum recreational contact with water, and maximum availability of crustacea in the marketplace. Primary transmission of the type indicated here would be expected to produce scattered, localized outbreaks with no link between them. As Chapter 3 of this book makes abundantly clear, this is exactly what happens in Bangladesh.

The demonstrated epidemiological patterns in endemic areas fit well a model of primary transmission from autochthonous aquatic V. cholerae 01 (CT[+]). What remains is to establish unequivocally that an environmental reservoir does indeed exist by determining the year-round presence of V. cholerae 01 (CT[+]) in the environmental niche(s) of brackish ponds and canals of Bangladesh, the bayous of Louisiana, and similar geographical locations throughout the world where cholera is either endemic or sporadic. A multi-year study that was undertaken in Bangladesh has just been completed and the data are now being analyzed. A number of questions are expected to be answered by this study (Colwell, Huq, and Russek-Cohen, unpublished data).

5. V. CHOLERAE ECOLOGY AND ITS IMPLICATIONS FOR CHOLERA EPIDEMIOLOGY

This subject is covered in Chapter 3, but our discussion of the ecology of V. cholerae is concluded by suggesting some of the broader implications raised with better understanding of cholera endemicity, seasonality, and control.

It is now quite clear that V. cholerae 01 (CT[+]) shares many characteristics with V.

cholerae 01 (CT$^-$) and non-01 that stem from evolution of the species *V. cholerae* as an autochthonous estuarine microorganism. Possession of characteristics demonstrated by *V. cholerae* discussed above provide the organism with the ability not only to exist permanently in the natural aquatic environment, but to perform its appropriate functions as an auto-chthonous species of brackish water, estuaries, and coastal waters. In temperature/salinity relationships, adherence to surfaces, colonization of chitinaceous macrobiota, the dorman-cy/dwarfing response to nutrient deprivation, and the viable but nonculturable phenomenon, no significant difference between *V. cholerae* 01 (CT$^+$) and the other members of the species *V. cholerae* has been detected.

Therefore, while the syllogism is not perfect, the argument by analogy is that *V. cholerae* 01 (CT$^+$) exists permanently, i.e., autochthonously, in the estuarine environment.

ACKNOWLEDGMENTS. The work reported here from the laboratory of R.R. Colwell was supported, in part, by NIH Grant No. 5ROIAI14242-09, NSF Grant No. BSR-8806509, and Environmental Protection Agency Cooperative Agreement No. CR812246. The authors gratefully acknowledge Dr. Anwarul Huq for his careful review of the manuscript.

REFERENCES

1. Felsenfeld O: The survival of cholera vibrios, in Barua D, Burrows W (eds): *Cholera.* Philadelphia, W.B. Saunders, 1974, pp 359–366
2. Koch R: An address on cholera and its bacillus. *Br Med J* 2:403–407, 453–459, 1884
3. MacDonell MT, Colwell RR: Identical 5S rRNA nucleotide sequence of *Vibrio cholerae* strains representing temporal, geographical, and ecological diversity. *Appl Environ Microbiol* 48:119–121, 1984
4. MacDonell MT, Colwell RR: Nucleotide base sequence of vibrionaceae 5S rRNA. *FEMS Microbiol Lett* 175:183–188, 1984
5. Citarella RV, Colwell RR: Polyphasic taxonomy of the genus *Vibrio:* polynucleotide sequence relationships among selected *Vibrio species. J Bacteriol* 104:434–442, 1970
6. Hugh R, Feeley JC: Report (1966–1970) of the subcommittee on taxonomy of vibrios to the International Committee on Nomenclature of Bacteria. *Int J Sys Bacteriol* 22:123, 1972
7. West PA, Colwell RR: Identification and classification of Vibrionaceae—An Overview, in Colwell RR (ed): *Vibrios in the Environment.* John Wlley and Sons, New York, 1984, pp 285–363
8. Colwell RR, Brayton P: Abstract, Proceedings of the International Union of Microbiology Societies Congress, Manchester, U K, 1986
9. Colwell RR, Brayton PR, Grimes DJ, Roszak DR, Huq SA, Palmer LM: Viable, but non-culturable *Vibrio cholerae* and related pathogens in the environment: implications for release of genetically engineered micro-organisms. *Bio/Technology* 3:817–820, 1985
10. Colwell RR, Kaper J, Joseph SW: *Vibrio cholerae, Vibrio parahaemolyticus* and other Vibrios: Occurrence and distribution in Chesapeake Bay. *Science* 198:394–396, 1977
11. Huq A, Colwell RR, Rahman R, Ali A, Chowdhury MAR, Parveen S, Sack DA, Russek-Cohen E: Detection of *Vibrio cholerae* 01 in the aquatic environment by fluorescent-monoclonal antibody and culture methods. *Appl Environ Microbiol* 56:2370–2373, 1990
12. Roszak DB, Grimes DJ, Colwell RR: Viable but nonrecoverable stage of *Salmonella enteritidis* in aquatic systems. *Can J Microbiol* 30:334–338, 1984
13. Pollitzer R: *Cholera,* Monograph No. 43. Geneva, World Health Organization, 1959
14. Feacham R, Miller C, Drasar B: Environmental aspects of cholera epidemiology. II. Occurrence and survival of *Vibrio cholerae* in the environment. *Trop Dis Bull* 78:865–880, 1981
15. Finkelstein RA: Cholera. *Crit Rev Microbiol* 2:553–623, 1973
16. Litsky W: Gut critters are stressed in the environment, more stressed by isolation procedures, in Colwell RR, Foster J, (eds): *Aquatic Microbial Ecology.* Proceedings of the Conference Sponsored by the American Society for Microbiology. Maryland Sea Grant Publication UM-SG-TS-80-03. University of Maryland, College Park, MD, 1979, pp 345–347
17. Grieg EDW: On the vitality of the cholera vibrio outside the human body. *Indian J Med Res* 1:481–504, 1914

18. Forbes GI, Lockhart JDF, Bowman RK: Cholera and nightsoil infection in Hong Kong, 1966. *Bull. WHO* 36:367–373, 1967

19. Sinha R, Deb BC, De SP, Abou-Gareeb AH, Shrivastava DL: Cholera carrier studies in Calcutta in 1966–67. *Bull. WHO* 37:89–100, 1967

20. Pesigan TP, Plantilla J, Rolda M: Applied studies on the viability of El Tor vibrios. *Bull. WHO* 37:779–786, 1967

21. Gerichter CB, Sechter I, Gavish A, Cahan D: Viability of *Vibrio cholerae* El Tor and of cholera phage on vegetables. *Israeli J Med Sci* 11:889–895, 1975

22. Felsenfeld O: Notes on food, beverages, and fomites contaminated with *Vibrio cholerae*. *Bull. WHO* 33:725–734, 1965

23. Prescott LM, Bhattacharjee NK: Viability of El Tor vibrios in common foodstuffs found in an endemic cholera area. *Bull. WHO* 40:980–982, 1969

24. McCormack WM, Islam MS, Fahimuddin M, Mosley WH: Endemic cholera in rural East Pakistan. *Amer J Epid* 89:393–404, 1969

25. Xu H-S, Roberts N, Singleton FL, Attwell RW, Grimes DJ, Colwell RR: Survival and viability of non-culturable *Escherichia coli* and *Vibrio cholerae* in the estuarine and marine environment. *Microb Ecol* 8:313–323, 1982

26. Brayton PR, Colwell RR: Fluorescent antibody staining method for enumeration of viable environmental *Vibrio cholerae* 01. *J Microbial Meth* 6:309–314, 1987

27. Singleton FL, Attwell RW, Jangi MS, Colwell RR: Influence of salinity and nutrient concentration on survival and growth of *Vibrio cholerae* in aquatic microcosms. *Appl Environ Microbiol* 43:1080–1085, 1982

28. Novitsky JS, Morita RY: Morphological characterization of small cells resulting from nutrient starvation of a psychrophilic marine vibrio. *Appl Environ Microbiol* 32:617–622, 1976

29. Novitsky JS, Morita RY: Survival of a psychrophilic marine vibrio under long-term nutrient starvation. *Appl Environ Microbiol* 33:635–641, 1977

30. Novitsky JA, Morita RY: Possible strategy for the survival of marine bacteria under starvation conditions. *Mar Biol* 48:289–295, 1978

31. Jones KL, Rhodes-Roberts ME: The survival of marine bacteria under starvation conditions. *Appl Bacteriol* 50:247–258, 1981

32. Torrella F, Morita RY: Microcultural study of bacterial size changes and microcolony and ultramicrocolony formation by heterotrophic bacteria in seawater. *Appl Environ Microbiol* 41:518–527, 1981

33. Kjelleberg S, Humphrey BA, Marshall KC: Initial phases of starvation and activity of bacteria at surfaces. *Appl Environ Microbiol* 46:978–984, 1983

34. Amy PS, Morita RY: Protein patterns of growing and starved cells of a marine *Vibrio* sp. *Appl Environ Microbiol* 45:1748–1752, 1983

35. Amy PS, Pauling C, Morita RY: Starvation-survival processes of a marine vibrio. *Appl Environ Microbiol* 45:1685–1690, 1983

36. Amy PS, Pauling C, Morita RY: Recovery from nutrient starvation by a marine *Vibrio* sp. *Appl Environ Microbiol* 46:930–940, 1983

37. Oliver JD, Stringer WF: Lipid composition of a psychrophilic marine *Vibrio* sp. during starvation-induced morphogenesis. *Appl Environ Microbiol* 47:461–466, 1984

38. Schaechter M: Patterns of cellular control during unbalanced growth. *Cold Spring Harbor Symp Quant Biol* 26:53–62, 1961

39. MacDonell MT, Hood MA: Ultramicrovibrios in Gulf Coast estuarine waters: Isolation, characterization and incidence, in Colwell RR (ed): *Vibrios in the Environment.* New York, John Wiley and Sons, 1984, pp 551–562

40. Anderson JIW, Heffernan WP: Isolation and characterization of filterable marine bacteria. *J Bacteriol* 90:1713–1718, 1965.

41. Casida LW Jr: Small cells in pure cultures of *Agromyces ramosus* and in natural soil. *Can J Microbiol* 23:214–216, 1977

42. Boylen DW, Ensign JC: Long-term starvation survival of rod and spherical stage cells of *Arthrobacter crystallopoietes*. *J Bacteriol* 103:569–577, 1970

43. Roszak DB, Grimes DJ, Colwell RR: Viable but non-recoverable stage of *Salmonella enteritidis* in aquatic systems. *Can J Microbiol* 30:334–338, 1984

44. Rollins DM, Colwell RR: Viable but nonculturable stage of *Campylobacter jejuni* and its role in survival in the natural aquatic environment. *Appl Environ Microbiol* 52:531–538, 1986

45. Byrd J, Colwell RR: Maintenance of plasmids pBR322 and pUC8 in non-culturable *Escherichia coli* in the marine environment. *Appl Environ Microbiol* 56:2104–2107, 1990

46. Francisco DE, Mah RA, Rabin AC: Acridine orange epifluorescence technique for counting bacteria in natural waters. *Trans Am Microscop Soc* 92:416–421, 1973

47. Daley RJ, Hobbie JE: Direct counts of aquatic bacteria by a modified epi-fluorescent technique. *Limnol Oceanogr* 20:875–882, 1975

48. Floodgate GD: The assessment of marine microbial biomass and activity, in Colwell RR, Foster J, (eds.): *Aquatic Microbial Ecology.* Proceedings of the Conference Sponsored by the American Society for Microbiology. Maryland Sea Grant Publication UM-SG-TS-80-03. University of Maryland, College Park, MD, 1979, pp 217–252

49. Korgaonkar KS, Ranade SS: Evaluation of acridine orange fluorescence test in inability studies on *Escherichia coli. Can J Microbiol* 12:185–190, 1966

50. Kogure K, Simidu U, Taga N: A tentative direct microscopic method for counting living marine bacteria. *Can J Microbiol* 25:415–420, 1979

51. Kosinski RJ, Singleton FL, Foster BG: Sampling culturable heterotrophs from microcosms: a statistical analysis. *Appl Environ Microbiol* 38:906–910, 1979

52. Postgate JR: Death in macrobes and microbes. *Symp Soc Gen Microbiol* 26:1–18, 1967

53. Chan K: Responses of marine bacteria to nutrient addition and secondary heat stress in relation to starvation. *Microbios Lett* 6:137–144, 1977

54. Stevenson LH: A case for bacterial dormancy in aquatic systems. *Microb Ecol* 4:127–133, 1978

55. Singleton FL, Colwell RR: Use of microcosm to determine the effects of environmental parameters on growth of *Vibrio cholerae.* 1981 Abs. 81st Annual Meeting of Amer Soc Microbiol

56. Felter RA, Colwell RR, Chapman GB: Morphology and round body formation of *Vibrio marinus. J Bacteriol* 99:326–335, 1969

57. Nicholls KM, Lee JV, Donovan TJ: An evaluation of commercial thiosulphate citrate–bile–salt sucrose agar. *J Appl Bacteriol* 41:265–269, 1976

58. Hood MA, Ness GE: Survival of *Vibrio cholerae* and *Exherichia coli* in estuarine waters and sediments. *Appl Environ Microbiol* 43:678–584, 1982

59. Baker RM, Singleton FL, Hood MA: Effects of nutrient deprivation on *Vibrio cholerae. Appl Environ Microbiol* 46:930–940, 1983

60. Kennedy SF, Colwell RR, Chapman GB: Ultra-structure of a psychrophilic marine vibrio. *Can J Microbiol* 16:1027–1032, 1970

61. Amy PS, Morita RY: Starvation-survival patterns of sixteen freshly isolated open-ocean bacteria. *Appl Environ Microbiol* 45:1109–1115, 1983

62. Hood MA, Guckert JB, White DC, Deck F: Effect of nutrient deprivation on lipid, carbohydrate, DNA, RNA, and protein levels in *Vibrio cholerae. Appl Environ Microbiol* 52:788–793, 1986

63. Guckert JB, Hood MA, White DC: Phospholipid ester-linked fatty acid profile changes during nutrient deprivation of *Vibrio cholerae:* Increases in the *trans/cis* ratio and proportions of cyclopropyl fatty acids. *Appl Environ Microbiol* 52:794–801, 1986

64. Colwell RR, Brayton PR, Grimes DJ, Roszak DR, Huq SA, Palmer LM: Viable, but non-culturable *Vibrio cholerae* and related pathogens in the environment: implications for release of genetically engineered microorganisms. *Bio/Technology* 3:817–820, 1985

65. Colwell RR: Polyphasic taxonomy of the genus *Vibrio:* numerical taxonomy of *Vibrio cholerae, Vibrio parahaemolyticus,* and related *Vibrio* species. *J Bacteriol* 104:410–433, 1970

66. Colwell RR, Kaper J, Joseph SW: *Vibrio cholerae, Vibrio parahaemolyticus,* and other vibrios: occurrence and distribution in Chesapeake Bay. *Science* 198:394–396, 1977

67. Kaper JB, Lockman H, Colwell RR, Joseph SW: Ecology, serology, and enterotoxin production of *Vibrio cholerae* in Chesapeake Bay. *Appl Environ Microbiol* 37:91–103, 1979

68. Colwell RR, West PA, Maneval D, Remmers EF, Elliott EL, Carlson NE: Ecology of pathogenic *Vibrios* in Chesapeake Bay, in Colwell RR (ed.): *Vibrios in the Environment.* New York, John Wiley and Sons, 1984, pp 367–387

69. Colwell RR, Seidler R, Kaper J, Joseph S, Garges S, Lockman H, Maneval D, Bradford H, Roberts N, Remmers E, Huq I, Huq A: Occurrence of *Vibrio cholerae* 0-group 1 in Maryland and Louisiana estuaries. *Appl Environ Microbiol* 41:555–558, 1981

70. Craig JP, Yamamoto K, Takeda Y, Miwatani T: Production of cholera-like enterotoxin by a *Vibrio cholerae* non-01 strain isolated from environment. *Infect Immun* 34:90–97, 1981

71. Hood MA, Ness GE, Rodrick GE, Blake NJ: Distribution of *Vibrio cholerae* in two Florida estuaries. *Microb Ecol* 9:65–75, 1983

72. Hood MA, Ness GE, Rodrick GE, Blake NJ: The ecology of *Vibrio cholerae* in two Florida estuaries, in Colwell RR (ed.): *Vibrios in the Environment*. New York, John Wiley and Sons, 1984, pp 399–409

73. Bashford DJ, Donovan TJ, Furniss AL, Lee JV: *Vibrio cholerae* in Kent. *Lancet* i:436–437, 1979

74. West PA, Lee JV: Ecology of *Vibrio* species, including *Vibrio cholerae*, in natural waters of Kent, England. *J Appl Microbiol* 52:435–448, 1982

75. W.H.O. Scientific Working Group: Cholera and other vibrio-associated diarrhoeas. *Bull WHO* 58:353–374, 1980

76. Kenyon JE, Gillies DC, Peixoto DR, Austin B: *Vibrio cholerae* (non-01) isolated from California coastal waters. *Appl Environ Microbiol* 46:1232–1233, 1983

77. Seidler RJ, Evans TM: Computer-assisted analysis of *Vibrio* field data: four coastal areas, in Colwell RR (ed.): *Vibrios in the Environment*. New York, John Wiley and Sons, 1984, pp 411–425

78. Singleton FL, Atwell RW, Jangi MS, Colwell RR: Effects of temperature and salinity on *Vibrio cholerae* growth. *Appl Environ Microbiol* 44:1047–1058, 1984

79. Miller CJ, Drasar BS, Feacham RG: Response of toxigenic *Vibrio cholerae* 01 to physico-chemical stresses in aquatic environments. *J Hyg Camb* 93:475–495, 1984

80. Miller CJ, Drasar BS, Feacham RG, Hayes RJ: The impact of physico-chemico stress on the toxigenicity of *Vibrio cholerae*. *J Hyg Camb* 96:49–57, 1986

81. Tamplin ML, Colwell RR: Effects of microcosm salinity and organic substrate concentration on production of *Vibrio cholerae* enterotoxin. *Appl Environ Microbiol* 52:297–301, 1986

82. Marshall KC: *Interfaces in Microbial Ecology*. Cambridge, MA, Harvard University Press, 1976

83. Dastidar SG, Nayaranaswami A: The occurrence of chitinase in vibrios. *Indian J Med Res* 56:654–658, 1968

84. Nalin D, Daya V, Reid A, Levine MM, Cisneros L: Adsorption and growth of *Vibrio cholerae* on chitin. *Infect Immun* 25:768–770, 1979

85. Kaneko T, Colwell RR: Ecology of *Vibrio parahaemolyticus* in Chesapeake Bay. *J Bacteriol* 113:24–32, 1973

86. Kaneko T, Colwell RR: Adsorption of *Vibrio parahaemolyticus* onto chitin and copepods. *Appl Microbiol* 29:269–274, 1975

87. Kaneko T, Colwell RR: The annual cycle of *Vibrio parahaemolyticus* in Chesapeake Bay. *Microb Ecol* 4:135–155, 1978

88. Belas MR, Colwell RR: Adsorption kinetics of laterally and polarly flagellated *Vibrio*. *J Bacteriol* 151:1568–1580, 1982

89. Kjelleberg S, Hermansson M: Starvation-induced effects on bacterial surface characteristics. *Appl Environ Microbiol* 48:497–503, 1984

90. Spira WM, Huq A, Ahmed QS, Saeed YA: Uptake of *Vibrio cholerae* biotype El Tor from contaminated water by water hyacinth (*Eichornia crassipes*). *Appl Environ Microbiol* 42:550–553, 1981

91. Daniel RR, Lloyd BJ: A note on the fate of El Tor cholera and other vibrios in percolating filters. *J Appl Bacteriol* 48:207–210, 1980

92. Huq A, Small EB, West PA, Huq MI, Rahman R, Colwell RR: Ecological relationships between *Vibrio cholerae* and planktonic crustacean copepods. *Appl Environ Microbiol* 45:275–283, 1983

93. Huq A, West PA, Small EB, Huq MI, Colwell RR: Influence of water temperature, salinity, and pH on survival and growth of toxigenic *Vibrio cholerae* serovar 01 associated with live copepods in laboratory microcosms. *Appl Environ Microbiol* 48:420–424, 1984

94. Huq A, Huq SA, Grimes DJ, O'Brien M, Chu KH, McDowell Capuzzo J, Colwell RR: Colonization of the gut of the blue crab (*Callinectes sapidus*) by *Vibrio cholerae*. *Appl Environ Microbiol* 52:586–588, 1986

95. Tamplin ML, Colwell RR, Hall S, Kogure K, Strichartz GS: Sodium-channel inhibitors produced by entero-pathogenic *Vibrio cholerae* and *Aeromonas hydrophila*. *Lancet* 1:975, 1987

96. Miller CJ, Feacham RG, Drasar BS: Cholera epidemiology in developed and developing countries: New thoughts on transmission, seasonality, and control. *Lancet* i:261–263, 1985

97. Spira WM, Daniel RR: Biotype clusters formed on the basis of virulence characteristics in non-0 group 1 *Vibrio cholerae*, in *Proceedings of the Fifteenth Joint Conference on Cholera, US–Japan, July 23–25, 1979*. NIH Publication No. 80-2003, Bethesda, MD, National Institutes of Health, 1980, pp 440–454

98. Kaper JB, Moseley SL, Falkow S: Molecular characterization of environmental and non-toxigenic strains of *Vibrio cholerae*. *Infect Immun* 32:661–667, 1981

99. Kaper JB, Bradford HB, Roberts NC, Falkow S: Molecular epidemiology of *Vibrio cholerae* in the U.S. Gulf coast. *J Clin Microbiol* 16:129–134, 1982

100. Spira WM, Khan MU, Saeed YA, Sattar MA: Microbiological surveillance of intra-neighborhood El Tor cholera transmission in rural Bangladesh. *Bull WHO* 58:731–740, 1980

101. Oppenheimer JR, Ahmad MG, Huq A, Haque KA, Alim AKMA, Aziz KMS, Ali S, Haque ASM: Limnological studies of three ponds in Dacca, Bangladesh. *Bangladesh J Fisheries* 1:1–28, 1978

102. Miller, CJ, Drasar BS, Feacham RG: Cholera and estuarine salinity in Calcutta and London. *Lancet* i:1216–1218, 1982

103. Colwell RR, West PA, Maneval D, Remmers EF, Elliot EL, Carlson NE: Ecology of pathogenic vibrios in Chesapeake Bay, in Colwell RR (ed.): *Vibrios in the Environment*. New York, John Wiley and Sons, 1984, pp 367–387

104. Tamplin ML, Gauzens AL, Huq A, Sack DA, Colwell RR: Attachment of *Vibrio cholerae* Serogroup 01 to zooplankton and phytoplankton of Bangladesh waters. *Appl Environ Microbiol* 56:1977–1980, 1990

7

The Epidemiology of Cholera

Roger I. Glass and Robert E. Black

1. INTRODUCTION

1.1. Epidemiologic Lessons from the Early Pandemics and Epidemics

Since the first pandemic of cholera in 1817 spread through the Middle East to Europe, cholera has been among the most feared of the classic epidemic diseases.[1] Cholera was highly virulent, decimating entire communities within weeks of its introduction. The disease had a high case–fatality ratio that approached 50% in some areas and spread relentlessly in worldwide pandemics from endemic foci in Asia to the Middle East, Europe, East Africa, and the Americas. While cholera epidemics have been extensively described and studied, epidemiologic understanding of the transmission of V. cholerae 01 is still too inadequate to permit effective control measures that would contain the disease and prevent its emergence and spread.[2] Proper and timely rehydration therapy can reduce mortality to less than 1%, and antibiotic treatment can decrease shedding of vibrios, but neither of these treatment measures has significantly altered the spread of disease.

Public health measures to control the spread of cholera have been based, until recently, on epidemiologic insights drawn from observations made in the nineteenth century. Preventive measures included the provision of good, safe drinking water, proper disposal of human waste, education and attention to personal hygiene, the quarantine of goods and travelers from infected countries, and vaccination. These measures may be useful at times but have been inadequate to prevent the spread of cholera. These inadequacies underscore the need to understand the epidemiology of cholera more completely.

During the early pandemics, the spread of cholera from Asia to Europe followed the routes of travelers and merchants, which suggested that man was an important reservoir of infection. International spread of cholera by ships led to International Sanitary Conventions

Cholera, edited by Dhiman Barua and William B. Greenough III. Plenum Medical Book Company, New York, 1992.

and to the establishment of International Health Regulations including quarantine services to prevent the disembarkation of cargos and individuals in ports. These quarantine measures may have slowed the introduction of disease in some areas but they also caused much inconvenience and economic losses. They were mostly ineffective, perhaps because either many individuals were mild cases or asymptomatically infected or other modes of transmission were involved.

The fecal–oral route of transmission of cholera was identified by early pioneers working with cholera including John Snow[3] and Robert Koch.[4] Each recognized that some agent or poison in human feces was the etiologic cause of disease. Snow demonstrated that cholera was spread by drinking water that was contaminated with fecal wastes. Koch identified the cholera vibrio in intestinal contents of victims who died during outbreaks in Egypt and in India. Rudolph Emmerich, a student of Pettenkoffer, attempted to disprove the etiologic role of cholera vibrios by swallowing a pure culture of the organism. He came down with a severe case of cholera, thereby fulfilling Koch's postulates and confirming both the causative role of the organism and its oral route of inoculation.[5]

Early observers noted that when cholera returned to areas that had previously been infected, the population suffered illnesses of lesser severity and decreased fatality. These observations supported concepts of immunity to disease, which were new in the late nineteenth century, and experiments conducted in Spain by Jaime Ferran in 1892.[6]

1.2. New Concepts in the Epidemiology of Cholera

In the past 30 years, results of laboratory and epidemiologic studies have led to a major evolution in thinking about the epidemiology of cholera. First, while humans were long believed to be the only reservoir of *V. cholerae* 01, the organism now appears to have a free-living cycle with a natural reservoir in the environment.[7,8] This means that the control of cholera will not be achieved merely by containing the movement of infected individuals, but will require either altering man's exposure to this previously undetected reservoir of infection or placing more emphasis on control of the secondary spread of disease. Second, cholera was long felt to be spread primarily by drinking contaminated water. Investigations of recent outbreaks have identified raw bivalves (clams, oysters, and mussels) and undercooked shellfish (shrimp, crabs) to be important vehicles of transmission.[9–14] Some of these creatures have been harvested at some distance offshore, suggesting that the vibrios maintain a lifecycle that does not require continuous inoculation with human feces. Furthermore, in arid and inland areas of Africa that should be inhospitable to the marine vibrios, the disease has also taken hold, indicating that the organisms may survive under a much broader range of environmental conditions[15,16] and that transmission may occur by other routes such as person-to-person contact,[17,18,19] nosocomial spread,[18,20] or consumption of foods other than seafoods that are contaminated.[21] Third, numerous studies of family contacts of cholera patients have documented the high rates of asymptomatic infection in many cholera-endemic areas.[5] This makes it nearly impossible to identify the index case responsible for beginning an epidemic or introducing the organism into a new environment. Finally, although much has been learned about cholera transmission from studies of epidemics, similar studies of traditional endemic disease have failed to identify a single predominant mode of spread. This may be due to the presence of multiple routes of transmission, confounding factors such as immunity and asymptomatic infections and the occurrence of transient inocula (e.g., sporadic fecal contamination of food and running water) that are difficult to identify and quantify retrospectively. The following questions remain to be answered before control measures will be completely effective: What conditions favor the creation and maintenance of endemicity? Why have pandemic strains naturally disappeared?

2. CHOLERA IN THE SEVENTH PANDEMIC

The seventh pandemic of cholera that was caused by the El Tor biotype of *V. cholerae* 01 began in Sulawesi in 1961[21,22] (see Figure 1). It extended in yearly waves to the Pacific Islands and Southeast Asia, the Middle East, and the U.S.S.R. In the 1970s, the disease continued to spread through Africa, outbreaks occurred in Europe,[10,13] and isolated cases were identified in coastal areas of the United States bordering on the Gulf of Mexico[9,23,24] and in Mexico in 1983.[25] During this pandemic, more than 100 countries have reported cholera and no sign of remission is visible[26] (see Figure 2). (See Chapter 1.)

As the seventh pandemic of cholera has spread, the El Tor biotype of *Vibrio cholerae* 01 has completely replaced its predecessor, the classical biotype. The complete replacement of one strain by another led to much speculation about the biologic advantages of the El Tor vibrio and the higher rates of asymptomatic infections of the new strain. In 1979, 6 years after El Tor cholera had completely replaced classical cholera in Bangladesh, the classical strain reemerged.[27,28] The reappearance of the classical strain after years of absence suggests its long-term survival in the country at levels below the threshold of detection. Reasons for its reappearance and current coexistence with El Tor strains are as poorly understood as reasons for its original displacement.

The World Health Organization (WHO) monitors countries reporting cholera in order to follow trends in the disease over time.[26] This surveillance is quite incomplete since many countries with major cholera problems do not report their cases for political, economic, or other reasons including the lack of facilities for surveillance. Even in countries with nation-wide surveillance, reporting is incomplete both because of problems of reporting and difficulties in field diagnosis of a disease with a clinical spectrum that ranges from mild, nonspecific diarrhea to severe purging with dehydration. In 1991, WHO was notified of more than 400,000 cases of cholera from more than 45 countries, with 386,805 cases being reported from Latin America (see Figure 3).

In 1985, an alternative estimate of the disease burden of cholera was made by a review panel of experts brought together by the National Academy of Sciences of the United States.[29] This panel, using a Delphi method, estimated from their own experience and from a review of the literature that about 5.5 million cases of cholera occur annually in Asia and Africa, 8% of these cases are sufficiently severe to require hospitalization, and 20% of the severe cases would result in deaths totaling approximately 120,000 per year.

In endemic settings, the prevalence of severe, dehydrating cholera may appear to be relatively low, as in Bangladesh where the incidence of hospitalization has been 1.0–3.0 cases per thousand people per year for the past 20 years.[30] Such figures must be interpreted with care. First, this incidence occurs for the entire population from the age of 2 years to mid-adult life, so a person's cumulative risk of severe cholera in the first 20 years of life is about 6%. Given a 20% case–fatality rate, roughly 1% of people living in Bangladesh and exposed to cholera might die if left untreated. Second, studies of family contacts of diarrhea cases demonstrate the broad spectrum of infection and disease. For every individual with severe disease, more than ten will have mild to moderate diarrhea and an equal number will have an asymptomatic infection. The rates of severe disease reported do not properly reflect the more

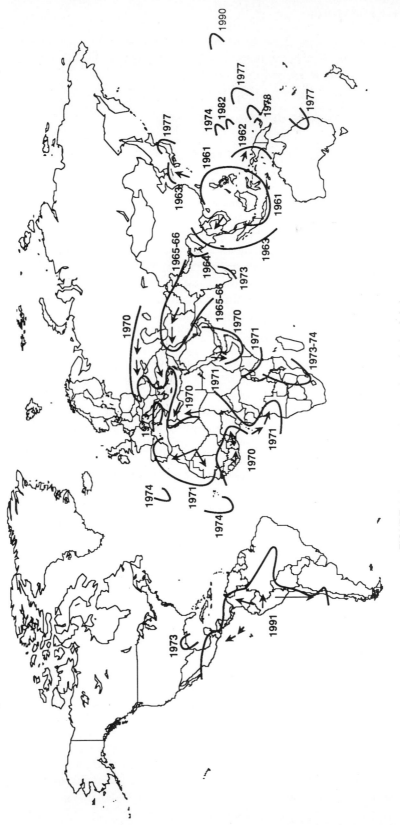

FIGURE 1. The spread of the seventh pandemic of cholera.

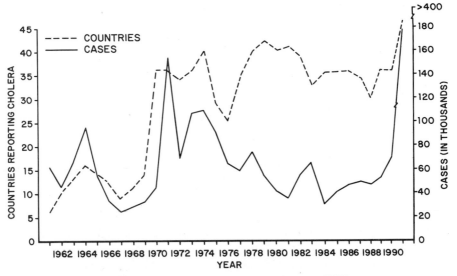

FIGURE 2. Countries reporting cholera. Source: WHO.

prevalent milder cases. Finally, epidemics of cholera in developing countries without endemic cholera may be associated with higher case–fatality rates, both because of the lack of pre-existing immunity in the population and inexperience in administering rehydration therapy. Since the epidemics occur sporadically and unpredictably, their contribution to estimates of disease burden have not been addressed.

The case–fatality rates for cholera must be interpreted carefully in view of this known spectrum of disease and the effectiveness of proper rehydration therapy. Case–fatality rates have often been reported as the death rate among patients who were hospitalized (Table 1).[31]

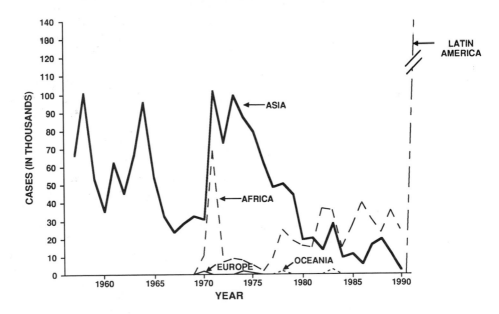

FIGURE 3. Cases of cholera reported by region. Source: WHO.

TABLE 1
Case–Fatality Ratio Due to Cholera in Selected African Countries

Country	Year	Cases	Deaths	Case–fatality ratio
Mozambique	1986	62	7	11.3
Nigeria	1984	3788	304	8.0
Senegal	1984	601	70	11.6
Mauritania	1984	109	15	13.8
Mali	1984	1803	408	22.6
Zambia	1983	1380	122	8.8
Tanzania	1977	69	38	55.0
Tanzania	1977	184	3	1.6

When hospitalization comes late in the illness and rehydration therapy is inadequate or not given, fatality has approached 50% of cases. Appropriate rehydration therapy can decrease case–fatality rates in outbreaks to less than 1%.[32,33] High case–fatality rates in recent epidemics in Africa in excess of 10% suggest difficulties in providing rapid, adequate, and timely rehydration therapy rather than an increased severity of disease.[34]

3. EPIDEMIOLOGIC AND LABORATORY TOOLS IN THE STUDY OF CHOLERA

3.1. Laboratory Markers of *V. cholerae* 01 Strains

In tracing the introduction and spread of *V. cholerae* 01, markers of the strain can help in interpreting epidemiologic results. The initial classification of *V. cholerae* into two biotypes and three serotypes was of limited usefulness in studying the spread of disease because a single biotype and serotype would often persist for a prolonged period and was insensitive to variations in the epidemiology of disease.[35] Phage typing developed initially by Mukerjee[36] and later by Takeya[37] and Lee[38] produced new strain markers that could reproducibly distinguish stable characteristics within a single biotype and serotype. In Tanzania[39] and Bangladesh,[40] the emergence of antibiotic-resistant strains of *V. cholerae* mediated by group C plasmids provided an additional marker to help in tracing the outbreak. More recently, molecular methods have been introduced to examine strain similarities and differences.[41] Autoradiography of Hind III digested chromosomal DNA that has been hybridized with P32-labeled DNA coding for cholera toxin subunit A has been used to examine the homology of the toxin genes between strains that appear to be the same. All of the strains found in waters of the Gulf of Mexico have had similar patterns on hybridization compared with those patterns seen from strains isolated in Bangladesh and the Cameroon.[25]

The usefulness of strain markers varies greatly between settings where cholera is abundant and endemic versus other settings where cholera is newly introduced or a rare event. Cholera vibrios isolated from patients from different coastal areas in the Gulf of Mexico over a 10-year period have uniformly been of a single biotype, serotype, phage type, and toxin profile.[25,42] This suggests that the strain comes from a stable, uniform reservoir that has persisted in the area over time and that new cases were not introduced by travelers or people infected outside the region. In Bangladesh, the cholera season begins each year with many patients from different locations, each having *V. cholerae* of different phage types.[43] The diversity of strains appearing at the same time but at distinct locations supports the hypothesis that an environmental reservoir for vibrios exists.

The usefulness and interpretation of epidemiologic results based upon strain markers are not clear-cut in settings when infection with multiple organisms can occur. In Bangladesh, family contacts of cholera patients who become infected with *V. cholerae* are equally as likely to be infected with strains of the same and of different phage types as those strains of the index case. Infection with the same strain might suggest a common source exposure or infection directly from the index case, whereas infection with a different strain would suggest exposure from a distinct source. Given the abundance of phage types circulating and the tendency to test only a single isolate, exact conclusions are difficult to reach. Consequently, the variety of molecular and phage typing methods available to distinguish strains has been of greater help in documenting that the isolates in a new outbreak are all the same or in tracing the introduction and spread of a new strain, rather than in elucidating the more interesting patterns of endemic disease.

3.2. Serologic Tools for the Study of Cholera

Infection with *V. cholerae* 01 —is associated with a rise in a variety of circulating antibodies, including vibriocidal antibodies[44] and antibodies to cholera toxin[45] and its A and B subunits,[46] cell wall lipopolysaccharide and nonlipopolysaccharides,[47] and outer membrane protein.[48] Early studies with vibriocidal antibodies in Bangladesh documented the clear association between elevated titers and protection against cholera.[49] Serosurveys were able to document further the nearly universal acquisition of antibodies in Bangladeshis by the age of 20 years, which confirmed the high incidence of infection in this population.[49,50] Finally, seroconversions among family contacts of cholera patients in the absence of disease documented the importance of asymptomatic infections and suggested the possible role of these silent infections in the transmission of cholera.[51]

Antibodies to cholera toxin are a simpler and often more sensitive indicator of recent cholera infection. Because cholera toxin (CT) is immunogenically similar to the heat-labile toxin (LT) of *Escherichia coli,* patients with cholera will raise their titers to both CT and LT toxin. In countries where enterotoxigenic *E. coli* and cholera coexist, it may be difficult to discriminate between infections with one organism or the other. The epidemiologic usefulness of these serologic indicators has been documented in several settings. In an investigation of a cholera outbreak on the mid-Pacific islands of Truk, Harris[52] demonstrated that *V. cholerae* 01 had been newly introduced to the islands because serum from none of 57 Truk residents sampled in 1964 before the outbreak, but that from 64% of 242 sampled in 1982 after the outbreak, had elevated levels of vibriocidal antibody. Furthermore, while 30 and 40% of residents had antibodies to CT and LT in 1964, respectively, after the 1982 outbreak those rates rose to 80% and 84%, respectively, and the ratio of anti-CT/anti-LT was significantly elevated.

Svennerholm[45,46] improved on the ability to discriminate between cholera and enterotoxigenic *E. coli* (ETEC) infections in an endemic setting by using more purified reagents and examining the antibodies response to cholera toxin subunits A and B. Bangladeshi patients convalescing from cholera had a significantly decreased ratio of toxin antibodies (LT/CT) when compared to patients convalescing from ETEC LT disease. Moreover, the cholera patients experienced a 17-fold increase in their mean titer to the cholera B subunit but no rise to the A subunit. American volunteers challenged with *V. cholerae* 01 and Americans who were infected naturally had similar vibriocidal and antitoxin antibody responses.[53–55]

Serologic studies have been used to extend case-finding to individuals suspected of having cholera and to identify contacts who have been asymtomatically infected.[56,57] They have also helped interpret hypotheses concerning immunity and transmission. For example, Bangladeshi mothers who have high titer antibodies to cholera that should be protective are nonetheless at high risk of disease when their small children become infected.[50] Although antibodies are associated with protection against disease, this immunity can be overwhelmed by ingestion of a large inoculum of vibrios. The child's infected feces can contaminate the mother's hand and clothing[58] so that she becomes ill in spite of her immunity.

3.3. Epidemiologic Methods for the Study of Cholera

3.3.1. Case–Control Studies in Epidemic Settings and Family Studies in Endemic Settings

In both epidemic and endemic settings, severe cholera is usually an uncommon event, affecting only a small portion of the total population. It is usually impossible to determine how the organism is specifically introduced into a new environment and how first cases become infected. In investigations of new epidemics and sporadic endemic cases, however, case–control studies have enjoyed a unique success in identifying risk factors for the transmission of cholera. In these studies index cases, i.e., patients with cholera that has usually been confirmed by culture, are matched by age and sex with controls who have had no diarrhea in the recent past. Controls of the same sex and approximate age as the cases can be chosen from other patients in the hospital or from neighbors of the case, depending on the risk factors being examined. This type of study is particularly powerful when cholera is spread by a single mode of transmission or where a single mode of transmission or where a single, identifiable and predominant source of infection exists in the community (e.g., contaminated well, bottled-water, shellfish). In endemic settings in developing countries, case–control studies have been notoriously unsuccessful, due perhaps to the existence of multiple modes of transmission or vehicles of infection, high rates of asymptomatic infection among controls, or exposures that are transient or poorly defined in time or place.

In cholera-endemic areas where hygiene is poor, family contacts of cholera patients often have a risk of infection in the subsequent 10–14 days that can approach 50%.[5] The family study, i.e., the intense follow-up of family contacts for colonization and disease, has become a useful epidemiologic technique to prospectively examine risk factors for disease and consider modes of prevention.[59] Risk factors that have been established from family studies include the predisposition of people of blood group O for severe disease, the protection afforded by breast-feeding and serum antibodies, and the lack of association between chronic malnutrition in children and the disease risk. The efficacy of two interventions for cholera were demonstrated from family studies: tetracycline prophylaxis protected family contacts of cholera patients from infection with *V. cholerae* 01[60] and, in Calcutta, the introduction of closed-mouth water jugs (Sorai) decreased intrafamilial spread of cholera and documented the importance of contaminated household water in transmitting the disease.[61] Family studies provide much information on the secondary spread of disease within the family unit but are limited in their ability to extrapolate these results to other modes of transmission that might be more important in the larger community.

3.3.2. Environmental Sampling in the Study of Cholera

An important adjunct to the epidemiologic investigation of cholera has been the ability to sample the environment in search of reservoirs of cholera vibrios. *V. cholerae* 01 have been found in drinking water, sewage, shellfish and seafoods, human sweat, soil, night soil, and crops.[7] Methods to identify vibrios have usually involved enrichment of the sample in a medium such as alkaline peptone broth followed by routine bacterial culture. Moore swabs have been routinely used to concentrate vibrios from water supplies and sewage where they may exist in low concentration.[62] These swabs of gauze pads are dropped into water sources (wells, rivers, tanks) or sewage for 24 h and then placed into an enrichment broth. Alternatively, cholera vibrios can be isolated from the filamentous roots of floating plants or from filters used to purify large volumes of water.[63] (See Chapters 2 and 12.)

4. EPIDEMIOLOGIC PATTERNS OF CHOLERA

The epidemiology of cholera varies greatly between epidemic areas where cholera has been newly introduced and endemic areas where cholera has persisted for years (Table 2).[64] These endemic and epidemic settings differ in the presence of reservoirs of cholera vibrios, cultural and behavioral practices particularly regarding food and water, modes of transmission of disease, and the immune status of the population that affects both the age of people affected and the ratio of people who are symptomatically versus asymptomatically infected. These distinctions are important because for epidemic cholera and for endemic cholera in areas with little secondary transmission, case–control studies have frequently been able to identify a single mode of transmission suitable for control. In areas with poor sanitation and hygiene, once cholera becomes endemic, control and prevention of further spread becomes difficult. With the seventh pandemic, cholera has spread through small and big epidemics to large

TABLE 2
Comparison of Epidemiologic Features of Epidemic vs. Endemic Cholera

Features	Epidemic	Endemic	
		Developing country	Developed country
Age at greatest risk	All ages (if exposed)	Children 2–15	All ages (if exposed)
Modes of transmission	Single introduction and fecal–oral spread	Multiple (water, food, fecal–oral contamination)	Single (often shellfish/seafood)
Reservoir	Absent	Aquatic reservoirs,[a] asymptomatically infected people	Aquatic reservoir
Asymptomatic infections	Less common	More common	Less common
Immune status of population	Seronegative, no preexisting immunity	Seropositive acquisition with increasing age	Seronegative, no preexisting immunity
Secondary spread	Variable	Present	Less common
Special epidemiologic methods most helpful for study	Case–control	Family study	Case–control

[a]Includes water, shellfish, aquatic plants, etc.

parts of Asia and Africa and Latin America. In many areas, this has led to the establishment of an endemic pattern where the vibrios continue to persist. For example, in South Africa and Malawi, cholera was first introduced in the early 1970s. For the past 10 years, all *V. cholerae* 01 isolated have had a single phage type, indicating that this single strain has become endemic and persistent in this area. The transition from epidemic introduction to endemic persistence must be accompanied by the establishment of natural reservoirs of infection in the locality or environment and spread of disease by several different routes. Where rates of cholera infection are high with much secondary spread, endemic cholera may be associated with the development of some immunity in the population, leading to higher rates of asymptomatic infection and a shift in the age distribution toward younger children and away from immune adults.

4.1. Endemic Cholera

Endemic cholera describes a pattern of disease that recurs in the same area over time. Until recently, endemic areas of cholera were considered to be localized to estuarine deltas in tropical or semitropical areas such as the Ganges basin, where a densely crowded population lived with elemental water and sewage facilities near water used for washing, bathing, defecation, and drinking. In this setting, human feces containing vibrios were felt to seed the environment and contaminate water that, if consumed, would perpetuate transmission of the organism. The recognition of repeated cases of cholera caused by the El Tor biotype in areas of the United States bordering the Gulf of Mexico has led to an appreciation that vibrios can maintain a free-living cycle in the aquatic environment and that endemicity may not require continual or recurrent seeding from human sewage. Cholera has also become endemic in areas of Africa that are distant from coastal waters, suggesting that the vibrios have adapted to survive in a broader range of environmental conditions. Hence, as the area where cholera is endemic has expanded, conventional views of the reservoirs and modes of transmission have been challenged and altered.

Cholera traditionally was observed to follow the routes of travellers, which suggested that humans were an essential reservoir of infection. This hypothesis received further support from many studies documenting the high rates of asymptomatic infection among family contacts and neighbors of cholera patients. These silent carriers with asymptomatic infections were of great public health importance since they could unknowingly transmit their infection during travel, and they made it impossible to trace the first introduction of cholera into new outbreak settings. While people with asymptomatic infections provided a potentially important focus of transmission during the cholera season, 90% of these individuals were vibrio-free within 8–10 days, and rarely does excretion go beyond 2 weeks.[5,65] Outside the cholera season, studies to identify chronic carriers of cholera vibrios through cultivation of large groups of people have yielded extremely low rates of infection.[66] Prolonged excretion of vibrios is unusual but has been documented in the Philippines[65] and Calcutta[67] with individuals who shed the organism for months. A single Philippine woman, Delores M., became renowned in the literature of cholera because she excreted vibrios at irregular intervals for a 10-year period following her initial infection in 1962.[68] Her *V. cholerae* 01 was distinct from strains circulating locally at the time, thereby excluding the possibility that she was reinfected and downplaying her role in transmitting her infection back into the community. The role of long-term carriers of *V. cholerae* 01 has consequently never been substantiated.

Identification of an aquatic reservoir for cholera that persists independently of continual fecal contamination has prompted a rethinking about the epidemiology and control of cholera. *V. cholerae* 01 survives well in warm water with marginal salinity, and with a rich supply of biological nutrients and oxygen. Vibrios are found on the roots of plants, on the shells of crabs and copepods, in shellfish, and on plankton. Some investigators have suggested that *V. cholerae* 01 goes into a dormant, noncultivatable state in the off-season and blooms with seasonable changes in these environmental conditions.[69] The environment could be further enriched with vibrios excreted by infected humans.

In the Gulf waters of the Southeastern United States, the presence of a natural marine environment for cholera and the persistence of a single strain of *V. cholerae* 01 biotype El Tor over a 14-year period suggests that eradication of this organism from these endemic areas may be difficult, if not impossible. Cholera has been spread by eating raw or poorly cooked shellfish or seafood collected with contaminated water. No large outbreaks have occurred, secondary transmission has been of little importance, and the disease is more a curiosity than a major public-health concern. In areas such as the Philippines or Bangladesh, the aquatic reservoir of cholera may be responsible for the yearly recurrence of cholera outbreaks. When the cholera season begins in Bangladesh, early cases occur in widely divergent areas within days of each other and with different phage types, a yearly coincidence that is consistent with multiple reservoirs of *V. cholerae* 01 in the aquatic environment or neighborhood. Once ingested, vibrios can be amplified in the guts of infected individuals and spread due to the numerous breaches of food and water hygiene that occur in many endemic settings in developing countries. Prevention of cholera can no longer be aimed at preventing the introduction of vibrios once the environment has been seeded. Rather, control must be directed at interrupting the secondary spread of disease through interventions to ensure clean household drinking water, improvements in hygienic practices and food safety, and separation of infected feces from water used for bathing and cooking.

In endemic areas where hygiene is poor, cholera primarily affects children 2–15 years of age, many of whom are experiencing their initial infection.[30] These first infections can be severe but rarely are people hospitalized twice for the disease suggesting that immunity is longlasting and protects against severe illness. Once immunity develops, exposure to *V. cholerae* can still lead to asymptomatic infections, which play a critical role in spreading disease and in maintaining an infective reservoir. The ratio of symptomatic to asymptomatic infections has been reported to vary from 1:2 to 1:100, but this variation undoubtedly relates to conditions of sampling, population density, prevalence of immunity in the population, blood group distribution, biotype, and many other factors. Occasionally, epidemics of cholera do occur in endemic settings. This may represent exposure of cases to an unusually heavy inoculum of vibrios, a change in the growth properties or virulence of the strain, or alteration of the normal cycle of transmission. In Bangladesh, epidemics of cholera in adult men who are usually at low risk can be a potent indicator of such an event.

4.2. Epidemic Cholera

The introduction of cholera into a new area has many epidemiologic features that distinguish the disease. First, since the population has no pre-existing immunity, all people exposed are theoretically at equal risk of disease. Consequently, cholera in this setting is not a disease primarily of children but a disease that affects adults as well. The occurrence of epidemic diarrheal disease in adults associated with severe dehydration and death at a time or place where cholera may exist must be investigated as a potential cholera outbreak. Second, when cholera is first introduced, it has no pre-existing reservoir in the environment so the vibrios are often localized to a single water source or food exposure and transmission takes place by a single, predominant route. In some settings, this has been easy to identify through case–control studies and, in many instances, control of the disease has been effective. Third, the infected individual has pre-existing immunity to disease but it is often dose-related. One practical approach to the epidemiological study of cholera in newly endemic areas is to try to examine patterns of disease transmission in marginal areas as the disease spreads. In Indonesia and in parts of Africa, for example, cholera is endemic in many coastal areas but sporadic and epidemic as one goes inland. Examination of the rare cases of epidemic disease inland may provide more clear-cut clues to transmission than study of many endemic cases drawn from the coastal plains.

5. PATTERNS OF TRANSMISSION

5.1. Fecal–Oral Route

Vibrio cholerae 01 are transmitted only by the fecal–oral route, i.e., the organisms are excreted in the feces and must be ingested by a susceptible host to cause disease. The number of organisms in the feces of an individual with cholera is 10^7 per ml or more,[69] and the copious stool output of up to 20 liters per day can result in massive environmental contamination. A high number of *V. cholerae* 01 may also be found in vomitus during illness and presumably represents refluxed small-bowel fluids.

5.2. Infectious Dose and Gastric Acidity

V. cholerae 01 are extremely sensitive to an acidic environment and are killed within minutes in gastric juice with pH < 2.4.[70,71] Since ingested *V. cholerae* 01 must survive and transit through the gastric acid of the stomach to colonize the intestine, the relationships among the ingested number of organisms, the stomach acidity, and the vehicle of transmission are of interest. In normochlorhydric adult volunteers, doses of up to 10^{11} pathogenic *V. cholerae* 01 given without buffer or food did not reliably cause illness, whereas doses of 10^4–10^8 organisms given with 2g of $NaHCO_3$ resulted in diarrhea in 90% of individuals.[72] Furthermore, the severity of diarrhea was greater with doses of 10^6 than with 10^4 viable organisms and the spectrum of illness with the 10^6 dose was similar to that of cholera. In similar volunteer studies, doses of 10^5, 10^4, and even 10^3 resulted in at least a 60% attack rate, although the diarrheal illnesses at the two lower doses were milder and appeared to have a somewhat longer incubation period.[73] In studies in which gastric acidity (pH < 2.0) was neutralized by 2g of $NaCHO_3$, some had gastric contents that remained at pH ≥ 5.0 for 30 min, while others returned to baseline acidity by 30 min.[72] Those individuals who maintained a neutralized gastric environment longer seemed to have a higher attack rate on challenge with 10^6 *V. cholerae* 01.

Hypochlorhydria, which has been found in patients with cholera, apparently predisposes to the development of illness, rather than resulting from cholera.[71,74–77] Hypochlorhydria has been associated with malnutrition, with B_{12} deficiency, and with gastritis, but occurs for unknown reasons in many cases.[78,79] In addition, stomach acid production may be relatively lower in normal infants than in adults. Thus, it has been hypothesized that hypochlorhydria is an important risk factor in the occurrence and severity of illness with *V. cholerae* 01 infection.[71,74–77] Epidemiologic evidence has supported this hypothesis by finding that a history of gastric resection was associated with any illness and with severe illness in a raw shellfish-borne cholera outbreak in Italy in 1973.[77] Further determinants of resting gastric acid or of acid production when stimulated need also be considered in regard to risk of disease. Medications that reduce acid secretion, such as cimetidine,[80] or that neutralize acid, such as antacids, could put individuals at higher risk of enteric diseases such as cholera. The regular use of cannabis has been reported to be associated with low acid production and with more severe diarrhea in cholera studies in adult volunteers.[81]

In endemic or epidemic settings, the infectious dose of *V. cholerae* 01 may be substantially less than that used to achieve a high attack rate in adult volunteers. In endemic areas, only a minority (20–40%) of infections with *V. cholerae* 01 El Tor results in any illness, and in these settings, the attack rate among exposed individuals is probably even lower.[28,82] Among persons exposed to *V. cholerae* 01-contaminated household water in rural Bangladesh, the incidence of infection was only 11% and only about half of the infected individuals had any illness.[83] In the same study the range of concentrations of *V. cholerae* 01 in contaminated water was up to 500 colony-forming units (cfu) per ml, but approximately 90% of positive household water samples were found to contain *V. cholerae* 01 only on enrichment cultures, representing a probable range of concentrations from 1–500 cfu per 100 ml of water. Although the true level of inocula resulting in illness cannot be determined precisely, it is likely to be only 10^2–10^3 organisms.

Since *V. cholerae* 01 are usually ingested with water or food, it is important to consider the potential of these vehicles for enhancing the survival of the organisms through the gastric acidity. It has been postulated that vibrios taken with a large volume of water might pass quickly through the stomach, the so-called "splash-through" effect, and thus be spared from destruction in the acidic environment. Further, it has been postulated that food might protect the vibrios either by buffering gastric acid or by sequestering the organisms inside a mass of food. In a specific evaluation of these hypotheses in adult volunteers, individuals ingested 10^6 *V. cholerae* 01 El Tor with 2g of $NaHCO_3$, in 300 ml of water, or in a meal of fish, rice, milk, and custard.[73] While none of the volunteers who ingested the vibrios in water alone developed illness or even infection, all of the other volunteers became infected and all but one (who took the vibrios with $NaHCO_3$) became ill. The individuals who ingested organisms with a meal had cholera of similar severity to those who had buffered gastric acidity with $NaHCO_3$. Thus, food may serve to protect the pathogens from destruction, and a comparable inoculum taken with water will not cause illness, as was previously demonstrated in earlier volunteer studies with classical *V. cholerae* 01.

5.3. Incubation Period

The incubation period for cholera is determined by both the size of the inoculum and host factors such as the level of gastric acid. In field settings, exposures precede symptoms by about 24–48 h, although this can range from 14 h to as long as 5 days. This time may be determined by the requirements that the vibrios colonize and multiply in the gut before they elaborate cholera toxin.

5.4. Waterborne Transmission

Since the classic investigations of a cholera epidemic by John Snow in London in 1854,[3] water has been considered an important vehicle of transmission for *V. cholerae* 01. Indeed, further demonstration of the potential for water to transmit the infection was furnished by Koch, who first isolated and characterized the *Vibrio* and was able to find the organisms in pond water used by an Indian community experiencing a cholera outbreak.[4] Thus, in the earlier pandemics water from public waterworks was implicated in transmission, especially in Europe, and other types of water were suggested as sources of transmission in endemic areas.[84]

In discussing waterborne transmission, one should distinguish transmission by ingesting water alone from ingesting water in contaminated foods; contaminated waterways may even be important in facilitating the spread of infection from one area to another.[85] Concerning the latter aspect, one observer said that cholera "travels as man travels, stops where he stops, and proceeds again at the time, and in the direction, in which he resumes his journey."[1] Diffusion of cholera is thus along routes of trade and travel, which in the last century were mostly sea or river routes. Spread through sea or river ports continues to occur during the seventh pandemic and may have played a particularly significant role in Africa in the 1970s.[15,16,21,86] Likewise, in a cholera-endemic area, Bangladesh, boatmen have been implicated in the geographical spread of the disease.[87] Furthermore, endemic areas have traditionally been riverine deltas or brackish rivers, although cholera has apparently become endemic since 1970 in dry areas of Africa.[16,21] Although these observations are relevant for the diffusion of cholera, they do not indicate that cholera is transmitted by ingestion of water.

Transmission by consumption of water from contaminated waterworks appears to be uncommon during the seventh pandemic, either in countries with newly introduced cholera or in endemic areas. In contrast, water used without treatment from rivers, tanks, ponds, irrigation channels, or even wells probably has had and continues to have an important role in transmission.[84,88,89] A rather common observation was that dug or drilled wells that became contaminated by seepage of fecally contaminated water or by washing of soiled clothing on or near the well were implicated in family or community outbreaks. Although the investigations at the time included descriptive epidemiology and sometimes demonstration of *V. cholerae* 01 in the water, they rarely included more rigorous epidemiologic methods that would more clearly implicate drinking water from these origins as the cause of the epidemic.

In cholera-endemic areas of developing countries, the importance of precisely how water is related to transmission is still unclear. Most of these areas have a high population density, extreme poverty, elemental or no sanitation facilities, and frequently and heavily contaminated water supplies. In these areas, people may use a variety of water sources for drinking, washing, bathing, or cooking, and this use may vary by age, sex, wealth, season, or other factors. A particularly illuminating study in rural Bangladesh found that factors, such as distance and quarrels among neighbors were important determinants of the selection of water sources among the poor and that other factors such as water taste, odor, or color and purdah of women, were important among the wealthier residents.[88] Thus, the precise role of consumption of contaminated water is difficult to determine.

A series of studies has been conducted in which sanitary wells have been installed in communities in endemic areas and the effect on cholera and other diarrhea measured. The results have generally been disappointing in finding no reduction in the incidence of cholera or diarrhea in users of sanitary wells.[90,91] Aside from the documented occasional *V. cholerae* 01 contamination of such wells, the water was generally of better bacteriologic quality than surface water. To explain this apparent paradox, i.e., that drinking less contaminated water failed to reduce cholera incidence, investigators hypothesized that the continued consumption of surface water, which was often preferred for reasons of taste, convenience, or local beliefs about water "quality," in addition to use of well water may have overcome any protective effect.[92] The continued use of surface water for all purposes by children, who have a high rate of cholera, and by adults for bathing, washing utensils, and cooking may also have played an important role. A family and neighborhood study of cholera transmission provided further evidence to support this hypothesis.[89] In addition to generally implicating water in transmission of *V. cholerae* 01, this study demonstrated the importance of water use other than for drinking. Persons who used culture-positive water sources for cooking, bathing, or washing but culture-negative sources for drinking had the same rate of infection as persons who used culture-positive water for drinking. Bathing in contaminated surface water may have been particularly important in this setting since Muslims commonly rinse the mouth with handfuls of water as part of the bathing ritual.

Studies in the rural Matlab area of Bangladesh also evaluated incidence rates of cholera by village between 1968 and 1977 to determine high- or low-risk areas.[30] Areas that were not adjacent to the main river, but were on small canals, had higher rates of disease, and no distinct pattern of spread from a single focus or following the flow of the river was noted. In fact, the early cases of each cholera season began almost simultaneously at distant villages in the Matlab area and, at least in 1979, isolates from these early cases were of various phage types. Furthermore, no correlations were observed between the seasonality of cholera and the timing of environmental parameters, such as onset or peak of the monsoon, river water levels, or ambient temperature. These findings are consistent with the introduction of *V. cholerae* 01 by multiple individuals or with the "blooming" of vibrios persistent in the environment when unstudied ecological factors, such as water salinity, become appropriate.

The variation in risk by use of sources of surface water has also been studied by others in Bangladesh. Some, but not all, studies suggested that users of water from canals had a higher attack rate than users of other sources, such as tanks and rivers.[93] Canals may be more heavily contaminated due to the direct discharge of fecal waste from a community into the canals and the sluggish movement of water that may spread, but not dilute or "wash away," contamination. Another study also suggested higher rates for users of canals and the lowest rates for users of "tanks," small ponds for one or a few families. This apparent relationship may be due to protection from the use of relatively protected tanks or enhanced risk from use of more contaminated canals, since these are often alternative sources of water.

The results indicating that cholera incidence does not substantially decline following introduction of protected sources of drinking water, even assuming it is safer and is used, do not necessarily suggest that transmission of *V. cholerae* 01 by consumption of water is not an important route. As Briscoe illustrated, when the dose–response relationship between the organism and disease is log-linear, as it is with *V. cholerae* 01, and when there are multiple transmission routes, as there clearly are with cholera, the improvement in only one transmission route may result in little or no reduction in disease.[94] Thus, in Bangladesh, use of safer water for drinking, even if consumption of contaminated water were the predominant route of transmission, would have little effect on disease rates until improvements in other routes also occurred, such as ingestion of water during bathing, consumption of contaminated food, or person-to-person spread.

As a further complication, it must be recognized that the use of water from a relatively protected and less contaminated source does not ensure that the actual water consumed will be uncontaminated. Water is rarely ingested directly from the source, but instead is collected in a variety of ways, in a variety of containers, and stored in different manners for one or more days in the household. This is true in both rural areas and in urban areas where drinking from household taps is not the rule or where the supply is intermittent. This collection and storage provides ample opportunity for contamination of the water prior to consumption. Although data from Bangladesh indicate that *V. cholerae* 01-positive water in the household was usually associated with a culture-positive water source,[83] data from Calcutta, India demonstrate the contrary.[95] These studies suggested that *V. cholerae* 01-infected persons, often asymptomatic, contaminated household water by putting fingers or utensils in the water, which was stored in wide-mouthed vessels in the house. As a further demonstration of the role of household contamination, the introduction of a narrow-necked earthenware vessel for storing the water in this setting reduced the *V. cholerae* 01 infection rate by 75%.[61]

Supporting the importance of environmental sanitation in transmission of cholera is a controlled field intervention in a cholera-endemic area of the Philippines.[96] In this study, either provision of improved water supply (piped from an artesian well) or improved toilet facilities (communal water-seal latrines) appeared to reduce incidence of cholera by 68–73%. As mentioned previously, other studies involving the provision of wells failed to demonstrate reduction in the incidence of cholera or diarrhea.

During the seventh pandemic, waterborne transmission has been suggested in several outbreaks. In Queensland, Australia, inadequately treated river water, which was used as an auxiliary town water supply, was implicated in a case of cholera occurring in 1977.[97] River water was positive for *V. cholerae* 01 intermittently over a 22-month period suggesting persistence and multiplication of the organism in the river water. In an outbreak of cholera on the Maldive Islands in 1978, contamination of subsurface groundwater from which drinking and domestic water was obtained was suggested as the cause (Centers for Disease Control, unpublished observation). In Aceh Province, Indonesia in 1982, a cholera outbreak occurred; an epidemiologic investigation suggested, but could not definitively prove, that river water and ice made from that water were important vehicles for transmission.[98] In a rather unusual instance of transmission by ingested water, an outbreak in Portugal in 1974 was partially attributed to consumption of bottled noncarbonated water taken from a *V. cholerae* 01-positive spring.[99] Carbonated water of the same brand and from the same source was not implicated in transmission, suggesting that the carbonation reduced vibrio survival, as has been demonstrated in the laboratory.

5.5. Foodborne Transmission

The probable role of food in transmission of cholera has reviewed by Pollitzer in many cholera outbreaks.[100] The likelihood of food serving as an important transmission route is enhanced by: (1) the potential for some foods to become contaminated, (2) the ability of the vibrio to survive and multiply in foods, resulting in higher ingested doses, and (3) the gastric-acid buffering effect of food, which may permit low numbers of organisms to pass unharmed through the stomach.

Early observers noted that fish and shellfish were frequent vehicles in cholera transmission.[100] These foods are apt to be contaminated by the waters in which they live, and *V. cholerae* 01 may even have an affinity for certain shellfish. Furthermore, these foods are often eaten raw or after cooking that is inadequate to destroy the vibrios.

Much of the evidence for the importance of fish and shellfish as vehicles for *V. cholerae* 01 comes from epidemiologic investigations of cholera outbreaks in newly infected areas of the seventh pandemic. These investigations have identified seafood products, such as raw shrimp, mussels, raw oysters, salted fish, and inadequately steamed crabs, as causes of outbreaks (Table 3). In these areas a single exposure is sufficient, and, due to the short incubation period, this exposure can usually be recalled at the time of the epidemiologic studies.

Seafood must serve as an important vehicle in endemic areas, such as the Asian subcontinent, where it is a major part of the diet and where contamination of water and harvested shellfish can be readily demonstrated.[12] However, it is often not possible to implicate a single food or exposure in this setting because of multiple potentially infectious exposures to a variety of possible routes of transmission and to the presence of immunity in portions of the population. Some investigators have hypothesized, but not yet demonstrated, that in estuarine environments, consumption of seafood rather than water is the important risk factor for cholera. V. cholerae 01 in these areas can be isolated from brackish water (0.5–3.0% salinity), which may vary by time of year, perhaps providing one reason for the often striking seasonality of cholera.[64] Since water is unpalatable for drinking at salinities above 0.1%, other routes of transmission must be implicated in many settings. One proposal is that seafood is the most likely vehicle for transmitting V. cholerae 01 from the aquatic reservoir to the local population. Once cholera is introduced into communities, other routes of transmission including water and food could occur. In developing countries with poor sanitation and hygiene, this secondary transmission may be extensive, whereas in areas such as the United States or Australia, little or no secondary transmission is likely.[9,24,97]

Other foods have also been implicated. In Israel, raw vegetables irrigated with inadequately treated wastewater caused an outbreak in 1970.[102] In Bahrain, bottle-feeding, as opposed to breast-feeding, was a risk factor for cholera in infants; however, this may have been due to a protective effect of breastfeeding, rather than to contamination of the bottle feedings.[109–111] In an outbreak in Micronesia, illness appeared to be spread through food contaminated in the home.[108] Although no specific food could be implicated, food prepared by a person who had recently been ill was associated with subsequent illness

TABLE 3
Outbreaks of Cholera Traced to a Food Source[a]

Country	Year	Exposure	References
Philippines	1961	Raw shrimp	13
Malaysia	1963	Seafood/shellfish	101
Israel	1970	Raw vegetables	102
Bahrain–Sydney flight	1972	Hors d'oeuvres	103
Italy	1973	Mussels	10
Portugal	1974	Raw cockles/bottled mineral water	14,99
Guam	1974	Salted fish	104
Gilbert Islands	1977	Raw shellfish/salted fish	105,106
USA (Louisiana)	1980	Inadequately steamed crabs	9
Sardinia	1980	Shellfish	11
Singapore	1982	Seafood	107
USA (Gulf of Mexico	1983	Water-contaminated rice	24
Micronesia	1984	Food	108

[a]Many anecdotal reports of foodborne larvae spread remain unconfirmed.

in family members. Persons who had tended an ill person were not at increased risk of cholera, suggesting that foodborne transmission rather than person-to-person spread was more important.

The contamination of food in the household may play a major role in transmission of cholera in unhygienic developing country settings. In Bangladesh, water kept in the house and used for cooking had a higher rate of contamination with *V. cholerae* 01 than water for drinking.[83] Regardless of whether this water became contaminated at the source or in the home, it could serve as a means to further contaminate food during or after preparation. Only 0.13% of foods cultured in the Bangladesh study households were positive for *V. cholerae* 01, suggesting that the risk of contamination may be small, but when it occurs the risk may be high due to multiplication of vibrios and the acid-buffering effect of food. As an illustration of how such contamination might occur, one can refer to an outbreak on an oil rig in the Gulf of Mexico.[24] The outbreak was associated with consumption of rice, which had been rinsed in contaminated water after cooking and maintained for most of the day at a temperature that permitted *V. cholerae* 01 to multiply. The high attack rate in this outbreak (93% of infected persons were ill) suggests that a large inoculum was ingested and that gastric acid was buffered, presumably by the meal consumed. The conditions of food preparation, storage at ambient temperatures, and consumption without further cooking are very common in households in developing countries and may greatly contribute to transmission of enteric pathogens through food.[112]

The transmission by food-service establishments in endemic areas should also be considered. In Hong Kong, consumption of Chinese "moonsalus" were linked to transmission.[113] In Bangladesh during the urban Dhaka outbreak in 1974 and 1975, cholera was associated with eating in places outside the home, especially charitable feeding centers set up to provide free food during a famine.[114]

5.6. Person-to-Person Transmission

Although person-to-person transmission of infection may be considered broadly as resulting from contact with an ill individual, either directly or via secondary contamination of household water, food, or fomites, it seems most logical to consider here only possible direct routes of transmission from one person to another. The indirect routes or means of contamination are considered separately. Direct transmission of *V. cholerae* 01 would then consist of the introduction of the organisms into the mouth by fingers contaminated with feces of infected individuals. In Bangladesh, the higher attack rate of cholera in young women compared with men of the same age could be explained by exposure of mothers to a large number of *V. cholerae* 01 organisms while caring for an ill child, although other explanations are also possible.[30] Likewise, the higher attack rate among family members of cholera cases could be from direct spread, but indirect routes seem more likely.[82,115–117] Investigations that have suggested person-to-person transmission often have failed to demonstrate that water or food were responsible and then have proposed direct transmission by exclusion.[17,118]

Person-to-person transmission has been conjectured to be important in the dry Sahelian area of Africa and among gold miners in South Africa. In both settings the possible role of sweat was suggested. Sweat will apparently support the survival and multiplication of *V. cholerae* 01 for prolonged periods.[119] Although the organism has not been found in sweat on the skin, it was postulated that profuse sweating could rinse vibrios from the perianal region of infected persons and contaminate the floor or other surfaces.[119–121] One rather unique setting where this was suggested was in rooms where newly recruited miners underwent heat acclimatization.[120,121]

One of the settings in which person-to-person transmission has been reported is in hospitals.[18,122,123] These outbreaks clearly have the characteristics of common-source outbreaks. Thus, contamination of food or water in the hospital seems the most likely explanation, although direct cross-infection cannot be excluded. The latter would certainly be favored by the poor hygiene, overcrowding and handwashing practices among children, attendants, and staff in the reported outbreaks, as well as the habit of eating with fingers from a communal plate.

Transmission at the time of burial ceremonies has also been postulated. This possibility was noted by John Snow who observed: "the duties performed about the body, such as laying it out, when done by women of the working class, who make the occasion one of eating and drinking, are often followed by an attack of cholera; and persons who merely attend the funeral, and have no connection with the body, frequently contract the disease in consequence, apparently, of partaking of food which has been prepared or handled by those having duties about the cholera patient, or his linen and bedding." In the present day, burial ceremonies have also been implicated.[34] Of particular note is a Muslim custom in some parts of the world in which friends and relatives gather after a death. According to local practice, the dead body is cleaned before burial, including squeezing out all of the intestinal contents followed by rinsing of the intestine with water. After burial the participants are provided with meals and drinks in the deceased's home. In some areas eating is done with fingers from a communal plate. In this situation the actual transmission may be by means of food or drinks contaminated in the home.

5.7. Fomites

Fomites are inanimate objects that might become contaminated and serve to transmit infection. During early cholera pandemics it was commonly believed that fomites could spread the disease.[124] Thus, it was common practice to insist on disinfection of articles, even letters, being sent out of affected communities. These concepts also served as the basis for embargoes of goods as a means of limiting the spread of the epidemic. In light of more recent evidence that *V. cholerae* 01 survive poorly on dry surfaces, it is very unlikely that such fomites could facilitate the transmission of infection, and disinfection or embargo of goods would seem inappropriate. Cooking or eating utensils have the potential to be contaminated by washing in *V. cholerae* 01-containing water but this should not be a problem if utensils are dried before use. On the other hand, fecally contaminated bed-linen or clothing could contain large numbers of vibrios, which could survive for some time on moist cloth.[7] Such materials could pose a risk to others and should be laundered without further contaminating the environment.

5.8. Flies

The role of flies in transmission of enteric pathogens has been rather controversial.[125,126] A variety of enteric pathogens has been cultured from flies, and flies may become contaminated from feces of an ill person and subsequently land on and inoculate food with the vibrios.[95,125] Multiplication of the organisms in food could then result in sufficient organisms to cause disease. Although this means of transmission is conceivable, it is probably relatively unimportant compared with other routes in developing countries. Nevertheless, proper disposal of cholera stools is advisable and should prevent contact by flies.

6. RISK FACTORS ASSOCIATED WITH CHOLERA TRANSMISSION

6.1. Blood Group

In 1977, Barua[127] and Chaudhuri[128] each noted that patients hospitalized with cholera were more likely to be of O blood group than a control population. Levine[129] subsequently observed that U.S. volunteers with O blood group who were challenged with *V. cholerae* 01 tended to purge more severely than volunteers of other blood groups. These observations were confirmed in a large study in Bangladesh and the basis of this association was explored.[130] Of 682 patients hospitalized for diarrhea with an identified pathogen, cholera patients were nearly twice as likely as non-cholera controls with diarrhea and controls who were healthy blood donors to have O blood group (57% versus 30%) and one-ninth as likely to have AB. Neither patients with non-O group 1 vibrios nor patients with strains of enterotoxigenic *E. coli* (ETEC), which produce a heat-labile toxin that is antigenically similar to cholera toxin, differed in the distribution of their blood groups from the control population. Blood group was not related to risk of colonization with *V. cholerae* 01 since the distribution of blood groups was similar in family contacts of cholera patients who became infected with *V. cholerae* 01 and those who did not. Among family contacts infected with *V. cholerae* 01, the prevalence of O blood group increased directly and significantly with the severity of diarrhea. The mechanism of this O group predisposition for cholera is unclear but seems to be unrelated to secretor status. People living in the Ganges Delta have the lowest prevalence of O blood group genes. This may reflect long-term genetic selection of O group individuals from the population where (1) cholera has long been endemic, (2) the lifetime incidence is high, and (3) people die prematurely, before their reproductive age.

6.2. Breast Feeding

Breast-feeding appears to protect infants against cholera in both epidemic and endemic settings. During an outbreak of cholera in Bahrain,[109] Gunn found that cholera was more common in infants who were bottle-fed than those who were breast-fed. He was not able to distinguish whether this risk was due to contamination of the infant formula or to a protective effect of the breast milk itself. In endemic areas like Bangladesh, breast-feeding appears to protect against cholera in infancy. Cholera generally spares children in their first 2 years of life, and children seen with cholera in Dhaka were less likely to be breast-fed than children seen for diarrhea with any other agent except shigella.[131]

The importance of breast-milk antibodies in protecting children against cholera was demonstrated in a prospective study of family contacts of cholera cases.[111] Antibodies to cholera were assayed in breast milk of lactating mothers at the start of each family study, and infection and disease in breast-fed infants were monitored daily over the subsequent 10-day period. IgA antibodies in breast milk did not appear to protect children against colonization with *V. cholerae* 01 but did protect those children colonized from developing diarrhea.

6.3. Nutritional Status

Although undernutrition or malnutrition have often been considered risk factors for diarrheal diseases, little evidence is available to suggest that individuals who are poorly nourished have an increased risk for disease or severity of disease with cholera. In 1962–1963, Rosenberg[132] was unable to detect any difference in levels of thiamine, ascorbic acid, folate, or B_{12} between cholera patients and a healthy control population. Gangerosa,[133] on biopsy, demonstrated histological evidence of malabsorption in a group of Thai patients with acute cholera, but these changes were subsequently found to be nonspecific, chronic, and common among Thais and others in South and Southeast Asia.[134] While searching for the most effective antibiotic treatment for cholera in children, Lindenbaum[135] and Karchmer[136] noted that those children in the lowest weight-quartile, who received tetracycline, nonetheless had an increased duration of diarrhea. These differences were small and were not found in children who did not receive tetracycline. Palmer[137] measured the severity and nutritional status prospectively in 97 patients hospitalized for cholera in Dhaka. He noted that the duration but not volume of stool/hour was prolonged by 30–70% in those adults and children suffering from more severe malnutrition. In a prospective family study in Bangladesh, children with chronic malnutrition had no increased risk of infection with V. cholerae 01 or disease compared with children who were well nourished.[58]

6.4. Gastric Acidity

The relationship between the infectious dose and level of gastric acidity was discussed earlier in this chapter. Hypochlorhydria places an individual exposed to V. cholerae 01 at increased risk of disease. Low acid production may be due to malnutrition or gastritis or secondary to gastric surgery or medications that reduce or neutralize stomach acid. The importance of gastric hypoacidity has not only been demonstrated in volunteer studies but also in investigations of cholera epidemics. In Italy, for example, index patients with cholera were 5.8 times more likely to have had a history of gastric surgery than controls ($P < 0.0005$).[10]

6.5. Risks to Family Contacts

In many cholera-infected areas where the level of hygiene is poor, family contacts of cholera cases are at great risk of contracting cholera themselves.[5] This may be due either to sharing of a common exposure (e.g., contaminated water) or to secondary spread of V. cholerae 01 from the index case to other contacts. Appreciation of the high rates of infection among family contacts has led in some instances to recommendations for prophylactic treatment of family contacts. (See Chapter 15.)

In Bangladesh, the incidence of cholera has a secondary peak among women of child-bearing age despite the presence of protective levels of antibody in these women. Both mothers and caretakers of small children may be exposed to an overwhelming inoculum of vibrios by unhygienic practices, e.g., use of a sari to cleanse feces from an infected child, and are at increased risk of cholera.[139]

6.6. Traveler's Diarrhea

Cholera in the nineteenth century was a classic disease of long-distance travelers. In recent years, long-distance travelers from North America and Europe who visit endemic areas have rarely contracted cholera, with a rate on the order of 1 case per 500,000 travelers.[138] This low risk is probably more related to lack of exposure to vibrios in the local environment and to effective hygienic practices by the traveler and not to protection afforded by vaccination.

REFERENCES

1. Pollitizer R: *Cholera.* Monograph No. 43, Geneva, World Health Organization, 1959
2. World Health Organization: *Guidelines for Control of Cholera.* Programme for Control of Diarrhoeal Diseases. WHO CDD SER 80.4 Rev.2, Geneva, 1991
3. Snow J: *Snow on Cholera.* Hafner Publications Co., New York, 1962
4. Koch R: An address on cholera and its bacillus. *Br Med J* 2:403–407, 453–459, 1884
5. Feachem RG: Environmental aspects of cholera epidemiology. III. Transmission and control. *Trop Dis Bull* 79:1–47, 1982
6. Borneside GH: Jaime Ferran and preventive inoculation against cholera. *Bull Hist Med* 55:516–532, 1981
7. Feachem RG: Environmental aspects of cholera epidemiology. II. Occurrence and survival of *Vibrio cholerae* in the environment. *Trop Dis Bull* 78:865–880, 1981
8. Colwell RR, Seidler RJ, Kaper J, Joseph SW, et al: Occurrence of *Vibrio cholerae* serotype 01 in Maryland and Louisiana estuaries. *Appl Environ Microbiol* 42:555–558, 1981
9. Blake PA, Allegra DT, Snyder JD, et al: Cholera-A possible endemic focus in the United States. *N Engl J Med* 302:305–309, 1980
10. Baine WB, Zampieri A, Mazzotti M, et al: Epidemiology of cholera in Italy in 1973. *Lancet* ii:1370–1376, 1974
11. Salamaso S, Greco D, Bonfiglio B, et al: Recurrence of pelecypod-associated cholera in Sardinia. *Lancet* ii:1124–1128, 1980
12. Joseph PR, Tamayo JF, Mosley WH, et al: Studies of cholera El Tor in the Philippines. 2. A retrospective investigation of an explosive outbreak in Bacalod City and Talisay, November 1961. *Bull WHO* 33:637–643, 1965
13. Blake PA, Rosenberg ML, Bandeira Costa J, et al: Cholera in Portugal, 1974. I. Modes of transmission. *Am J Epidemiol* 105:337–343, 1977
14. Pavia AT, Smith JD, Campbell JF, et al: Cholera from raw oysters shipped interstate. *JAMA* 258:2374, 1987
15. Goodgame RW, Greenough WB: Cholera in Africa: A message for the west. *Ann Intern Med* 82:101–106, 1975
16. Stock RF: *Cholera in Africa: Diffusion of the Disease 1970–1975 with Particular Emphasis on West Africa.* African Environmental Special Report 3. London, International African Institute, 1976
17. Sitas F: Some observations on a cholera outbreak at the Umvoti Mission Reserve, Natal. *S Afr Med J* 70:215–218, 1986
18. Mhalu FS, Mtango FDE, Msengi AE: Hospital outbreaks of cholera transmitted through close person-to-person contact. *Lancet* ii:82–84, 1984
19. Felize H: Le development de l'epidemic de cholera en Afrique de l'Ouest. *Bull Soc Pathol Exot* 64:561–586, 1971
20. Cliff JL, Zinkin P, Martell A: A hospital outbreak of cholera in Maputo, Mozambique. *Trans R Soc Trop Med Hyg* 80:473–476, 1986
21. Barua D: The global epidemiology of cholera in recent years. *Proc Soc Med* 65:423–432, 1972
22. Kamal AM: The seventh pandemic of cholera. in Barua D, Burrows W (eds.): *Cholera* Philadelphia, W.B. Saunders Co., 1974, pp 1–14
23. Weissman JB, DeWitt WE, Thompson J, et al: A case of cholera in Texas, 1973. *Am J Epidemiol* 100:487–498, 1974
24. Johnston JM, Martin DL, Perdue J, et al. Cholera on a Gulf Coast oil rig. *New Engl J Med* 309:523–526, 1983
25. Blake PA, Wachsmuth K, Davis BR: Toxigenic *Vibrio cholerae 01* strains from Mexico identical to United States isolates. *Lancet* ii:912, 1983

26. World Health Organization: *Weekly Epidemiol Rep* 1991:55–70
27. Huq MI, Glass RI, Stoll BJ: Epidemiology of cholera. *N Engl J Med* 303:643–644, 1980
28. Shahid NS, Samadi AR, Khan MU, et al: Classical vs. El Tor cholera. A prospective family study of a concurrent outbreak. *J Diarrhoeal Dis Res* 2:73, 1984
29. Institute of Medicine: *New Vaccine Development: Establishing Priorities. Volume II, Diseases of Importance in Developing Countries*. Washington, DC, National Academy Press, 1986
30. Glass RI, Becker S, Huq MI, et al: Endemic cholera in rural Bangladesh. *Am J Epidemiol* 116:959–970, 1982
31. Black RE: The epidemiology of cholera and enterotoxigenic *Escherichia coli* diarrheal disease, in Holmgren J, Lindberg A, Mollby R (eds.): *Development of Vaccines and Drugs against Diarrhea. Eleventh Nobel Conference. Stockholm 1985*. Lund, Sweden, Studentliteratur, 1986, pp 23–32
32. Mahalanabis D, Brayton J, Mondal A, and Pierce NF: The use of Ringer's lactate in the treatment of children with cholera and non-cholera diarrhea. *Bull WHO* 46:311–319, 1972
33. Baqui AH, Yunus M, Zaman K: Community-operated treatment centres prevented many cholera deaths. *J Diarrhoeal Dis Res* 2:92–98, 1984
34. Mandara MP, Mhalu FS: Cholera control in an inaccessible district in Tanzania: Importance of temporary rural centers. *Med J Zambia* 15:10–13, 1980
35. Barua D: Laboratory diagnosis of cholera, in Barua D, Burrows W (eds.): *Cholera*. Philadelphia, WB Saunders, 1974, pp 85–128
36. Mukerjee S, Takeya K: Vibrio-phages and vibriocins, in Barua D, Burrows W (eds.): *Cholera*. Philadelphia, WB Saunders, 1974, pp 61–83
37. Takeya K, Shimodori S, Gomez CZ: Kappa-type phage detection as a method for the tracing of cholera El Tor carriers. *Bull WHO* 37:806–810, 1967
38. Lee JH, Furniss AL: Discussion 1: the phage-typing of *Vibrio cholerae* serovar 01, in Holme T, Holmgren J, Merson MH, Mollby R, (eds.): *Acute Enteric Infections in Children. New Prospects for Treatment and Prevention*. Amsterdam, Elsevier/North Holland, 1981, pp 119–122
39. Mhalu FS, Mmari PW, Ijumga J: Rapid emergence of El Tor *Vibrio cholerae* resistant to antimicrobial agents during first six months of fourth cholera epidemic in Tanzania. *Lancet* i:345–347, 1979
40. Glass RI, Huq MI, Lee JV, et al: Plasmid-borne multiple drug resistance in *Vibrio cholerae* serogroup 01, biotype El Tor: evidence for a point-source outbreak in Bangladesh. *J Infect Dis* 147:204–209, 1983
41. Kaper JB, Bradford HB, Roberts NC, Falkow S: Molecular epidemiology of *Vibrio cholerae* in the U.S. Gulf Coast. *J Clin Microbiol* 16:129–134, 1982
42. Shandera WX, Hafkin B, Martin DL, et al: Persistence of cholera in the United States. *Am J Trop Med Hyg* 32:812–817, 1983
43. Glass RI, Lee JV, Huq MI, et al: Phage types of *Vibrio cholerae* 01 biotype El Tor isolated from patients and family contacts in Bangladesh: epidemiologic implications. *J Infect Dis* 148:998–1004, 1983
44. Finkelstein RA: Vibriocidal antibody inhibition (VA1) analysis: a technique for the identification of the predominant vibriocidal antibodies in serum and for the detection and identification of *Vibrio cholerae* antigens. *J Immunol* 89:264–271, 1962
45. Svennerholm A-M, Holmgren J, Black R, et al: Serologic differentiation between antitoxin responses to infection with *Vibrio cholerae* and enterotoxin-producing *Escherichia coli*. *J Infect Dis* 47:514–522, 1983
46. Svennerholm A-M, Wikstrom M, Lindblad M, and Holmgren J: Monoclonal antibodies to *Escherichia coli* heat labile enterotoxins: neutralizing activity and differentiation of human and porcine LTs and cholera toxin. *Med Biol* 64:23–30, 1986
47. Levine MM, Nalin DR, Craig JP, et al: Immunity of cholera in man: relative role of antibacterial versus toxic immunity. *Trans R Soc Trop Med Hyg* 73:3–9, 1979
48. Sears SD, Richardson K, Young C, et al: Evaluation of the human immune response to outer membrane proteins of *Vibrio cholerae*. *Infect Immun* 44:439–444, 1984
49. Mosley, WH: The role of immunity in cholera: A review of epidemiological and serological studies. *Texas Rev of Biol Med* 27(suppl. 1):227–241, 1969
50. Glass RI, Svennerholm AM, Khan MR, et al: Seroepidemiological studies of El Tor cholera in Bangladesh: implications for vaccine development and field trials. *J Infect Dis* 151:236–242
51. Mosley WH: Epidemiology of cholera, in *Principles and Practice of Cholera Control*. Public Health Papers No. 40. Geneva, World Health Organization, 1970, pp 23–27
52. Harris JR, Holmberg SD, Parker RDR, et al: Impact of epidemic cholera in a previously uninfected island population: Evaluation of a new seroepidemiologic method. *Am J Epidemiol* 123:424–430, 1986
53. Levine MM, Young CR, Hughes TP, et al: Duration of serum antitoxin response following *Vibrio cholerae* infection in North Americans: relevance for seroepidemiology. *Am J Epidemiol* 114:348–354, 1981

54. Snyder JD, Allegra DT, Levine MM, et al: Serologic studies of naturally acquired infection with *Vibrio cholerae* serogroup 01 in the United States. *J Infect Dis* 143:182–187, 1981
55. Clements ML, Levine MM, Young CR, et al: Magnitude, kinetics, and duration of vibriocidal antibody responses in North Americans after ingestion of *Vibrio cholerae*. *J Infect Dis* 145:465–473, 1982
56. Dizon JJ, Fukumi H, Barua D, et al: Studies on cholera carriers. *Bull WHO* 37:737–743, 1967
57. Woodward WE, Moseley WH: The spectrum of cholera in rural Bangladesh. II. Comparison of El Tor Ogawa and classical Inaba infection. *Am J Epidemiol* 96:342–351, 1971
58. Stanton BF, Clemens JD: Soiled saris: a vector of disease transmission. *Trans R Soc Trop Med Hyg* 80:485–488, 1986
59. Glass RI, Greenough WB, Holmgren J, Khan MR: The use of family studies for prospective epidemiologic investigations of cholera, in Kuwahara S, Pierce NF, (eds.): *Advances in Research on Cholera and Related Diarrheas*. Tokyo, KTK Scientific Publishers, 1986, pp 25–33
60. McCormack WM, Chowdhury AM, Gahanger N, et al: Tetracycline prophylaxis in families of cholera patients. *Bull WHO* 38:787–797, 1968
61. Deb BC, Sircar BK, Sengupta PG, et al: Studies on interventions to prevent El Tor cholera transmission in urban slums. *Bull WHO* 64:127–131
62. Barrett TJ, Blake PA, Morris GK, et al: Use of Moore swabs for isolating *Vibrio cholerae* from sewage. *J Clin Microbiol* II:385–388, 1980
63. Spira WM, Ahmed QS: Gauze filtration and enrichment procedures for recovery of *Vibrio cholerae* from contaminated waters. *Appl Environ Microbiol* 42:731–733, 1981
64. Miller CJ, Feachem RG, Drasar BS: Cholera epidemiology in developed and developing countries: New thoughts on transmission, seasonality and control. *Lancet* i:261–263, 1985
65. Dizon JJ: Cholera carriers, in Barua D, Burrows W (eds.): *Cholera*. Philadelphia, WB Saunders, 1974, pp 367–380
66. McCormick WM, Isam MS, Fahimuddin M, et al: A community study of inapparent cholera infections. *Am J Epidemiol* 89:658–664, 1969
67. Pierce NF, Banwell JG, Sack RB, et al: Convalescent carriers of *Vibrio cholerae*. Detection and detailed investigation. *Ann Intern Med* 72:357–364, 1970
68. Azurin JC, Kobari K, Barua D, et al: A long-term carrier of cholera: Cholera Dolores. *Bull WHO* 37:745–749, 1967
69. Miller CJ, Drasar BS, Feachem RG: Cholera and estuarine salinity in Calcutta and London. *Lancet* i:1216–1218, 1982
70. Levine MM, Black RE, Clements ML, et al: Evaluation in humans of attenuated *Vibrio cholerae* El Tor Ogawa strain Texas Star-SR as a live oral vaccine. *Infect Immun* 43:515–522, 1984
71. Nalin DR, Levine RJ, Levine MM, et al: Cholera, non-vibrio cholera, and stomach acid. *Lancet* ii:856–859, 1978
72. Cash RA, Music SI, Libonati JP, et al: Response of man to infection with *Vibrio cholerae*. I. Clinical, serologic, and bacteriologic responses to a known inoculum. *J Infect Dis* 129:45–52, 1974
73. Levine MM, Black RE, Clements ML, et al: Volunteer studies in development of vaccines against cholera and enterotoxigenic *Escherichia coli:* A review, in Holme T, Holmgren J, Merson MH, Mollby R (eds): *Acute Enteric Infections in Children, New Prospects for Treatment and Prevention*. Elsevier/North-Holland Biomedical Press, 1981, pp 443–459
74. Abdou S: Susceptibility to cholera. *Lancet* i:903, 1948
75. Gitelson S: Gastrectomy, achlorhydria and cholera. *Israel J Med Sci* 7:663–667, 1971
76. Sack GH, Pierce NF, Hennessey KN, et al: Gastric acidity in cholera and noncholera diarrhoea. *Bull WHO* 47:31–36, 1972
77. Schiraldi O, Benvestito V, Di Bari C, et al: Gastric abnormalities in cholera: epidemiological and clinical considerations. *Bull WHO* 51:349–352, 1974
78. Thomason H, Burke V, Gracey M: Impaired gastric function in experimental malnutrition. *Am J Clin Nutr* 34:1278–1280, 1981
79. MacDonald WC, Rubin CE: Cancer, benign tumors, gastritis, and other gastric diseases, in Petersdorf RG, Adams RD, Braunwald E, et al (eds): *Harrison's Principles of Internal Medicine*, 10th Edition. New York, McGraw-Hill Book Co., 1983, p 1717
80. Ruddell WSJ, Losowsky MS: Severe diarrhoea due to small intestinal colonisation during cimetidine treatment. *Br Med J* 281:273, 1980
81. Nalin DR, Levine MM, Rhead J, et al: Cannabis, hypochlorhydria, and cholera. *Lancet* ii:859–861, 1978

82. Bart KJ, Huq Z, Khan M, et al: Seroepidemiologic studies during a simultaneous epidemic of infection with El Tor Ogawa and classical Inaba *Vibrio cholerae*. *J Infect Dis* 121:S17–S24, 1970

83. Spira WM, Khan MU, Saeed YA, et al: Microbiological surveillance of intra-neighbourhood El Tor cholera transmission in rural Bangladesh. *Bull WHO* 58:731–740, 1980

84. Pollitzer R: *Cholera*. Geneva, World Health Organization, 1959, pp 820–857

85. Pollitzer R: *Cholera*. Geneva, World Health Organization, 1959, pp 51–56

86. Webber RH, Mwakalukwa J: The epidemiology of cholera in South-West Tanzania. *E Afr Med J* 60:848–856, 1983

87. Khan M, Mosley WH: The role of boatman in the transmission of cholera. *E Pak Med J* 11:61–65, 1967

88. Briscoe J, Ahmed S, Chakraborty M: Domestic water use in a village in Bangladesh, I. A methodology and a preliminary analysis of use patterns during the "cholera season." *Prog Wat Tech* 11:131–141, 1978

89. Hughes JM, Boyce JM, Levine RJ, et al: Epidemiology of El Tor cholera in rural Bangladesh: importance of surface water in transmission. *Bull WHO* 60:395–404, 1982

90. Sommer A, Woodward WE: The influence of protected water supplies on the spread of classical/inaba and El Tor/Ogawa cholera in Rural East Bengal. *Lancet* ii:985–987, 1972

91. Levine RJ, Khan MR, D'Souza S, et al: Failure of sanitary wells to protect against cholera and other diarrhoeas in Bangladesh. *Lancet* ii:86–89, 1976

92. Briscoe J: The role of water supply in improving health in poor countries (with special reference to Bangladesh). *Am J Clin Nutr* 31:2100–2113, 1978

93. Khan M, Mosley WH, Chakraborty J, et al: The relationship of cholera to water source and use in rural Bangladesh. *Int J Epidemiol* 10:23–25, 1981

94. Briscoe J: Intervention studies and the definition of dominant transmission routes. *Am J Epidemiol* 120:449–455, 1984

95. Deb BC, Sircar BK, Sengupta PG, et al: Intra-familial transmission of *Vibrio cholerae* biotype El Tor in Calcutta slums. *Ind J Med Res* 76:814–819, 1982

96. Azurin JC, Alvero M: Field evaluation of environmental sanitation measures against cholera. *Bull WHO* 51:19–26, 1974

97. Rogers RC, Cuffe RGCJ, Cossins YM, et al: The Queensland cholera incident of 1977. 2. The epidemiological investigation. *Bull WHO* 58:665–669, 1980

98. Glass RI, Alim ARMA, Eusof A, et al: Cholera in Indonesia: Epidemiologic studies of transmission in Aceh Province. *Am J Trop Med Hyg* 33:933–939, 1984

99. Blake PA, Rosenberg ML, Florencia J, et al: Cholera in Portugal, 1974. II. Transmission by bottled mineral water. *Am J Epidemiol* 105:344–348, 1977

100. Pollitzer R: *Cholera*. Geneva, World Health Organization, 1959, pp 857–862

101. Dutt AK, Alwi S, Velauthan T: A shellfish-borne cholera outbreak in Malaysia. *Trans R Soc Trop Med Hyg* 65:815–818, 1971

102. Cohen J, Schwartz T, Klasmer R, et al: Epidemiological aspects of cholera El Tor outbreak in a non-endemic area. *Lancet* ii:86–89, 1971

103. Sutton RGA: An outbreak of cholera in Australia due to food served in flight on an international aircraft. *J Hyg* 72:441–451, 1974

104. Merson MH, Martin WT, Craig JP, et al: Cholera on Guam, 1974: Epidemiologic findings and isolation of non-toxinogenic strains. *Am J Epidmiol* 105:349–361, 1977

105. McIntrye RC, Tira T, Flood T, et al: Modes of transmission of cholera in a newly infected population on an atoll: implications for control measures. *Lancet* i:311–314, 1979

106. Kuberski T, Flood T, Tera T, et al: Cholera in the Gilbert Islands. I. Epidemiological features. *Am J Trop Med Hyg* 28:677–684, 1979

107. Goh KT, Lam S, Kumarapathy S, et al: A common source foodborne outbreak of cholera in Singapore. *Int J Epidemiol* 13:210–215, 1984

108. Holmberg SD, Harris JR, Kay DE, et al: Foodborne transmission of cholera in Micronesian households. *Lancet* i:325–327, 1984

109. Gunn RA, Kimball AM, Pollard RA, et al: Bottle feeding as a risk factor for cholera in infants. *Lancet* ii:730–732, 1979

110. Gunn RA, Kimball AM, Mathew PP, et al: Cholera in Bahrain: epidemiological characteristics of an outbreak. *Bull WHO* 59:61–66, 1981

111. Glass RI, Svennerholm A-M, Stoll BJ, et al: Protection against cholera in breast-fed children by antibodies in breast milk. *New Engl J Med* 308:1389–1392, 1983

112. Black RE, Brown KH, Becker S, et al: Contamination of weaning foods and transmission of enterotoxigenic *Escherichia coli* diarrhoea in children in rural Bangladesh. *Trans R Soc Trop Med Hyg* 76:259–264, 1982

113. Pan American Health Organization: Epidemiol Bull 12:1–12, 1991

114. Khan MU, Shahidullah M, Ahmed WU, et al: The El Tor cholera epidemic in Dhaka in 1974 and 1975. *Bull WHO* 61:653–659, 1983

115. Oseasohn RS, Ahmad S, Islan M, et al: Clinical and bacteriological findings among families of cholera patients. *Lancet* i:340–342, 1966

116. Bart KJ, Huq Z, Khan M, et al: Seroepidemiologic studies during a simultaneous epidemic of infection with El Tor Ogawa and classical Inaba *Vibrio cholerae*. *J Infect Dis* 121:S17–S24, 1970

117. Tamayo JF, Mosley WH, Alvero MG, et al: Studies of cholera El Tor in the Philippines. 3. Transmission of infection among household contacts of cholera patients. *Bull WHO* 33:645–649, 1965

118. Kuberski T: Cholera on Nauru: possible non-point source transmission. *Med J Aust* 2:563–566, 1980

119. Dobin A, Felix H: Du role de la sueur dans l'epidemiologie du cholera en pays sec. *Bull Acad Natl Med (Paris)* 156:845–852, 1972

120. Isaacson M, Clarke KR, Ellacombe GH, et al: The recent cholera outbreak in the South African gold mining industry: A preliminary report. *S Afr Med J* 48:2557–2560, 1974

121. Isaacson M, Smit P: The survival and transmission of *V. cholerae* in an artificial tropical environment. *Prog Water Tech* 11:89–96, 1979

122. Abrutyn E, Gangarosa E, Forrest J, et al: Cholera in a vaccinated American: Immunological response to vaccination and disease. *Ann Intern Med* 74:228–231, 1971

123. Ryder RW, Mizanur Rahman ASM, Alim ARMA: An outbreak of nosocomial cholera in a rural Bangladesh hospital. *J Hosp Inf* 8:275–282, 1986

124. Pollitzer R: *Cholera*. Geneva, World Health Organization, 1959, pp 862–863

125. Pollitzer R: *Cholera*. Geneva, World Health Organization, 1959, pp 863–865

126. Gangarosa EJ, Mosley WH: Epidemiology and surveillance of cholera, in Barua D, Burrows W. (eds.): *Cholera*. Philadelphia, W.B. Saunders, 1974

127. Barua D, Paguio AS: ABO blood groups and cholera. *Ann Human Biol* 4:489–492, 1977

128. Chandhuri A: Cholera and blood-group. *Lancet* ii:404–405, 1977

129. Levine MM, Nalin DR, Rennels MB, et al: Genetic susceptibility to cholera. *Ann Hum Biol* 6:369–374, 1979

130. Glass RI, Holmgren J, Haley CE, et al: Predisposition for cholera of individuals with O blood group: possible evolutionary significance. *Am J Epidemiol* 121:791–796, 1985

131. Glass RI, Stoll BJ, Wyatt RG, et al: Observations questioning a protective role for breast-feeding in severe rotavirus diarrhea. *Acta Paediatr Scand* 75:713–718, 1986

132. Rosenberg IH, Greenough WB, Lindenbaum J, Gordon RS: Nutritional studies in cholera, in *Proceedings of the Cholera Research Symposium (Jan. 24–29, 1965, Honolulu)*. PHS Publication No. 1328, Washington, DC, U.S. Government Printing Office

133. Gangarosa EJ, Beisel WR, Benyajati C, et al: The nature of the gastrointestinal lesion in Asiatic cholera and its relation to pathogenesis. A biopsy study. *Am J Trop M* 9:125–135, 1960

134. Sprinz H, Sribbhibhadh R, Gangarosa EJ, et al: Biopsy of small bowel of Thai people with special reference to recovery from Asiatic cholera and to an internal malabsorption syndrome. *Am J Clin Pathol* 38:43–51, 1962

135. Lindenbaum J, Greenough WB, Islam MR: Antibiotic therapy of cholera in children. *Bull WHO* 37:529–538, 1967

136. Karchner AW, Curlin GT, Huq MI, Hirschhorn N: Furazolidone in pediatric cholera. *Bull WHO* 43:373–378, 1970

137. Palmer DL, Koster AK, Alam MT, and Islam MR: Nutritional status: a determinant of the severity of diarrhea in patients with cholera. *J Infect Dis* 134:8–14, 1976

138. Snyder JD, Blake PA: Is cholera a problem for U.S. travelers? *JAMA* 247:2268–2269, 1982

8

Cholera Enterotoxin (Choleragen)
A Historical Perspective

Richard A. Finkelstein

An important scientific innovation rarely makes its way by gradually winning over and converting its opponents: it rarely happens that Saul becomes Paul. What does happen is that its opponents gradually die out and that the growing generation is familiarized with the idea from the beginning.

Max Planck
The Philosophy of Physics [1936]

1. KOCH'S POSTULATES

Slightly over a century ago, during the period from 1883 to 1885, Robert Koch summarized his masterful studies on the etiology of cholera in a series of reports[1-8] which presented the first convincing evidence that a particular distinctive microorganism, which he isolated in pure culture and called "comma-bacillus" (now known as *Vibrio cholerae* O group 1), was:

1. Consistently present during the disease (chiefly in the intestines and the dejecta of the victims)

The cholera enterotoxin (now enterotoxins) was hypothesized in 1884, discovered in 1959, recognized in 1962, and purified in 1969—eighty-five years after its conception. It has since "fathered" an ever-increasing number of cholera toxin-related enterotoxins. The literature has become voluminous—especially if one considers the many applications of cholera toxin, because of its broad spectrum of biologic effects, in research unrelated to cholera. In keeping with the editors' charge, the author, who has been involved in cholera research since 1952, will not attempt an all-encompassing review, but will rather try to point out the highlights so that "*the growing generation may be familiar with the idea from the beginning.*" In an effort to reduce citations to the essential minimum, a large number of references which are primarily confirmatory, slight modifications of existing information, irrelevant, or incorrect have intentionally been omitted. The author apologizes, in advance, to those authors not directly cited who feel, correctly or not, that their omitted contribution was one of those highlights. More comprehensive reviews are cited in the text.

Cholera, edited by Dhiman Barua and William B. Greenough III. Plenum Medical Book Company, New York, 1992.

2. Not found in the environment, other than in association with cholera patients

3. Routinely able to cause in guinea pigs, inoculated intraduodenally with *in vitro*-grown pure cultures, a process analogous to cholera in man

4. Present in (practically) pure culture in the small intestine of the diseased guinea pigs

and, thus, satisfied the four criteria of etiology, "Koch's Postulates," which he had established in his studies on anthrax and tuberculosis.[9] [In the course of these investigations, Koch demonstrated the bactericidal and protective effect of gastric acid (which could be neutralized by carbonate of soda) and the protective effect of peristaltic movement (which could be inhibited by tincture of opium, thus allowing the comma-bacilli to remain longer and gain a footing in the intestine of an unnatural host). He also deduced that convalescents from cholera had acquired a degree of immunity. Although he noted that there were examples of individual cholera cases who were attacked again in a later epidemic, he also observed that "it is often seen that, when a place has been attacked by cholera, and been thoroughly infected by it, this place is often spared the next year, or it only suffers slightly, when the cholera returns."]

2. KOCH'S FIFTH POSTULATE

In 1884, Koch proposed:

> That comma-bacilli produce a special poison, the effect of which shows itself partly in an immediate manner, the epithelium, and in the worst cases also the upper layers of the mucus membrane, being mortified thereby; it is partly reabsorbed and acts on the organism as a whole, but especially on the organs of circulation, which are as it were paralysed. The complex of symptoms of the attack proper of cholera, which is generally looked upon as a consequence of loss of water and the inspissation of the blood, is, according to my opinion, to be regarded essentially as a poisoning.[7]

He also alluded, in the same paper, to studies of "Mr. Richards, a medical man at Goalundo, in India,"[7] who fed some dogs large quantities of cholera dejecta without producing any effects. He then did the same experiment in pigs, which died in cramps a very short time after being fed. Koch concluded that this was a case of poisoning and not artificial cholera infection, because the contents of the intestines of a pig, killed by being fed on cholera dejecta, did not affect a second pig. "If genuine cholera could be produced amongst pigs, it would then be possible to infect a second pig with the contents of the intestine of the first, and a third with those from the second, and so on."[7]

Although the time of onset of symptoms in the pigs was suspiciously short, Mr. Richards's could have been the first demonstration of the cholera enterotoxin, which waited [patiently (?)] for three quarters of a century to be discovered. In fact, in 1959, the year of the "discovery" of cholera enterotoxin (independently and practically simultaneously) by two groups of Indian investigators, Pollitzer's encyclopedic summation of the cholera literature concluded that "the cholera vibrio does not secrete a true soluble exotoxin," that "Koch erred when assuming that the cholera vibrios produced an exotoxin," and that "it is generally accepted that the intestinal manifestations of cholera are due to the action of the *endotoxin* [*emphasis added*] of *V. cholerae*.[10]

3. THE "DRY YEARS"

In the "dry years" which intervened between the enunciation of "Koch's Fifth Postulate" and the discoveries of cholera enterotoxin, investigations using cholera vibrios yielded many observations which were fundamental to the evolving subdisciplines of microbiology and immunology, but are not particularly germane to the present chapter on cholera toxin. These included the discovery, by Pfeiffer, of the "Pfeiffer phenomenon," the immobilization and lysis of cholera vibrios in the peritoneum of guinea pigs previously immunized with killed cholera vibrios, which in turn led to the discovery of complement. Using *V. cholerae*, Pfeiffer was also the first to recognize heat-stable (lipopolysaccharide) endotoxin. And the phenomenon of specific bacterial agglutination by antibody was discovered through studies with cholera vibrios and typhoid bacilli. Although experimental animal models were introduced which were subsequently to prove useful in the discoveries of cholera toxin, the cholera toxin–related enterotoxins,* and other enterotoxins, and in their isolation and characterization, little (if any) enduring information directly pertinent to the subject of this chapter emerged in the 75 dry years—in this sense, the years were largely wasted.

The reason(s) why cholera enterotoxin was not discovered earlier is (are) not entirely clear. van Heyningen and Seal[11] considered that Koch's intimation that "the poison is partly reabsorbed and acts on the organism as a whole, but especially on the organs of circulation" inhibited the recognition of cholera toxin, by misdirecting subsequent investigators into seeking a poison which would act following parenteral rather than enteral administration. Indeed, the ensuing literature [see Pollitzer[10]] is full of irrelevant observations by innumerable investigators, who caused the death of a wide variety of experimental animals inoculated by various parenteral routes with various products of cholera vibrios and with the vibrios themselves, a reflection predominantly of their endotoxin content, as discovered earlier by Pfeiffer. In addition, the dogma (now obviously false) that, with the possible exception of the "neurotoxin" of the *Shiga* bacillus, gram-negative bacteria did not elaborate exotoxins may have had an inhibiting effect. To this reviewer, however, what was lacking was the recognition and the simultaneous demonstration that a suitable experimental animal model would respond with *diarrhea* (the cardinal manifestation of cholera) following the *enteral* administration of an appropriate cholera toxin–containing preparation. The use of the enteral route was of cardinal importance because that is the way by which cholera vibrios, which are not invasive, are obliged to deliver the toxin to the host. As we shall see, although the models were available, and the concept probably was at various times, not all cultures of *V. cholerae* produce sufficient cholera toxin to be detectable in animal models. The two conditions came together first in 1959.

4. THE "DISCOVERIES" OF CHOLERA ENTEROTOXIN

In 1959, two separate groups of investigators in India practically simultaneously reported the production of relevant symptoms, viz., diarrhea or outpouring of fluid into the lumen of the gut, in experimental animal models following the enteral administration of sterile cell-free products of cholera vibrios. S.N. De, a pathologist in Calcutta, in a note that appeared in the May 30 issue of *Nature,*[12] demonstrated that sterile filtrates of two Ogawa and two Inaba serotype *V. cholerae* strains grown in 5% peptone, 0.5% NaCl broth, pH 7.6, caused outpouring of fluid and distension of surgically isolated ileal loops in adult rabbits. Filtrates of the same strains grown in Dunham's (1%) peptone water medium were inactive. De used the word "enterotoxicity" to describe the activity. He also mentioned histo-

---

*Cholera toxin's relatives have frequently been called "cholera-like toxins," a misnomer in that they are not like cholera but like cholera *toxin*. This reviewer has been guilty of the same offense in the past, but it is time to be more correct.

pathological changes, including denudation of distended loops, which are now known to be artifacts produced by ischemia in the closed loop system. False-positive reactions occasionally encountered in control loops in the rabbit ileal loop model were attributed by De[13] to the use of loops shorter than four inches, or to too-rapid injection of samples. At the beginning of his work with live *V. cholerae*,[14] enteropathogenic *Escherichia coli*,[15] and *V. cholerae* culture filtrates, De was unaware that the experimental model had been introduced earlier, most notably by Violle and Crendiropoulo in 1915.[10,16] Subsequently, De and his colleagues[17,18] produced evidence dissociating the enterotoxicity from other factors (e.g., mucinase, lecithinase-C, and receptor-destroying enzyme) which had been described earlier, and also indicated that "somatic filtrate" of bacterial bodies had little or no activity.

Meanwhile, N.K. Dutta, a pharmacologist at the Haffkine Institute in Bombay, and his colleagues reported, in a note submitted in February, 1959 which appeared in the October issue of the *Journal of Bacteriology*,[19] that they could produce fatal choleraic diarrhea in infant rabbits fed multiple doses of sterile lysates of dense suspensions of *V. cholerae* strain 569B Inaba after gastric lavage. This strain had been used by Dutta earlier[20] to cause choleraic diarrhea in infant rabbits inoculated intraintestinally with live vibrios. In the earlier study, the virulence of the strain was found to have been enhanced following its reisolation from the heart blood of a dead infected infant rabbit. The derived strain caused fatal diarrhea in 100% of infant rabbits inoculated with 10^3 viable organisms. (In all probability, Dutta, by this procedure, succeeded in isolating a smooth virulent variant from a population of vibrios which had become degraded to become predominantly serologically rough and avirulent, following repeated serial passages in artificial culture media in the laboratory over a long period of time. In the author's experience, cholera vibrios freshly isolated from patients are invariably virulent in Dutta's model and retain this property when preserved by lyophilization.) It turns out that 569B is an exceptionally good strain for producing the cholera enterotoxin (CT) [it is now universally used for that purpose by laboratories that produce substantial quantities of CT, like the PW-8 strain of *Corynebacterium diphtheriae* is for production of diphtheria toxin], but the method used by Dutta to extract it is exceptionally poor. Additionally, because the preparations used by Dutta were rich in endotoxic lipopolysaccharide, he tended to equate the enterotoxic activity with the endotoxin.

The two groups, De's and Dutta's, were intensely competitive for a time—each maintaining that their's was the only truly relevant model for cholera. In fact, over ten years later the validity of Dutta's model was challenged by De's group,[21] which claimed that the large amount of fluid that soils the ventral surface of choleraic infant rabbit was urinary rather than intestinal in origin, a notion that was rendered untenable by a subsequent study.[22]

5. THE "RECOGNITION" OF CHOLERA ENTEROTOXIN

This author's interest in cholera began in 1952 with his doctoral research, conducted at the University of Texas, Austin, under the guidance of Professor Charles E. Lankford, which culminated in 1955 with the development of a completely chemically defined culture medium that permitted luxurious growth (to 2×10^{10} viable cells/ml) from small inocula of recently isolated *V. cholerae* strains.[23,24] After a postdoctoral interlude, that interest was rekindled in 1958 when he took a position as a civilian scientist at the Walter Reed Army Institute of Research (WRAIR) in Washington, D.C. When, practically simultaneously, cholera broke out in Bangkok, Thailand, his administrative superiors indicated that if he would work again on cholera he would be sent to Bangkok to collect specimens and perform studies. He kept his part of the bargain, but they did not, and he was not sent to Southeast Asia until El Tor biotype cholera broke out in the Philippines in 1961, early in the present pandemic.

His first years at WRAIR resulted in a rapid diagnostic test for cholera[25,26]; a series of publications on nonspecific resistance and experimental *V. cholerae* infections in chick embryos[27,28]; the introduction of an assay system for complement-dependent vibriocidal antibody in serum of cholera convalescents and vaccinees[29]; and the recognition of the cell-associated hemagglutinin of *V. cholerae* biotype El Tor,[30] which were not directly pertinent to the subject of this chapter. A part of the time was spent, futilely, trying to develop a reliable and reproducible system for infecting infant rabbits (Dutta's model) with *V. cholerae* by the oral route. [The reason that this does not result uniformly or predictably in infection is still not clear, but may relate to observations of H. Williams Smith[31] on the antimicrobial activity of infant rabbit stomach contents.]

The light dawned when the author first saw cholera patients, practically devoid of vital signs on admission, sitting up happily an hour later after rapid and vigorous intravenous fluid therapy, which had been introduced and championed by (U.S.) Navy Captain Robert Allan (Bob) Phillips[32] and his Naval Medical Research Unit (NAMRU) team in the San Lazaro Hospital in Manila. The patients continued to stool at a rate of ten or more liters a day for three or more days without any systemic manifestations, provided they were properly hydrated. *There must be a cholera toxin. It should be secreted by the vibrios. And, it must act locally. The 1959 observations of De and Dutta may indeed be relevant.*

Work on this exciting prospect was delayed and interrupted, however, while the author finished studies initiated in the Philippines,[26,33] and went to Calcutta in the summer of 1962 to continue efforts applying the vibriocidal antibody assay to detect *V. cholerae* somatic antigen[34] and to investigate the presence of the cell-associated *V. cholerae* hemagglutinin in classical biotype strains.[30] During the Indian visit his interest in the potential of Dutta's model was reinforced by seeing it utilized in Dutta's laboratory at the Haffkine Institute. In the autumn of 1962, Dutta visited WRAIR and Chicago to work, briefly, with Dr. Samuel Formal (chief of the author's department at WRAIR) and Dr. William Burrows (University of Chicago). Dutta and Formal were primarily trying to evaluate the activity of Dutta's sonic lysates of vibrios in De's ileal loop model, which Formal had used[35] to dispel the notion advanced by Jenkin and Rowley[36] that the outpouring of fluid in De's infected ileal loops was the result of lactic acid, mucinase, and endotoxin acting in concert. During Dutta's visit, however, a collaborative effort resulted in a brief presentation which showed that, while both live *V. cholerae* and Dutta's lysates produced experimental cholera in infant rabbits, purified *V. cholerae* endotoxin did not.[37] Endotoxin was thus ruled out (at least) as the sole factor responsible for the experimental choleraic diarrhea. The results were presented by Norris, a pathologist, who had done the histopathology on the intestines of the baby rabbits prepared in the author's laboratory.

Following Dutta's departure, Formal, still unable to reproduce De's findings that *V. cholerae* culture filtrates would produce positive ileal loops,[11] discontinued those studies to return to his enduring interest in the pathogenic mechanisms of *Shigellae*. The author then proceeded to evaluate his presumption that Dutta's infant rabbit model was a useful tool but that Dutta was looking in the wrong place for the active principle: it should be in the culture supernatants and not in the bodies of the vibrios. The first experiment to test the hypothesis was successful: sterile filtrates of shaken brain–heart infusion broth cultures of *V. cholerae* strain 569B (Dutta's "rabbit-passaged" strain) produced fatal choleraic diarrhea following perioral administration in infant rabbits. Not only that, the filtrates were active in a single dose, instead of the multiple doses used by Dutta, and were still active after dilution.[38] The supernatants were clearly a better source of the choleragenic principle, which was called "choleragen,"* than the bodies of the vibrios. Viewed retrospectively, several components of the successful experiment were fortuitous. The choice of strain 569B, while a rational one to provide continuity and comparison to Dutta's observations, was lucky since virtually all other strains produce less toxin, and some other virulent strains (as noted[38]) failed to produce active filtrates under the same conditions. Brain–heart infusion broth was selected as a rich, complex medium which provides luxuriant growth of *V. cholerae,* especially (from the author's earlier dissertation research) when the cultures are aerated by shaking. Had another medium or culture condition been selected, the results might not have been so encouraging. In fact, choleragen was not detected in filtrates of cultures grown in the completely defined basal medium which was the subject of the author's dissertation research, although it was produced when the synthetic medium was supplemented with casamino acids ("syncase medium"),[38] which seems to be optimal and is still used universally for production of cholera toxin. It is also providential that cholera vibrios do secrete most of their toxin into the culture medium, a property that is not as well expressed by other diarrheagenic enteropathogens which produce cholera toxin–related enterotoxins. The first indications that the cholera enterotoxin was immunogenic were also summarized in the same paper,[38] which was submitted in October, 1963. Dutta, who was not present during the experimental work, was included as an author,[38] at Formal's insistence, because of the stimulus his model had provided to the work.

Adsorption of antisera against choleragen with living vibrios did not remove their neutralizing activity, again indicating that the vibrios themselves did not contain much of the toxin.[39] This procedure also generated adsorbed sera which gave only a single precipitin band in Ouchterlony tests with concentrated mixtures containing choleragen,[39] an observation that would prove useful subsequently in the purification of the enterotoxin to homogeneity and in the recognition of another product, "choleragenoid." This product would later provide essential insight into the structure, function, and immunology of what was to be recognized as the prototype among the families of enzymatically active bipartite toxins.

Meanwhile, the 1958 outbreak of cholera in Thailand (which had subsided by 1960) and the subsequent emergence in 1961 of pandemic cholera caused by the El Tor biotype, manifest overtly first in Hong Kong and then the Philippines (and subsequently in much of the rest of the world, including Southeast Asia, Africa, Europe and North America), had stimulated an explosion of interest in basic and clinical research on the pathogenesis, immunology, and therapy of cholera, which had previously been restricted to a relatively few laboratories in the world. This in turn resulted in an information explosion, a great deal of rapid progress, and an equal, if not greater, accumulation of background noise and confusion. The list of investigators who entered the field would be a lengthy one indeed, the list of those whose contributions have been enduring and central is far shorter.

For some insight into the process, the interested reader might examine the *Proceedings of the SEATO Conference on Cholera,*[40] held in the "pre-toxin era" in Dacca, East Pakistan (now Bangladesh) in December, 1960 [at which neither De nor Dutta were present (perhaps for reasons of international politics at the time) and, even more significantly, at which their works were not even mentioned], which focused on intestinal histopathology, renal pathophysiology, fluid replacement therapy, epidemiology, laboratory diagnosis, classical vaccines, and (even) the possible involvement of viruses in the etiology of cholera and

---

*A term synonymous with cholera enterotoxin and now included in medical dictionaries.

compare the contents with those of a similar meeting in Hawaii[41] less than five years later, and with subsequent reviews.[11,42-50] The chapter on cholera "toxins" in the previous edition of this volume,[43] published in 1974, concluded that there were three general kinds of cholera toxins: endotoxins, heat-labile exotoxins, and heat-stable exotoxins. The heat-labile exotoxins were considered to be present in a dissociable complex of enterotoxic and permeability factor (PF) activities (*see below*).

We perhaps added to the confusion, temporarily, with an erroneous interpretation of reproducible observations. When choleragen preparations were subjected to dialysis, the diarrheagenic activity (which was demonstrated to be heat labile) remained within the sac when the choleragen had been prepared in the complex brain–heart infusion broth, but not when sonicate of vibrios or syncase medium had been used. In the latter instances, activity was fully restored by adding back the diffusate (which was heat stable). We postulated the requirement, under certain cultural conditions, for two factors: "procholeragen A" (choleragen), which remained inside the sac; and "procholeragen B", which, it soon turned out,[51] was simply buffer that was required (and was present, probably as large proteins, in sufficient amount in the complex medium) to protect choleragen against destruction in the acid conditions of the stomach of baby rabbits. As few, if any, people were paying much attention to our observations at the time (see van Heyningen and Seal[11]), the misinterpretation had no lasting effect; but, in retrospect, we should also have tested the diffusate of control medium (a point which was also overlooked by the editors of the journal).

Results of the innumerable other studies in the mid-1960s using various experimental animal models and systems were, with few notable exceptions, more distracting than contributory of significant or enduring positive effects on the progress of research on cholera toxin *per se,* and will not be summarized here. (The reader desirous of further information is invited to more comprehensive summaries.[42-50]) The observations by Panse and Dutta[52] that choleragenic activity for infant rabbits could be found in stool filtrates of cholera patients, and those of Chanyo Benyajati,[53] obtained in March, 1964, that choleragen prepared in syncase medium caused a choleralike syndrome in adult Thai volunteers,* were stimulatory in suggesting that we were on the right track but, in retrospect, were not essential. More important observations on the subunit structure and mechanism of action were to come later.

Some mention must be made, however, of the observations of John Craig, who in 1965 reported[54,55] that 13 of 20 filtrates of stools of acute cholera patients produced a characteristic delayed, sustained, edematous induration, which was permeable to and delineated by pontamine sky blue 6XB dye, in the skin of rabbits or guinea pigs following intracutaneous inoculation. No induration was produced by filtrates from diarrhea cases from whom *V. cholerae* was not isolated. The same skin reaction was evoked by filtrates of *V. cholerae* cultures grown in De's 5% peptone medium. Sera from cholera convalescents neutralized the reactivity. Although Craig noted similarities (*e.g.,* medium and growth conditions and heat lability) to the enterotoxin of De, which suggested possible identity, he called the factor

---

*Subsequently, when purified cholera toxin became available, a similar experiment was performed by Levine *et al.*,[47] who found that 5 μg pure CT (administered with cimetidine and $NaHCO_3$ to reduce gastric acidity) caused between 1–6 L of diarrhea (5–33 loose stools) in 5 out of 6 American volunteers, whereas 25 μg CT caused over 20 L of diarrheal stools (47–50 loose stools), over the course of 31–94 hours, with an incubation period ranging from 5–13 hours. With his crude preparations, Dr. Chanyo had fortuitously bracketed the minimal effective dose and the maximal response dose in two Thai volunteers. This reviewer, who participated in that study with Dr. Chanyo and suggested the doses based on his experience in infant rabbits, was not allowed to be a co-author by the then-Director of WRAIR.

"skin-toxin" and cautiously indicated that at present "there is no evidence that the skin-toxin plays a part in the morbid sequence of cholera in man." It is of interest to note that Craig approached this work from his background of prior experience[54] with toxins of *Clostridia spp.*, which do cause skin reactions when injected intracutaneously, "although in natural infection with these organisms skin damage is never primary. . . The absence of skin lesions in clinical cholera certainly does not preclude the possibility that the noxa responsible for gut damage could also have a deleterious effect upon skin provided it is applied to skin in sufficient concentration."[54] Although he was correct in his assumption, and various modifications of his assay system for "skin-toxin" [later called "permeability factor" (PF)] and its antibody have subsequently been widely used for detection and titration of the cholera enterotoxin and the related enterotoxins, for some time confusion reigned over the question of the identity of "skin-toxin" with the cholera enterotoxin. This was finally resolved when the latter was isolated to homogeneity exclusively by virtue of its enterotoxicity in Dutta's model and shown to be exquisitely reactive in skin as well.[56] Part of the problem lay in the fact that much less enterotoxin is required to produce a skin reaction than is required to produce diarrhea. Thus, preparations which were active in skin were frequently not sufficiently concentrated to be enterotoxic.

6. ISOLATION AND PURIFICATION OF CHOLERA ENTEROTOXIN

In comparison with "older," more established classical toxins, such as the diphtheria, tetanus, and botulinus toxins, progress in the isolation and characterization of the cholera enterotoxin was much more rapid because of technological developments (e.g., ion exchange and gel filtration chromatography and membrane ultrafiltration) which had been introduced in time to be applied to the cholera problem (although, as we see later, an immunological solution to the cholera problem is still more elusive). The toxin was first isolated to homogeneity, as reported[56] in 1969, using a sequence involving $(NH_4)_2SO_4$ precipitation, ion exchange chromatography, and Agarose A-5m and Sephadex G-75 gel filtration of culture supernatants of *V. cholerae* strain 569 B grown in syncase medium in 10 L fermentors. The purification was monitored both by bioassays in suckling rabbits and immunoassays by the Ouchterlony technique. The latter procedure used antiserum prepared against crude choleragen and adsorbed with live vibrios, leaving a single antigen–antibody precipitin band (with crude choleragen), which was assumed (correctly) to represent the toxin–antitoxin reaction. [Later, it would become possible to produce specific antisera to the isolated protein[57] and to its component subunit proteins.[58]] Interestingly, at the final stage of purification (gel filtration on Sephadex G-75) two peaks reactive with the adsorbed serum were obtained: the first, the larger molecular weight species, was choleragenic in infant rabbits—it was the "choleragen"; the second, an apparently smaller protein, was not. This second peak was called "choleragenoid," and was later to be identified as the natural oligomer of the B-subunits of this bipartite toxin, which is responsible for its binding to a specific glycolipid host (or target) cell-membrane receptor. This was a fortuitous, rather than imaginative, choice of nomenclature,[58] since the protein was originally called "B" simply because it was the second peak to emerge from a gel filtration separation of dissociated toxin. The first peak, having been called "A," was subsequently recognized as the enzymatically active subunit. For some time choleragen and choleragenoid were mistakenly considered to be immunologically identical[59] because of the relatively low antigenicity of the A subunit in the holotoxin.

The purification was also, in a sense, fortuitous in its dependence on the unique property of choleragen and choleragenoid of interacting mildly with Agarose, thus, being retarded in their elution from Agarose gel columns, and, thus, being separated from similarly sized proteins that behaved normally in this menstruum. This property, which we shall see is even more exaggerated in some of the cholera toxin–related enterotoxins, finally enabled their purification after a frustrating interval following their first recognition.

Purified choleragen had the highest specific activity in Craig's permeability factor assay, thus, finally establishing the unitarian hypothesis that both skin reactivity and choleragenicity or enterotoxicity were properties of the same molecule,[56] as are an enormous number of other biological effects which have since been demonstrated. [See Finkelstein[44] and Bennett and Cuatrecasas,[60] for partial summaries.] Perhaps its recent, and unexpected, use to promote the *in vitro* growth of epidermal cells for transplantation in burn victims merits special mention.[61,62]

Although the relationship between choleragen and choleragenoid was not yet clear, the authors postulated in 1969 that

> if choleragenoid is a precursor of choleragen, it might be possible to isolate a stable mutant, which one might predict would be incapable of causing cholera, and which could potentially provide the ideal immunizing agent—a living attenuated vibrio, capable of multiplication in the gut and stimulation of both antibacterial and antitoxic immunity at the important local level.[56]

It would take nearly a decade before such a mutant A^-B^+ strain, called Texas Star, could be isolated and tested.[63,64] And then, although the principle was (is) sound, in practice it would not prove so simple: evaluation of the mutant vaccine candidate revealed that although synthesis of the complete cholera enterotoxin is essential for the causation of the severe diarrhea of cholera, the cholera vibrios have additional mechanisms for causing diarrhea (of a smaller magnitude). One might conclude that the main goal in life of cholera vibrios, in addition to making more cholera vibrios, is to cause diarrhea—it certainly seems to be a highly preserved capability. This would also prove true with subsequent genetically engineered *tox*⁻ and A^-B^+ mutants.[65] The diarrhea caused by the mutant candidate vaccines in volunteers, although certainly milder than true cholera, is considered sufficient to make them unacceptable for use on a large scale. There is still hope, however, in that earlier a mutant (M13) of strain 569B, originally considered to be nontoxigenic[66] but subsequently shown to be hypotoxinogenic, did produce immunity without side effects against challenge with the virulent parent strain in volunteers.[67] However, M13 was considered to be capable of reversion to toxicity and was not used further. (See Chapter 4 for a discussion of recent observations with genetically engineered mutants of *V. cholerae* strain 569B.)

The procedures for purification of choleragen and choleragenoid were subsequently refined and modified by ourselves and others.[68–71] The availability of purified toxin, in the largest measure distributed to individuals by our laboratory and through our contracts with N.I.H. and subsequently with industry, greatly accelerated the development of our understanding of its structure and mode of action (see Sections 7 and 8).

7. PROPERTIES OF THE CHOLERA ENTEROTOXINS

The essential chemical and physical properties of the choleragen and choleragenoid molecules were summarized in 1972[72] and both proteins were crystallized for the first time the same year.[73] The toxin was reported to have a 82,000–84,000 mol.wt., whereas choleragenoid was approximately 57,000–58,000 mol.wt., as determined by sedimentation velocity/diffusion and sedimentation equilibrium measurements.[72] These values differed from previous approximations[56] because of the atypical behavior of the proteins in gel filtration. Extinction coefficients ($E_{1cm}^{1\%}$ 280 nm) of 11.41 for choleragen and 9.56 for choleragenoid were established, and pI values of pH 6.60 for choleragen and 7.58–7.75 for choleragenoid were also established, as was the presence of disulfide bonds (5–6 in choleragen and 4–5 in choleragenoid).[72] The proteins were reversibly dissociable at low pH (ca. pH 3.6), and were free of detectable lipid and carbohydrate.

The presence in choleragen of a unique 28,000 mol.wt. fragment, not found in choleragenoid, had been demonstrated[74] in 1972, but the significance of this observation was not entirely clear until the proteins were dissociated (in urea at low pH) into their separate A and B subunits and then reconstituted from the separated parts[58] as reported in 1974. Neither of the separated subunits had any significant biologic activity by itself in either infant rabbit or skin test assays, but activity in both assays was restored when the subunits were mixed and neutralized. Under such conditions choleragen could be separated into both A and B subunits, whereas choleragenoid yielded only B subunits of approximately 10,000 mol.wt. which were not affected by treatment with 2-mercaptoethanol (2-ME). Further, it was demonstrated that when the unique 28,000-mol.wt. A subunit of choleragen was exposed to 2-ME, its disulfide bond was cleaved to yield two peptides: A_1, approximately 23,000 mol.wt., and A_2, approximately 5000 mol.wt. (as estimated by gel filtration). Later studies were to show that the A subunit is secreted as an unnicked protein, which is subsequently proteolytically cleaved into the two peptides, A_1 and A_2, which remain linked by their disulfide bond. This nicking is accomplished by a zinc- and calcium-dependent metalloendopeptidase,[75,76] the hemagglutinin/protease (HA/protease), which is also secreted by *V. cholerae* (and has some other interesting properties as well). Cholera toxin can be obtained with an intact A subunit if culture filtrates are processed rapidly or if the HA/protease is inhibited by zinc chelators. Elegant work by D. Michael Gill, to be discussed below, established that the A_1 peptide is enzymically active and solely responsible for the toxicity and biological activity of the holotoxin, whereas choleragenoid (the B region of the toxin) was shown by W.E. van Heyningen[11] to be responsible for binding of the toxin to host-cell membranes containing a particular glycolipid. The function of the A_2 peptide is not yet entirely clear: it may serve as a bridge to provide the noncovalent interaction between the A and B subunits, and may perhaps participate in the assembly of the holotoxin in and its transport out of the vibrios. The A_2 peptide may also serve to protect the vibrios themselves against an untethered intracellular ADP-ribosyltransferase (see Section 8.2).

Although it is now universally accepted that cholera toxin consists of two kinds of subunits, A and B, and the ratio of A to B subunits is widely accepted to be 1:5, it is not yet entirely certain that there are precisely five, and only five, B subunits in the holotoxin or in choleragenoid. It was earlier demonstrated that choleragenoid could be formed from purified choleragen following shaking[77] or heat treatment,[69] without apparent recovery of free A subunit. In fact, free choleragenoid seems to be a byproduct of the fermentation and purification procedure: it is not usually seen in fresh culture supernatants. A recent paper[78] has described isoelectric microheterogeneity in various preparations of cholera toxin and choleragenoid.

Heat treatment of choleragen under controlled conditions results in the formation of a large molecular weight aggregate, called "procholeragenoid," prior to the release of choleragenoid.[69] Fürer *et al.*[79] recently determined the molar ratios of subunit B to subunit A in choleragen and procholeragenoid by calculating the area of stained bands of the proteins in SDS-PAGE gels, and found it to be 5:1 for choleragen and 3.3:1 for procholeragenoid, indicating the subunit B is released from the cholera toxin molecule, with the consequent enrichment of subunit A in procholeragenoid. (Procholeragenoid will be discussed again later in the context of antitoxic immunity.) Results of Klapper et al.[80] based on quantitation of the amino acid residues in the N-terminal amino acid sequences of the A_1, A_2, and B chains suggested that there may be some heterogeneity in choleragen, in that their calculations indicated that there were more than 5 (but less than 6) B chains per toxin molecule. Lai et al.[81] similarly concluded that cholera toxin was synthesized and excreted into the medium in the form AB_6. During purification, it was hypothesized that some rearrangement occurs, and some molecules of composition AB_5 are formed, together with choleragenoid—a hexamer ("or pentamer") of B subunits. Gill[82] concluded, using the cross-linking reagent dimethylsuberimidate, that (our) choleragenoid and choleragen contained five B subunits; but recently, Ludwig et al.[83] presented evidence for the presence of both hexameric and pentameric forms of choleragenoid from different sources (called B subunit in that paper), which they obtained using both cross-linking and optical analysis of lipid layer two-dimensional crystals. These workers, too, agree that further work is needed to resolve the issue. The central hole observed in this study and in earlier electron micrographs[84] could plausibly contain the A subunit.

Partial amino acid sequences of the N-terminal residues of the A_1, A_2, and B peptides were determined by Klapper et al., [80] and the complete primary structure of the mature B subunit was elucidated practically simultaneously by two groups: Kurosky et al.[85,86] and C.-Y. Lai.[87] The formula weight of the B subunit was thus fixed at 11,604 mol.wt., consistent with the presence of five B subunits in choleragenoid, M_r 57,000–58,000, and in choleragen, M_r 84,000.[72] The B subunit sequence of 103 residues contains a single intrachain disulfide bond, between Cys residues 9 and 86, and a single tryptophan at position 88. The A subunit amino acid sequence was defined from the nucleotide sequence of the chromosomal gene by Mekalanos et al.[88] The mature subunit consists of 240 amino acid residues; the calculated molecular weights for A_1 (195 residues) and A_2 are 21,817 and 5398, respectively. The internal disulfide bond connects the nicked protein by the Cys residues at positions 187 in A_1 and 5 in A_2. Both A and B are synthesized in V. cholerae with hydrophobic amino-terminal signal sequences of 18 and 21 residues, respectively. The last four nucleotides (ATGA) of the A subunit gene, including its stop codon (TGA), overlap and encode the beginning Mct (ATG) of the 21 amino acid signal peptide of the B subunit. The ribosomal binding site for the B subunit promotes translation more efficiently than that of the A subunit, thus enabling B to be expressed in larger amounts than A.[89]

It is important to note that the B subunit sequence derived by Mekalanos et al.[87] differs in five residues from that of the B subunit protein of the toxin from classical biotype strain 569B. While these differences are probably the result of only single-base changes, they have immunologic consequences. The ctx B cistrons of V. cholerae El Tor Ogawa strain 3083 and its A^-B^+ mutant, Texas Star (mentioned earlier), have recently been sequenced by us[90] and found to be identical to that of strain 2125. Toxin from strain 3083, although related, differs immunologically from 569B toxin, as demonstrated by precipitin analyses,[66] neutralization tests,[91] and monoclonal antibodies,[92] and therefore it may safely be presumed that 2125 toxin does also. It may be important to mention (as summarized below) that field studies of toxoid immunization have invariably used toxin antigen derived from strain 569B against the prevailing epidemic strains, which were predominantly of the El Tor biotype. These immunological differences could be responsible, in part, for the low prophylactic efficacy of those toxoid vaccines. The sequence of the B subunit of strain 62746, also of the El Tor biotype, differs from that of strains 2125 and 3083 by one amino acid substitution.[93] It is not known whether that difference is immunologically significant, but it is clear that, in terms of B subunit sequence, there are at least three cholera enterotoxins. Although the other cholera toxin–related enterotoxins will be discussed further below, the B subunit sequences of four cholera toxin (CT)–related enterotoxins (LTs) from strains of *E. coli* are known. The reported differences between these and the cholera toxins are summarized in Table 1.

H-LT-1, from an *E. coli* strain (H74-114) of human (H) origin, and P-LT, from an *E. coli* strain of porcine (P) origin, which respectively differ from CT-1 in 19 and 21 residues, and from each other in two residues (at positions 46 and 102), can readily be differentiated immunologically. H-LT-2 (from strain H10407), which is identical to H-LT-1 except for having Arg^{13}, can be distinguished from H-LT-1 by monoclonal antibodies.[92] However, H-LT-3 (from strain 240-3, recently sequenced by Tsuji *et al.*[94]), which differs from H-LT-2 only by having the cholera toxin B-subunit residue Ala^{76}, could not be differentiated from H-LT-2. These observations (and others cited in Finkelstein *et al.*[92]) indicate that certain single amino acid substitutions can have significant immunologic effects. As noted particularly by Jacob *et al.*,[95] who have produced immunogenic synthetic peptides which generate cross-reactive neutralizing antibodies, the amino acid sequence of residues 45–69 is highly (if not perfectly) conserved among the members of the CT–related enterotoxin family sequenced thus far.

These observations suggest that this family of enterotoxins has undergone significant evolutionary divergence. Finkelstein *et al.*[92] hypothesized an evolutionary tree, based upon the B-subunit amino acid sequence relationships, which allows for the insertion of other CT-related enterotoxins yet to be discovered and sequenced. It is of interest to note, as elaborated by Yamamoto *et al.*,[96–98] that the G + C content of the *E. coli* plasmid *tox* (*elt*) genes is markedly different from that of *E. coli* chromosomal genes, and rather close to that of the *V. cholerae* chromosome (the chromosomal locus of the structural gene of cholera toxin was first established by Vasil *et al.*[99] in 1975). From these and other considerations, Yamamoto *et al.* concluded that the LT gene is a foreign gene which has been acquired relatively recently, evolutionarily speaking, whereas the CT gene was present, according to them, before the appearance of humans. For additional information, the interested reader is referred to recent reviews on the genetics and genetic regulation of toxinology.[89,100–102] Recent evidence suggests that the synthesis of CT by *V. cholerae* is "co-regulated" with other virulence-associated factors.[103]

8. MODE OF ACTION OF CHOLERA ENTEROTOXIN AND THE CHOLERA TOXIN-RELATED ENTEROTOXINS

The mechanism of action of the cholera enterotoxin and its relatives has been the subject of a number of authoritative reviews,[104–107] and therefore it will only be discussed in its "historical perspective," in keeping with the title of this chapter. There are two major aspects to be considered: the binding of cholera toxin through its choleragenoid or B region to host or target cell membranes; and the enzymic action of the A_1 peptide, an NADase and an ADP-ribosyl transferase, which results in the activation of host cell adenylate cyclase. Here again, fortune played a significant role—at least in opening up these areas of investigation and hastening their solution.

8.1. Binding of Cholera Toxin

The late W.E. van Heyningen, of St. Cross College of the University of Oxford, England, made the pioneering observations[11] that led to the recognition that CT binds

TABLE 1

Amino Acid Residue Differences[a] among the B Subunits of the Cholera Toxin–Related Enterotoxins

Toxin	Strain	Amino acid residue																						
		1	4	7	10	13	18	20	22	25	31	38	44	46	47	54	70	75	80	82	83	94	95	102
CT-1	569B[b]	Thr	Asn	Asp	Ala	His	His	Leu	Asn	Phe	Leu	Ala	Asn	Ala	Thr	Gly	Asn	Ala	Ala	Val	Glu	His	Ala	Ala
CT-2	3083[c]						Tyr		Asp						Ile	Ser	Asp							
CT-3	62746[d]															Gly								
CT-4	2125[e]															Ser								
H-Lt-1	H74-114[f]	Ala	Ser	Glu	Ser			Ile		Leu	Met	Val	Ser		Thr	Gly			Thr	Ile	Asp	Asn	Ser	Glu
H-LT-2	H10407[g]					Arg																		
H-LT-3	240-3[h]																	Ala						
P-LT	P307[i]		Thr											Glu				Thr						Lys

[a] Only residues that differ from those of the toxin immediately above are indicated.
[b] From Kurosky et al.[86] and Lai.[87]
[c] From Brickman, McIntosh and Finkelstein.[90]
[d] From Lockman and Kaper.[93]
[e] From Mekalanos et al.[88]
[f] From Leong et al.[63]
[g] From Yamamoto and Yokota.[171]
[h] From Tsuji et al.[94]
[i] From Dallas and Falkow[162] (corrected[163] for error at Lys[43] in the original reference).

through its B region to a particular glycolipid, the sialidase-resistant monosialosyl G_{M1} ganglioside (also known as GGnSLC), which is ubiquitous in most higher eukaryotic cell membranes. van Heyningen had worked on bacterial toxins, gas gangrene, dysentery, and tetanus since 1940, and had made the important observation that tetanus toxin was "fixed" by a water-soluble ganglioside, the sialidase-labile GGnSSLC, extractable from brain tissue. Because of his expertise as a toxinologist, he was invited to serve as a consultant to the various (primarily American) committees which had arisen to confront the emerging cholera problem. In 1970, he found that, like tetanus toxin, crude CT was "fixed" by brain tissue even better than by intestinal scrapings, as evaluated by Craig's skin test. Later the same year, with Greenough, Pierce, and Carpenter at Johns Hopkins University, he showed that mixed gangliosides inactivated pure choleragen, as measured both in rabbit intestinal loops and in rat epididymal fat cells[108] (another experimental system to be discussed below). They postulated that "fixation to gangliosides may play a role in the binding of cholera toxin to cell membranes."[108] These observations were subsequently extended by King and van Heyningen,[109] Bennett and Cuatrecasas,[60] Holmgren and Svennerholm, [110] and others (see Eidels et al.[111]) to establish that it is the G_{M1} ganglioside, and specifically the oligosaccharide portion of that glycolipid, that is the major CT-binding component of susceptible whole cells. Three key additional observations, however, are considered (by this author) to have contributed in a material way to the early establishment of that concept. First, was the early demonstration by van Heyningen[11] that purified choleragenoid flocculated with concentrated solutions of ganglioside, as did choleragen, thus suggesting that it was through this biologically inactive portion of the holotoxin that the toxin was bound. Second, was the demonstration by Pierce[112] (following our observations that choleragenoid, as well as choleragen, bound to membranes of intestinal epithelial cells[113]) that treatment of rabbit ileal loops with choleragenoid *prior* to enterotoxin inhibited the secretory response, whereas choleragenoid had little, if any, inhibitory effect when injected *following* the enterotoxin. The binding of choleragenoid to cellular binding sites is prolonged, suggesting that the enterotoxin may also exhibit prolonged binding to the cellular receptor. While ganglioside inhibited the action of CT, formalinized cholera toxoid did not, suggesting that the toxoid did not compete for the mucosal binding site. "These observations suggest that the properties of antigenicity, mucosal binding, and enterotoxicity (manifested by induction of gut secretion) belong to separate portions or characteristics of the active enterotoxin molecule."[112] Third, was the observation by Hollenberg et al.[114] that cultured mouse embryonic kidney cell lines which differed in their G_{M1} content also differed in parallel in their binding and their responsiveness to choleragen. Additional studies indicated that exogenous G_{M1} would induce toxin-responsiveness in G_{M1}-deficient cells, which are otherwise refractory.[115] As a consequence of all these observations and others, it became well established that G_{M1} ganglioside is the major functional cholera toxin receptor of susceptible cell surface membranes; other cell surface toxin-binding compounds, particularly glycoproteins, have negligible roles, if any. This is not so clear, however, for (some of) the CT-related enterotoxins.

The first purification to homogeneity[116] of a CT-related enterotoxin, the heat-labile toxin (LT) of an *E. coli* strain of porcine (P) origin, was (as mentioned earlier) dependent on its unique ability, as distinguished from the cholera toxins, of binding to agarose with a degree of firmness that resists elution except by galactose, the monosaccharide component of agarose (and also a component of G_{M1}). It was postulated that "this difference [between LT and choleragen] may reflect significant differences in the nature of the interaction of the two enterotoxins with host cell membrane receptors."[116] To be sure, earlier investigators (see Griffiths et al.[117]) had noted subtle differences in binding characteristics between the two toxins but, as they were working with crude LT preparations, their observations were not definitive. It now appears quite clear that LT and CT both recognize the same receptor, G_{M1}, in some host cell membranes, but LT can bind to additional nonganglioside rabbit brush-border galactoproteins,[117] an observation that may have biological significance.

The precise mechanism of the binding of G_{M1} by the B region of the holotoxins at the inframolecular level is not yet clear. Various amino acid residues have been incriminated in chemical derivatization studies [see Ludwig et al.[118]], but it seems more likely that several different portions of the (linear sequence of the) B subunit proteins may contribute cooperatively to binding, rather than a single residue: each may be essential but not sufficient.[92] The broader binding capability of the LTs may be dependent on a three-dimensional configuration that is altered, in relation to cholera toxin, by the amino acid substitutions noted (Table 1). Reactivity of certain monoclonal antibodies with some of the proteins is blocked specifically by G_{M1} or its oligosacharide, OS-G_{M1},[92,119] indicating that the binding site or sites can be recognized by specific antibody. As the antibodies had different specificities, multiple sites may be involved.

The mechanisms by which the binding of the B subunits perturbs the host-cell membrane and facilitates the entry of the A subunit is not entirely clear. Moss et al.[120] and Tosteson et al.[121] reported that choleragenoid or CT altered the permeability of lipid bilayers to small molecules, perhaps in that way allowing the penetration of A through host-cell membranes. However, this is still somewhat controversial (see discussion in Gill and Wool-kalis[122]). The fact that the reactions of toxin and choleragenoid with G_{M1} ganglioside in some cases enhances their reactivity with monoclonal antibodies[92] suggests that the conformation of the toxin may also be altered in the process.

The binding of choleragen and the entry of its A subunit is summarized diagramatically in Fig. 1.[123]

8.2. Cholera Toxin: An ADP-Ribosyltransferase

The recognition that CT (and subsequently its relatives) worked enzymically to activate host-cell adenylate cyclase was dependent on the independent contributions of several individuals. The fundamental notion that excessive intracellular levels of cAMP could result in inhibition of sodium absorption, and net secretion of chloride and bicarbonate accompanied by water, viz. the cholera stool, was generated by Michael Field and his associates, who first reported[124−125] in 1968 that cAMP or theophylline, an inhibitor of the phosphodiesterase which breaks down cAMP to 5'-AMP, could increase the short-circuit current, a measure of ion transport, of rabbit ileal mucosa, although Field was not at that time (directly) involved in cholera research. (This observation, of course, depended on the earlier contributions of Nobel Laureate Earl W. Sutherland,[126] the discover of the role of cAMP as a ubiquitous, hormone-regulated second messenger.) W.B. Greenough, III, who had been interested in cholera since his experience with it in Dacca, East Pakistan (now Bangladesh) in 1962, demonstrated while visiting in Field's laboratory that similar changes could be induced, after a lag period, by crude culture filtrates containing cholera toxin.[127] Subsequently, in 1969, Greenough and Martha Vaughan, who had earlier been working on hormone-regulated, cAMP-mediated lipolysis in rat epididymal fat cells (a system used by Sutherland), demonstrated that the same lipolytic effect was duplicated, after a lag period, by crude cholera toxin and by nanogram amounts of purified choleragen, which was then available, whereas choleragenoid had no effect at 10,000-fold higher doses.[128] Greenough et al.[129] then showed that

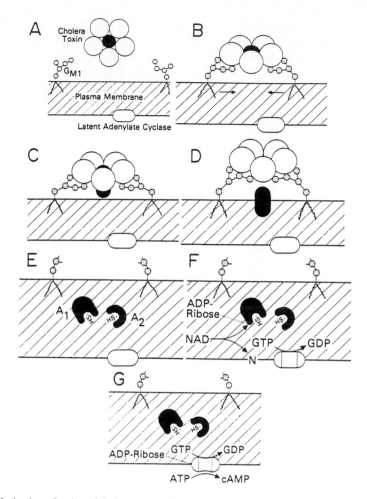

FIGURE 1. Mechanism of action of cholera enterotoxin (*modified from Fishman*[123]). (A) Cholera toxin approaching target cell surface. (B) Binding of B subunits to oligosaccharide of G_{M1} ganglioside. (C) Conformational alteration of holotoxin presenting A subunit (black) to cell surface. (D) Entry of A subunit. (E) Reduction of disulfide bond of A subunit by intracellular glutathione, freeing A_1 and A_2. (F) Cleavage of NAD by A_1 yielding ADP-ribose and nicotinamide. (G) ADP-ribosylation of G protein, inhibiting action of GTPase and "locking" adenylate cyclase in "on" mode.

the lipase-stimulating activity of pure enterotoxin was neutralized by antisera against crude cholera enterotoxin, thus, providing a useful *in vitro* assay for both cholera toxin and its antibody. These observations were also pioneering, in that they were the first demonstration that pure cholera toxin was active *in vitro* in extraintestinal tissue, thus paving the way for an endless variety of such demonstrations. (These included the use of mouse Y-1 adrenal tumor cells,[130,131] Chinese hamster ovary cells,[132] and nucleated erythrocytes,[133] each of which became widely used in studies of cholera toxin and its relatives.)

These observations were soon followed by reports of increased adenylate cyclase activity, or elevated cAMP levels, in experimental animal models treated with crude[134] or pure[135] CT, and in the intestinal mucosa of humans with naturally acquired cholera.[136] It was thus clear that cAMP was elevated and could account for the diarrhea of cholera. What was not clear was how CT accomplished this. The contributions of the late D. Michael Gill were essential to the solution of that problem.

Again, both prior experience and good fortune entered the picture. To some small extent, also, this reviewer feels some responsibility. Gill was just completing his exciting work with A.M. Pappenheimer[137] at Harvard. Gill, Pappenheimer, Uchida, Collier and others[137] had demonstrated that diphtheria toxin, synthesized by lysogenic *Corynebacterium diphtheriae* as a single polypeptide chain, when nicked by trypsinlike proteases yielded two large fragments, an amino-terminal A of 24,000 mol.wt. and a carboxy-terminal B of 38,000 mol.wt., which remain linked by a single disulfide bridge. The A fragment, after reduction, catalyzed the ADP-ribosylation of the elongation factor EF-2, thus inhibiting eukaryotic polypeptide chain formation (i.e., protein synthesis) and resulting in death of the intoxicated cell. The B moiety was responsible for binding to specific sites [not yet completely identified (*see* Eidels et al.[111])] on sensitive target cell membranes. The reviewer, while visiting his brother—a political scientist then at Harvard—gave an informal seminar to Pappenheimer's group at which Gill (rather vehemently) disagreed with the author's preliminary interpretations of the subunit structure of cholera enterotoxin. In part as a result of this experience, Gill applied his talents, fruitfully, to the cholera problem. Field had already demonstrated that cholera toxin activated adenylate cyclase in intact turkey erythrocytes, an effect which was blocked by pretreatment with choleragenoid,[133] and Zieve et al.[138] had earlier discovered that broken human platelets and liver cells responded to CT with increased glycogenolysis— a cAMP-mediated effect. Gill took a sabbatical in 1973* and, with Carolyn King, a postdoctoral fellow in van Heyningen's laboratory at Oxford, proceeded to demonstrate that whereas cholera toxin would elevate the adenylate cyclase activity of intact pigeon erythrocytes after a significant lag period, the adenylate cyclase activity of lysed (by a bacterial hemolysin or by freeze-thawing) cells started to rise immediately upon addition of toxin.[139] After demonstrating that most of the toxin's activity on lysed erythrocytes was retained after treatment with acid or with sodium dodecyl sulfate (SDS), it was shown that the activity was specifically associated with the A_1 peptide when the peptide was separated either by electrophoresis in SDS or by gel filtration in acid urea (as we had described[58]). Antiserum against both the A and B subunits prevented the toxin from acting on intact erythrocytes; anti-A neutralized the activity of both toxin and peptide A_1, and anti-B prevented the activity of intact toxin but not of A_1. A requirement for cytosolic factors [including NAD (*à la* diphtheria toxin)] was shown, as was a blocking effect of choleragenoid or ganglioside G_{M1} (obtained from van Heyningen). The fortuitous part was that if Gill had used turkey erythrocytes, as he originally intended, he might not have been so (immediately) successful, because pigeon erythrocytes have a relatively high NAD content due to their extremely low endogenous NAD glycohydrolase activity,[103] whereas turkey erythrocytes have a higher activity and a correspondingly lower NAD content. Turkeys were not available at Oxford, but pigeons were![11]

A number of investigators, including *inter alia* Gill, Moss, Vaughan, Cassel, Pfeiffer, and Selinger, contributed additional essential information (summarized in detail elsewhere[104−105]) leading to our current understanding of the mechanism of action of cholera toxin, probably vastly oversimplified (see Gilman[140]). In outline, the A_1 fragment of cholera toxin enzymically transfers ADP-ribose from cytosolic NAD covalently to (probably) an arginine residue on the GTP-binding protein then known as N_S (more recently called G_S or

---

*van Heyningen mistakenly [according to the author's recollection and Gill's (personal communication)] indicated that the year was 1975 on page 270 in his history,[11] perhaps because that was the year of Gill's first significant publication in the cholera field.

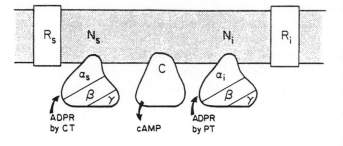

FIGURE 2. Comparison of activities of cholera enterotoxin (CT) with pertussis toxin (PT) (*modified from Gill and Woolkalis*[122]). Hormonally responsive stimulatory receptors (R_s) and regulatory components (N_s), and inhibitory receptors (R_i) and components (N_i). α-subunits of N_s and N_i, with GTP-binding sites, are ADP-ribosylated respectively by A_1 peptide of CT or by A subunit of PT, preventing respectively the hydrolysis of N_s-GTP to GDP or the responsiveness of N_i to inhibitory hormones, both effectively producing rises in adenylate cyclase activity.

αs [141]), which is a regulatory component of the adenyl cyclase system anchored in the plasma membrane of most mammalian cells and displayed on the cytoplasmic surface.[122] This results in a dramatic reduction in the hydrolysis to GDP of GTP bound to G_S. Since the catalytic component (C) of adenyl cyclase is dependent for its activity on a ternary complex with G_S and GTP (not GDP), this results in the continuous activation of adenyl cyclase, leading to the production of cAMP—probably for the duration of the life of the cell or turn over of its proteins. The precise mechanism by which cAMP effects fluid and electrolyte secretion remains to be clarified.[142] A recent study has suggested that prostaglandins may be involved.[143]

While the CT-related enterotoxins probably work in identical fashion, the pertussis toxin (also known as pertussigen), a "newer" ADP-ribosylating toxin, which is neither related to cholera toxin* nor an enterotoxin, interestingly transfers ADP-ribose to another G-protein, Ni (now called Gi) the negative regulatory protein of adenylate cyclase, and elevates cAMP by rendering the adenylate cyclase complex unresponsive to its inhibitory hormones, thus contributing to the pathogenesis of pertussis (whooping cough).[145]

Figure 2 (from Gill and Woolkalis[122]) illustrates schematically these relationships.

9. THE CHOLERA TOXIN-RELATED ENTEROTOXINS

The recognition that the diarrhea of cholera was mediated by an enterotoxin stimulated experimental inquiry into the possibility that other diarrheal diseases might similarly be mediated by enterotoxins. The result has been, as alluded to above, an ever-expanding list of bacteria—some not previously recognized to be enteropathogens—that cause diarrhea in man and animals by this means. Of these newly recognized enterotoxins, many are related to CT—structurally, functionally, and immunologically—while some are distinctly different. The families of the *Shiga* toxin-like toxins,† which in contrast to the CT-like toxins are cytotoxic,[146] are unrelated and will not be further considered. Similarly, the growing family of small-molecular-weight heat-stable enterotoxins (STs) related to the prototype first found

---

*While this was "true" at the time of writing, more recent information[143] indicates that there are regions of amino acid homology between the subunits of PT and CT (and, for that matter, among the A subunits of other ADP-ribosylating toxins such as diphtheria toxin, *Pseudomonas aeruginosa* exotoxin A, and the LTs from *E. coli*).
†Called "Shiga-like toxins" by those authors and others, which (for the same reason as noted for CT-like toxins) should be called "Shiga toxin-like toxins." They do not resemble Professor Shiga.

in *E. coli*,[147] although undoubtedly significant, are unrelated to cholera toxin and will not be discussed here.

In human medicine, the first recognition that gram-negative enteric bacteria other than *V. cholerae* could cause diarrheal disease by means of enterotoxins was probably that of Gorbach, Sack, and their associates.[148,149] Working in Calcutta in 1967–1968 during the cholera epidemic season, they observed that cholera vibrios could not be isolated even from the small bowels of many patients who presented with cholera-like symptoms—namely, severe secretory diarrhea, which was called "non-vibrio cholera." (On admission, it is clinically impossible to differentiate one kind of secretory diarrhea from another.) Although cholera was the expected diagnosis, and indeed was the presumptive clinical diagnosis, these patients generally recovered more rapidly and required less fluid rehydration therapy than those with bacteriologically confirmed cholera. Instead of *V. cholerae,* some of these patients yielded virtually pure cultures of *E. coli*. Further, these isolates were not among the so-called "enteropathogenic serotype *E. coli*" (EPEC), which had been recognized in the 1940s as having the potential for causing devastating outbreaks of diarrhea in babies, particularly in hospital nurseries. When these Calcutta *E. coli* isolates were tested in the bioassays developed for cholera toxins, particularly De's rabbit ileal loop model, they were found to produce enterotoxins. In fact, it should be remembered that De had earlier reported that *E. coli* strains from diarrheal patients could produce positive ileal loops in his model.[15]

Actually, it had been known since Theobald Smith's work in the 1920s that *E. coli* can cause economically highly significant diarrheal disease, known generally as "colibacillosis," in food supply animals.[150] In the 1960s, before the recognition of enterotoxigenic *E. coli* (ETEC) in humans, veterinary microbiologists were using De's ileal loop model to study strains of *E. coli* associated with enteric colibacillosis in pigs.[150] These observations culminated in the recognition in 1969 by Gyles and Barnum[151] of the remarkable similarities between a heat-labile enterotoxin (LT) produced by strains of *E. coli* that cause diarrhea in pigs and the (then) already-identified cholera enterotoxin. Interestingly, these workers used primarily whole-cell lysates (WCL) of the *E. coli* strains in their pig ileal loops (an observation that was largely overlooked by subsequent investigators), which required relatively large (approximately 50-mg) doses. They also used concentrated broth culture supernatants. Most significantly, Gyles and Barnum observed that the enterotoxicity was neutralized by antiserum against *V. cholerae* WCL (produced by W. Burrows), which was enterotoxic at doses larger than 1 mg. They also noted that *E. coli* strain P307 produced an ST, which had been described earlier by Smith and Halls.[152]

Smith and Gyles[153] subsequently demonstrated that both LT and ST were controlled by transmissible plasmids ("Ent"), and noted that ST was not antigenic. In that paper, however, they concluded that LT and ST "are probably two forms of essentially the same enterotoxin." This error was soon corrected by Gyles,[154] who went on to make the important observations that:

1. Antiserum against choleragenoid[57] neutralized LT from porcine and human strains of *E. coli,* thus establishing the antigenic relationship of the B regions of CT and the LTs (although in that study antisera against LT did not neutralize choleragen)
2. Sufficiently concentrated preparations of LT precipitated in Ouchterlony tests with anti-CT with a reaction of partial identity to that of CT. [After some years in the wilderness, this observation finally enabled us to purify LT to homogeneity.[116]]

Following the initial observations of Gyles and Gorbach and Sack, which suggested the production of the CT-related enterotoxin, LT, by strains of *E. coli,* innumerable investigators attempted to purify LT to homogeneity. This resulted in large numbers of "progress reports" (*see Finkelstein*[155] *for a summary*) describing products ranging in size from 20,000 to $>10^7$ mol.wt., with equally wide variations in specific activity in the bioassays used. Each product described was orders of magnitude less active than cholera toxin in the same assays. As recently as 1975, Dorner[156] and we[157] described "purified LTs"—apparently single peptides of *ca.* 100,000 mol.wt., that appeared to be similar but not identical to each other. Independent analysis of these products by Michael Gill (*personal communication*) revealed that the biological activity of these preparations (for pigeon erythrocyte lysates) was present in an unstained region of SDS-PAGE gels at *ca.* 28,000 mol.wt. (similar in size to cholera toxin A subunit). Apparently, both groups had isolated a large, irrelevant protein with a small amount of noncovalently associated *E. coli* LT A subunit.

The elusive real LT finally was purified to homogeneity two years later[116] and shown to be quite similar to CT in subunit structure and in activity, especially when the LT was treated with trypsin (as reported earlier for crude LT by Rappaport *et al.*[158]). Several critical factors finally led to the purification. One was the use of a transformed K-12 strain derivative, provided to us by Stanley Falkow, which carried the LT gene from the Ent plasmid of Gyles' strain P307. A second was the use of Ouchterlony tests with cholera antitoxin to follow the purification process. Although the starting material, concentrated crude LT, precipitated with the antibody, none of the fractions from an agarose column precipitated with the same antiserum, even when they were pooled and concentrated to the original volume applied. The LT had either been destroyed, or it was still stuck on the agarose gel. This led us to use galactose to elute the LT in virtually pure form. The third factor was the demonstration that *E. coli* whole cell lysates (used earlier by Gyles) are the richest source of LT: in contrast to *V. cholerae*, *E. coli* do not effectively transport their toxin (LT) to the external medium. In fact, Neill *et al.*[159] showed that both LT and CT are produced and secreted by genetically engineered *V. cholerae* carrying an LT plasmid, but CT produced in *E. coli* remains cell-associated. Additionally, unlike *V. cholerae*, which has an endogenous protease that nicks and activates the A subunit of its toxin,[76] *E. coli* lacks such protease activity and the A subunit of its LT is usually un-nicked. The N-terminal amino acid sequence of 20 residues of the LT B subunit was reported to differ from that of CT in 5 residues.[160] Also in 1979, Kunkel and Robertson reported[161] the purification of an LT produced by an *E. coli* strain of human origin, by procedures involving pH extraction, ultrafiltration, $(NH_4)_2SO_4$ fractionation, hydrophobic chromatography, and gel filtration.

In 1980, Dallas and Falkow[162] deduced the complete amino acid sequence of the mature (porcine) LT-B subunit, as well as its 21-amino acid leader sequence, from the nucleotide sequence of the cloned LT-B cistron (*elt B*). [An erroneously reported Met[43] (in lieu of Lys[43], as in cholera toxin) was corrected subsequently.[163]] The sequence of the mature B subunit protein differed in 21 residues (of 103) from that of CT-1 (Table 1). Of these, single-base changes in the *elt B* codon accounted for the overwhelming majority. The N-terminus was tentatively identified by comparison with the overall sequence of CT-B, and confirmed by comparison with the partial N-terminal sequence of LT-B.[160] To this reviewer's knowledge, this represents the first instance in which the amino acid sequence of a bacterial virulence factor was defined completely by application of molecular genetics, from the cloning of the gene through the determination of the nucleotide sequence.

From 1969 to the present, evidence of varying degrees of solidarity indicates that there is an increasingly large family of CT-related enterotoxins. Rare strains of non-01 *V. cholerae* [formerly called non-agglutinable vibrios (NAGs) or non-cholera vibrios (NCVs)], in some instances associated with diarrheal disease, may produce enterotoxins that are similar or identical to CT-1 from classical biotype/Inaba serotype strain 569B[164−166]; other strains may produce related but distinctive enterotoxins.[167] *V. cholerae* El Tor biotype/Ogawa serotype strain 3083 (isolated by the author in Vietnam in 1963), a hypertoxinogenic El Tor strain by usual standards (*see Craig*[168]), was first considered to produce a toxin (which we subsequently called CT-2[92]) identical to CT-1,[169] but was later recognized to produce a related but distinctive toxin, as somewhat more refined immunological reagents and techniques were applied.[65,91,169] CT-3 was only recognized to be distinctive (from CT-1) because of the sequencing of its B subunit,[92] as was CT-4[87] (which, it now turns out, is identical[89] with CT-2). As mentioned previously (*also see below*), these differences, which can be demonstrated by monoclonal antibodies[92] and by quantitative cross-neutralization assays,[91] may have important consequences on the efforts to develop protective toxoid vaccines.

Whereas three different H-LTs produced by *E. coli* strains isolated from humans have been defined by the DNA sequences of their B subunits (H-LT-1, from strain H74-114, Leong *et al*[163]; H-LT-2, from strain H10407, Yamamoto and Yokota[171]; and H-LT-3, from strain 240-3, Tsuji *et al.*[94]), only one P-LT from strains of porcine origin has been identified—that which was first used by Gyles and Barnum[151] and sequenced by Dallas and Falkow.[162] The structure of P-LTs from different sources appears to be highly conserved, at least as determined by partial restriction endonuclease analyses.[163] A mutant P-LT B subunit described by Tsuji *et al.*,[172] having Asp[33] in lieu of Gly[33], although still able to complex with the A subunit was unable to bind to G_{M1} ganglioside (and thus is not effective on intact cells), and also has altered immunologic reactivity. The *V. cholerae* Texas Star A⁻B⁺ mutant (of strain 3083, which produces CT-2) has an amino acid substitution at residue 173 in the mature A subunit, which apparently renders it nonfunctional and unable to complex with the B subunit for transport.[90] Additional studies using site-directed mutagenesis in the cholera family of enterotoxins should yield further insights into their assembly, transport, binding, penetration, and enzymic activity.

Additional toxins in the family include *Salmonella* LT (S-LT),[173–175] which has recently been cloned into *E. coli* by Peterson *et al.*[176] A toxin isolated from strains of *V. mimicus* was considered to be identical to CT-1, except that the A subunit was unnicked.[177] *Aeromonas hydrophila*[178–179] (which also produces cytotoxic factors[180]) and *Campylobacter jejuni*[181] also have been reported to produce CT-like toxins, as have *Klebsiella* and *Enterobacter*.[182] Whether expression of enterotoxin can always be equated with enteric virulence, however, is still problematical. For example, *Aeromonas* which produce CT-like cytotonic enterotoxin have been isolated frequently from children without diarrhea.[179]

An LT cloned from *E. coli* strain SA53 (isolated from a water buffalo in Thailand), which is structurally similar to the LTs and to CT and also activates adenylate cyclase by ADP-ribosylation, is not neutralized by antisera against the preceding toxins; apparently does not bind to G_{M1} avidly; and does not produce positive rabbit ileal loops.[183] DNA probes that react with previously recognized LTs and with CT did not hybridize with this new LT, which has been called LT-like toxin, type II LT, or LT-II, and which may be the prototype for a second major serogroup of LTs.[183]

10. IMMUNOLOGICAL ASPECTS

With the recognition and acceptance of the fact that cholera is a toxin-mediated disease came the hope, indeed the expectation, that a toxoid vaccine would do the same for cholera as it did for diphtheria and tetanus—diseases which were essentially controllable by toxoid vaccines before they were understood.

To date, this expectation remains unfulfilled, and we do not yet have an appropriate, safe, economical, and effective vaccine against cholera (and the related diarrheal diseases). The literature has been reviewed extensively and is summarized elsewhere,[46–48,184–189] but again in keeping with the intent of this chapter, some brief restatement of the highlights is appropriate.

First, by the beginning of the CT era, scientifically controlled field studies conducted in Bangladesh, the Philippines, and India in the 1960s and 1970s had revealed that the time-honored parenterally administered, killed whole-cell vaccines, used since the late 1800s, offered only limited protection against cholera in certain population groups. In general, they were primarily protective, and then only for limited time periods, in adult populations of heavily endemic regions, where cholera is largely a pediatric problem. They were not sufficiently protective to have a significant impact on the incidence, endemicity, or epidemicity of cholera to justify their (rather minimal) cost.[190] Subsequent field studies employing the partially purified lipopolysaccharide (LPS) somatic antigen (endotoxin) of the vibrios were similarly unencouraging (as might have been expected: if the intact cells did not work, why should a part of them?). While some improvement in the efficacy of whole-cell bacterins could be generated by appropriate attention to the selection of vaccine strains,[191] the method of killing, and the use of adjuvants, another approach was clearly desirable, if not essential.

Purified toxoids, also administered parenterally, were the next major thrust. After the unexpected finding that a formaldehyde toxoid preparation reverted partially to toxicity, causing unacceptable local reactions in volunteers inoculated with 25 μg doses, a stably nonreactogenic toxoid prepared by glutaraldehyde treatment was evaluated in about 93,000 people in Bangladesh.[192] The cumulative protection over a one-year period was marginal at best. Although glutaraldehyde treatment resulted in polymerization of the antigen (which might be advantageous), it also vastly reduced its immunogenicity.

The question then arose as to whether immunity to cholera, which is after all a very superficial disease involving only the epithelial cells of the surface of the small bowel, was an attainable goal. The decisive answer was provided by live *V. cholerae* challenges in American volunteers. Those who had recovered from induced cholera were found to be solidly (if not quite absolutely) immune to rechallenge for three years, the longest period tested.[47] The disease itself is an immunizing process, in which the host is presented with all of the products of cholera vibrios: lipopolysaccharide somatic antigen, flagellum, membrane proteins, colonization factors/adhesins, enzymes, and other products elaborated by vibrios growing *in vivo*. The putative immunogens are also presented at the local level, which prevailing opinion considers to be optimal for a secretory immune response to result in protection (although, to this reviewer, it is not yet entirely clear whether it is the manner of presentation, the nature of the antigens presented, or both that is of paramount importance).

[It may be important to mention that cholera vibrios growing *in vivo* produce (at least) different membrane proteins, particularly iron-regulated outer membrane proteins, than vibrios grown *in vitro* under normal growth conditions of iron-sufficiency.[193] Thus, different antigens are produced *in vivo*. It is also pertinent that there is wide phenotypic variation in the expression of various hemagglutinins (also likely to be immunogenic), which may be employed by the vibrios to adhere to the surface of the small intestinal microvilli.[194,195] Thus, cultural conditions may be important, especially in the case of nonviable antigens.]

In part because of the perceived deficiencies of the parenterally administered vaccines which have been tested (killed bacteria, LPS, and toxoid), and in large measure because of the success of the disease itself in inducing immunity, the prevailing thought has overwhelmingly shifted to favor perorally administered vaccines. One school has championed the use of living attenuated mutants, such as the A$^-$B$^+$ strain[56] proposed in 1969, which might simulate the immunogenicity of the disease without its undesirable side effects. Such vaccines would have the obvious advantage of economy (at a not-unreasonable dose of 10^8 live vibrios per person, one Petri dish of growth would be sufficient to immunize 1000 people), and the possible advantage of inducing herd immunity if they are transmitted in the environment (like virulent *V. cholerae* are). Thus, the unvaccinated population might receive, free, the benefits of the vaccine. (This may be a complicating factor, it should be pointed out, in controlled field studies to evaluate the efficacy of such vaccines.) The other school proposes the use of orally administered nonviable antigens. The proponents of both schools have made progress, but neither has achieved unqualified success.

As mentioned above, M13 (the hypotoxinogenic mutant of strain 569B) induced immunity (without side effects) against challenge in volunteers, but was regarded as unstable and was not further evaluated.[67] The Texas Star A⁻B⁺ strain[63] also induced immunity, but caused mild diarrhea as a side effect in 25% of the volunteers (the worst case had less than 1.5 liter diarrhea in 6 stools over the course of 3 days). This effect was not related to the dose administered over the extraordinary range of 10^5 through 5×10^{10} vibrios.[64] Subsequent genetically engineered strains, both *tox*⁻ and A⁻B⁺, induced somewhat more severe diarrhea in a larger proportion of the vaccine recipients.[195,197] Attempts are being made to identify and eliminate the factors responsible for the diarrhea. If these are not essential to colonization and replication in the gut, it should be possible to develop an appropriate attenuated vaccine strain through genetic engineering. (Presumably Dr. Kaper may have some new information in Chapter 4.)

The use of perorally administered killed whole-cell *V. cholerae* bacterins is not a new concept (*see Pollitzer*[10]), although in the past it has generally been agreed that parenteral vaccines (described above as defective) are better (!). For example, in 1974 Cash *et al.*[198] fed volunteers 1.6×10^{10} killed vibrios/day, with or without a booster course of five more doses, and found that the volunteers were significantly protected against a subsequent live vibrio challenge. However, the oral vaccine was not as protective as parenteral vaccine (8×10^9 vibrios/ml), and neither was as effective as recovery from the disease itself. The reason why perorally administered killed vibrio cells are so much less effective than live bacteria is not clear, but may reside (at least in part) in the fact that the specialized absorptive cells (M cells) in the epithelium overlaying the Peyer's patches in the small intestine preferentially sample viable *V. cholerae*.[199]

The concept that a combination of some form of toxin antigen with bacterial antigens might result in improved protection is also not new, although the earlier field studies were dedicated to ascertaining whether one or the other would suffice. In 1976, Svennerholm and Holmgren[200] reported a synergistic protective effect of combinations of choleragen or choleragenoid with vibrio LPS—the combinations provided more protection than the sum of the protections afforded by each of the individual components. As Rappaport and Bonde[201] subsequently showed that killed *E. coli* could substitute for the *V. cholerae* component, the mechanism of the synergistic effect is not quite clear. Nevertheless, the concept has recently matured into a large-scale field study in Bangladesh.[202] Approximately 20,000 people per group received either killed *V. cholerae* whole cells (WC); WC plus choleragenoid, which they called "B subunit* component" (BS-WC); or killed *E. coli* placebo. The whole cell

*A point of clarification is in order here. Choleragenoid, described earlier, is the natural polymer [pentamer (or hexamer)] of the subunits of the cholera holotoxin, or the reformed polymer of the B subunits after their separation from the A subunit. Although composed exclusively of B subunits, it is not in senso stricto "B subunit," which does not exist as such under physiological conditions. The phrase "B subunit component," in a mixture of different substances (e.g., as in a combination together with whole cells), is more acceptable nomenclature.

vaccine (10^{11} WC representing four different *V. cholerae* strains, killed by heat or formalin) was given *per os* together with $NaHCO_3$/citric acid buffer (75–155 ml), with or without 1 mg BS, on three occasions. The protective efficacy of choleragenoid alone was not tested. During the first six months after oral vaccination, the incidence of cholera in the three groups was 26 cases in the placebo group, 11 cases in the WC group (protective efficacy 58%), and 4 cases in the BS-WC group (protective efficacy 85%).[202] In contrast to the lasting immunity induced by infection, protection was declining at one year, and it was also less effective in children 5 years old and younger.[203] The difficult-to-administer and costly oral concoction offered little, if any, advantage over parenteral vaccine, which has now been discontinued by most of the developed countries of the world.

It is significant that whereas WC similar to the preparation used in this field study was protective with or without choleragenoid in previous tests with volunteers, another WC preparation containing similar numbers of killed vibrios of different strains mixed with procholeragenoid (50 or 200 µg) did not reduce the incidence of cholera in the challenged volunteers, but did significantly reduce the number and volume of diarrheal stools. Ergo, the second killed vibrio preparation was ineffective; however, relatively small doses of orally administered procholeragenoid elicited effective antitoxic immunity.[47,188,189] The experiments demonstrate that, clearly, we still know very little (nothing?) about how to choose the most appropriate strains, how to cultivate them, and how to kill them to prepare the most effective antigen. Further, there are no appropriate animal or *in vitro* assays to assess in the laboratory, and standardize, the potency of such whole-cell bacterins which, at this point, are really unreproducible "black magic concoctions."

Procholeragenoid is interesting and worthy of further consideration. As mentioned earlier, it is a high-molecular-weight, relatively nontoxic polymer (or polymers) enriched in A subunit, formed by controlled heating of pure cholera toxin. Shortly after its discovery[69] in 1971, Fujita *et al.*[204] found procholeragenoid to be the most effective form of toxin antigen in stimulating gut immunity (in mice) following parenteral administration, an observation which has been confirmed repeatedly since.[205–209] In fact, the Fujita study[204] showed, for the first time, that perorally administered toxin antigen was (also) effective in stimulating effective gut immunity. (Choleragenoid, by the way, was originally considered by us and by others to have great promise as "the natural toxoid" of cholera toxin, until we showed that, despite its immunologic dominance in the holotoxin, choleragenoid by itself was an "erratic" antigen in rats and mice.[210])

It is not clear precisely why the polymeric form, procholeragenoid, is such an effective antigen—it has even been demonstrated to produce effective cross-immunity against experimental salmonellosis in rabbits[207] and colibacillosis in pigs.[208] While it is certainly true that the B region is the immunodominant portion of the holotoxin (immunized animals and cholera convalescents respond with antibodies primarily to the B region), the holotoxin is a powerful immunomodulator, as revealed first by Robert Northrup and Anthony Fauci[211] and confirmed by many subsequent investigators (reviewed in Finkelstein[186]). It is not unlikely that the superior immunogenicity of the holotoxin and of procholeragenoid is due to the A subunit component, which is enriched in procholeragenoid.[79] Germanier and his colleagues demonstrated that the slight residual toxicity of procholeragenoid could be eliminated, without reducing its immunogenicity, by treatment with formaldehyde.[206] While it seems to this reviewer that an appropriate live vaccine would be most desirable (for reasons mentioned above), failing that, further attention to procholeragenoidlike products may be worthwhile. Similar products have been generated from CT-related toxins, H-LT, and P-LT[212] which might be even more effective because they generate specific immunity, instead of cross-reactions, against the homologous antigens.

Other promising possibilities might include such technological developments as the administration of antigens in enteric-coated capsules or microspheres, as advocated by Klipstein et al.,[213] perhaps accomplishing a more continuous presentation of antigen (as in the disease itself), and the use of synthetic peptides (mentioned earlier).

There are still other options (e.g., genetically engineering cholera antigens into established, safe, and effective live vaccines, such as the Ty 21a strain of *Salmonella typhi*[214]) which can be developed (summarized elsewhere[47,48,188,189]). However, special mention should be made of the prospect of passive immunity attained by oral administration of antibody. Breast feeding is already widely accepted as a natural means of providing passive protection to infants; however, the mechanisms of the protective effects (not clearly defined) must, in large measure, be dependent on the immunologic experience of individual mothers. Interestingly, the milk of Missouri mothers is inhibitory *in vitro* to *V. cholerae,* a pathogen not present in Missouri. The inhibitory effect is dependent on the interaction of secretory immunogloblin A (sIgA) and unsaturated lactoferrin.[215] The results suggest the presence of a cross-reactive antigenic stimulus. Human milk has a broad spectrum of inhibitory activity against other pediatric pathogens as well.[216–218]

It may be possible to complement and supplement the protective effects of breast milk, and to provide protection to infants and children who cannot be breast-fed, with appropriately supplemented infant feeding formulae. In particular, it should be noted that immunized newly parturient cows secrete into colostrum large quantities (300–800 g/cow[219]) of a relatively protease-resistant immunoglobulin (IgG_1) containing neutralizing activity against CT and LT, which has been shown to retain antibody activity during passage through human and other animal intestines.[220,221] While this is also not a new concept, recent studies suggesting the possibility of intervention and prophylaxis against rotavirus[222] and enterotoxigenic *E. coli* diarrhea[223] through passively administered bovine colostral and milk immunoglobulin have been encouraging. Additionally, consideration could be given to the inclusion of antigens in formula or milk for children old enough to mount an effective response.

If the editors, and readers, will forgive me, I might end this section by saying:

1. Live vaccines are not dead as potential solutions for the prevention of cholera and related diarrheas.
2. Dead vaccines are still alive (as a concept, similarly).
3. Parenteral vaccines are nearly dead (as a concept), but might deserve further consideration.
4. Passive bovine lactogenic immunity offers promise as a method of complementing and supplementing the protective effects of breast feeding in the prevention of diarrheal disease.
5. Finally it should be recognized that as the cholera vibrios have multiple, redundant mechanisms for causing diarrheal disease (as shown by studies with *V. cholerae* mutants in volunteers), one cannot expect effective antitoxic immunity to protect against *V. cholerae* diarrhea—the target of earlier field studies—although it might protect against the life-threatening aspects of cholera.

11. EPILOGUE

The reviewer has summarized what he considers to be the salient features in the history of cholera toxin research from Koch's Postulate to the present. He hopes he has conveyed the excitement and enthusiasm which characterized the period after the discoveries of cholera toxin independently by two groups of Indian investigators in 1959. It is undoubtedly disappointing to recognize that the enormous body of research has not (yet) resulted in a solution to the cholera problem. It has resulted, however, in perhaps the most significant advance in medical science in this century: the ability to treat (simply by oral fluid replacement therapy), and thus prevent the deaths of, countless millions of children and adults who annually suffer potentially fatal secretory diarrheal disease. It has also created a body of knowledge which will be applicable, soon it is to be hoped, to the prevention of secretory diarrheal disease, and to the solution of a myriad of other medical problems, which, at the outset, no sane person could have predicted would result from cholera research.

REFERENCES

1. Anonymous: Dr. Koch's newly described cholera-organism. *Brit Med J* 1883(2):828–829, 1883
2. Anonymous: Dr. Koch's fifth cholera report. *Brit Med J* 1884(1):375–376, 1884
3. Anonymous: Dr. Koch's sixth cholera report. *Brit Med J* 1884(1):568–569, 1884
4. Anonymous: The German Cholera Commission. *Brit Med J* 1884(1):740, 1884
5. Anonymous: Koch on cholera. *Brit Med J* 1884(2):427–428, 1884
6. Anonymous: Conferences in Berlin for the discussion of cholera. *Brit Med J* 1885(1):1011–1012, 1885
7. Koch R: An address on cholera and its bacillus. *Brit Med J* 1884(2):403–407, 1884
8. Koch R: Further researches on cholera. *Brit Med J* 1886(1):6–8, 62–66, 1886
9. Koch, R: Die Aetiologie der Tuberkulose. *Mittheilungen aus dem Kaiserlichen Gesundheitsamte* 2:1–88, 1884
10. Pollitzer R: *Cholera.* Geneva, World Health Organization, 1959
11. van Heyningen WE, Seal JR: *Cholera: The American Scientific Experience, 1947–1980.* Boulder, Westview Press, 1983
12. De SN: Enterotoxicity of bacteria-free culture-filtrate of *Vibrio cholerae. Nature* 183:1533–1534, 1959
13. De SN, Ghose ML: False reaction in ligated loop of rabbit intestine. *Indian J Pathol Bacteriol* 2:121–128, 1959
14. De SN, Chatterje DN: An experimental study of the mechanism of action of *Vibrio cholerae* on the intestinal mucous membrane. *J Pathol Bacteriol* 66:559–562, 1953
15. De SN, Bhattacharya K, Sarkar JK: A study of the pathogenicity of strains of *Bacterium coli* from acute and chronic enteritis. *J Pathol Bacteriol* 71:201–209, 1956
16. Violle H, Crendiropoulo: Note sur le cholèra experimental. *C R Soc Biolog (Paris)* 78:331, 1915
17. De SN, Ghose ML, Sen A: Activities of bacteria-free preparations from *Vibrio cholerae. J Pathol Bacteriol* 79:373–380, 1960
18. De SN: *Cholera: Its Pathology and Pathogenesis.* London, Oliver and Boyd, 1961
19. Dutta NK, Panse MW, Kulkarni DR: Role of cholera toxin in experimental cholera. *J Bacteriol* 78:594–595, 1959
20. Dutta NK, Habbu MK: Experimental cholera in infant rabbits: a method for chemotheurapeutic investigation. *Brit J Pharmacol Chemother* 10:153–159, 1955
21. Mukherjee B, Bhattacharjee KK, De SN: Observations on experiments on infant rabbits with *Vibrio cholerae. Indian J Med Res* 57:2205–2212, 1969
22. Finkelstein RA: Experimental cholera in infant rabbits: diarrhea or diuresis? *Indian J Med Res* 59:50-31, 1971
23. Finkelstein RA: *Nutrition of Vibrio cholerae,* Ph.D. dissertation. Austin, University of Texas, Austin, 1955
24. Finkelstein RA, Lankford CE: Nutrient requirements of *Vibrio cholerae. Bacteriol Proc* 1955:49, 1955
25. Finkelstein RA, LaBrec EH: Rapid identification of cholera vibrios with fluorescent antibody. *J Bacteriol* 78:886–891, 1959
26. Finkelstein RA, Gomez CZ: Comparison of methods for the rapid recognition of cholera vibrios. *Bull WHO* 28:327–332, 1963
27. Finkelstein RA, Ransom JP: Non-specific resistance to experimental cholera in embryonated eggs. *J Exp Med* 112:315–328, 1960
28. Finkelstein RA, Ramm GM: Effect of age on susceptibility to experimental cholera in embryonated eggs. *J · Infect Dis* 111:239–249, 1962
29. Finkelstein RA: Vibriocidal antibody inhibition (VAI) analysis: a technique for the identification of the predominant vibriocidal antibodies in serum and for the recognition and identification of *Vibrio cholerae* antigens. *J Immunol* 89:264–271, 1962

30. Finkelstein RA, Mukerjee S: Hemagglutination: a rapid method for differentiating *Vibrio cholerae* and El Tor vibrios. *Proc Soc Exp Biol Med* 112:355–359, 1963

31. Smith HW: The antimicrobial activity of the stomach contents of suckling rabbits. *J Pathol Bacteriol* 91:1–9, 1966

32. Phillips RA: Cholera in the perspective of 1966. *Ann Intern Med* 65:922–930, 1966

33. Basaca-Sevilla V, Pesigan TP, Finkelstein RA: Observations on serological responses to cholera immunization. *Am J Trop Med Hyg* 13:100–107, 1964

34. Finkelstein RA, Mukerjee S, Rudra BC: Demonstration and quantitation of antigen in cholera stool filtrates. *J Infect Dis* 113:99–104, 1963

35. Formal SB, Kundel D. Schneider H, et al: Studies with *Vibrio cholerae* in the ligated loop of the rabbit intestine. *Brit J Exp Pathol* 42:504–510, 1961

36. Jenkin CR, Rowley D: Possible factors in the pathogenesis of cholera. *Brit J Exp Pathol* 40:474–482, 1959

37. Norris HT, Dutta NK, Finkelstein RA, et al: Morphologic alterations of the intestine of ten day old rabbits given intact and ultrasonically disrupted cholera vibrios or cholera endotoxin. *Fed Proc* 22:512, 1963

38. Finkelstein RA, Norris HT, Dutta NK: Pathogenesis of experimental cholera in infant rabbits. I. Observations on the intraintestinal infection and experimental cholera produced with cell-free products. *J Infect Dis* 114:203–216, 1964

39. Finkelstein RA: Immunological aspects of experimental cholera, in *Proceedings of the Cholera Research Symposium, Honolulu, 1965*, US Public Health Service Publication No 1328. Washington DC, US Government Printing Office, 1965, pp 58–63

40. *SEATO Conference on Cholera, Dacca, East Pakistan, December 5–8, 1960*. Bangkok, Post Publishing Co Ltd, 1962

41. *Proceedings of the Cholera Research Symposium*, Honolulu, 1965, U.S. Public Health Service Publication No 1328. Washington DC, US Government Printing Office, 1965, pp. 1–397

42. Finkelstein RA: Cholera. *CRC Crit Rev Microbiol* 2:553–623, 1973

43. Burrows W, Kaur J: Cholera toxins, in Barua D, Burrows W (eds): *Cholera*. Philadelphia, WB Saunders, 1974, pp 143–167

44. Finkelstein RA: Progress in the study of cholera and related enterotoxins, in Bernheimer A (ed): *Mechanisms in Bacterial Toxinology*. New York, John Wiley and Sons, 1976, pp 53–84

45. Ouchterlony Ö, Holmgren J (eds): *Proceedings of the 43rd Nobel Symposium: Cholera and Related Diarrheas—Molecular Aspects of a Global Health Problem*, Stockholm, 1978. Basel, Switzerland, S Karger, 1980

46. Holmgren J: Actions of cholera toxin and the prevention and treatment of cholera. *Nature (London)* 292:413–417, 1981

47. Levine MM, Kaper JB, Black RE, et al: New knowledge on pathogenesis of bacterial enteric infection as applied to vaccine development. *Microbiol Rev* 1983:510–550, 1983

48. Finkelstein RA: Cholera, in Germanier R (ed): *Bacterial Vaccines*. New York, Academic Press, Inc., 1984, pp 107–136

49. Finkelstein RA, Dorner F: Cholera enterotoxin (choleragen), in Dorner F. Drews J (eds): *Pharmacology of Bacterial Toxins*. Oxford, Pergamon Press, 1986, pp 161–171

50. Finkelstein RA: Structure of the cholera enterotoxin (choleragen) and the immunologically related ADP-ribosylating heat-labile enterotoxins, in Hardegree MC, Habig WH, Tu A (eds): *Handbook of Natural Toxins, Vol II: Bacterial Toxins*. New York, Marcel Dekker Inc, 1988, pp. 1–38

51. Finkelstein RA, Atthasampunna P, Chulasamaya M, et al: Pathogenesis of experimental cholera: biologic activities of purified Procholeragen A. *J Immunol* 96:440–449, 1966

52. Panse MW, Dutta NK: Excretion of toxin with stools of cholera patients. *J Infect Dis* 109:81–84, 1961

53. Benyajati C: Experimental cholera in humans. *Brit Med J* 1:140–142, 1966

54. Craig JP: The effect of cholera stool and culture filtrates on the skin of guinea pigs and rabbits, in *Proceedings of the Cholera Research Symposium, Honolulu, 1965*, US Public Health Service Publication No 1328. Washington DC, US Government Printing Office, 1965, pp 153–158

55. Craig JP: A permeability factor (toxin) found in cholera stools and culture filtrates and its neutralization by convalescent cholera sera. *Nature* 207:614–616, 1965

56. Finkelstein RA, LoSpalluto JJ: Pathogenesis of experimental cholera: preparation and isolation of choleragen and choleragenoid. *J Exp Med* 130:185–202, 1969

57. Finkelstein RA: Monospecific equine antiserum against cholera exo-enterotoxin. *Infect Immun* 2:691–697, 1970

58. Finkelstein RA, Boesman M, Neoh SH, et al: Dissociation and recombination of the subunits of the cholera enterotoxin (choleragen). *J Immunol* 113:145–150, 1974

59. Lönnroth I, Holmgren J: Subunit structure of cholera toxin. *J Gen Microbiol* 76:417–427, 1973
60. Bennett V, Cuatrecasas P: Cholera toxin: membrane gangliosides and activation of adenylate cyclase, in Cuatrecasas, P (eds.): *The Specificity and Action of Animal, Bacterial and Plant Toxins*. London, Chapman and Hall, 1977, pp 3–66
61. Green H, Kehinde O, Thomas J: Growth of cultured human epidermal cells into multiple epithelia suitable for grafting. *Proc Natl Acad Sci USA* 76:5665–5668, 1979
62. Okada N, Kitano Y, Ichihara K: Effects of cholera toxin on proliferation of cultured human keratinocytes in relation to intracellular cyclic AMP levels. *J Invest Dermatol* 79:42–47, 1982
63. Honda T., Finkelstein RA: Selection and characteristics of a novel *Vibrio cholerae* mutant lacking the A (ADP-ribosylating) portion of the cholera enterotoxin. *Proc Natl Acad Sci USA* 76:2052–2056, 1979
64. Levine MM, Black RE, Clements ML, et al: Evaluation in humans of attenuated *Vibrio cholerae* El Tor Ogawa Strain Texas Star-SR as a live oral vaccine. *Infect Immun* 43:515–522, 1984
65. Kaper JB, Baldini MM, Chapter 4, this volume.
66. Finkelstein RA, Vasil ML, Holmes RK: Studies on toxinogenesis in *Vibrio cholerae*. I. Isolation of mutants with altered toxinogenicity. *J Infect Dis* 129:117–123, 1974
67. Woodward WE, Gilman RH, Hornick RB, et al: Efficacy of a live oral cholera vaccine in human volunteers. *Dev Biol Stand* 33:108–112, 1976
68. Finkelstein RA, LoSpalluto JJ: Production of highly purified choleragen and choleragenoid. *J Infect Dis* 121(Suppl):S63–S72, 1970
69. Finkelstein RA, Fujita K, LoSpalluto JJ: Procholeragenoid: an aggregated intermediate in the formation of choleragenoid. *J Immunol* 107:1043–1051, 1971
70. Mekalanos JJ, Collier RJ, Romig WR: Purification of cholera toxin and its subunits: new methods of preparation and the use of hypertoxinogenic mutants. *Infect Immun* 20:552–558, 1978
71. Tayot J-L, Tardy M: Isolation of cholera toxin by affinity chromatography on porous silica beads with covalently coupled ganglioside G$_{M1}$, in Svennerholm L, Dreyfus H, Urban P-F (eds): *Structure and Function of Gangliosides*. New York, Plenum Publishing Corp, 1980, pp 471–478
72. LoSpalluto JJ, Finkelstein RA: Chemical and physical properties of cholera exo-enterotoxin (choleragen) and its spontaneously formed toxoid (choleragenoid). *Biochim Biophys Acta* 257:158–166, 1972
73. Finkelstein RA, LoSpalluto JJ: Crystalline cholera toxin and toxoid. *Science* 175:529–530, 1972
74. Finkelstein RA, LaRue MK, LoSpalluto JJ: Properties of the cholera exo-enterotoxin: effects of dispersing agents and reducing agents in gel filtration and electrophoresis. *Infect Immun* 6:934–944, 1972
75. Finkelstein RA, Boesman-Finkelstein M, Holt P: *Vibrio cholerae* hemagglutinin/lectin/protease hydrolyzes fibronectin and ovomucin: FM Burnet revisited. *Proc Natl Acad Sci USA* 80:1092–1095, 1983
76. Booth BA, Boesman-Finkelstein M, Finkelstein RA: *Vibrio cholerae* hemagglutinin/protease nicks cholera enterotoxin. *Infect Immun* 45:558–560, 1984
77. Finkelstein RA, Peterson JW, LoSpalluto JJ: Conversion of cholera exo-enterotoxin (choleragen) to natural toxoid (choleragenoid). *J Immunol* 106:868–871, 1971
78. Spangler BD, Westbrook EM: Crystallization of isoelectrically homogenous cholera toxin. *Biochem* 28:1333–1340, 1989
79. Fürer E, Cryz SJ Jr, Germanier R: Protection of piglets against neonatal colibacillosis based on antitoxic immunity. *Dev Biol Stand* 53:151–167, 1983
80. Klapper DG, Finkelstein RA, Capra JD: Subunit structure and N-terminal amino acid sequence of the three chains of cholera enterotoxin. *Immunochemistry* 13:605–611, 1976
81. Lai C-Y, Mendez E, Chang D: Chemistry of cholera toxin: the subunit structure. *J Infect Dis* 133(Suppl):S23–S30, 1976
82. Gill DM: The arrangement of subunits in cholera toxin. *Biochemistry* 15:1242–1248, 1976
83. Ludwig DS, Ribi HO, Schoolnik GK, et al: Two-dimensional crystals of cholera toxin B subunit–receptor complexes: projected structure at 17A resolution. *Proc Natl Acad Sci USA* 83:8585–8588, 1986
84. Ohtomo N, Muraoka T, Tashio A, et al: Size and structure of the cholera toxin molecule and its subunits. *J Infect Dis* 133(Suppl):S31–S40, 1976
85. Kurosky A, Markel DE, Peterson JW, et al: Primary structure of cholera toxin α-chain: a glycoprotein hormone analog? *Science* 195:2299–2301, 1977
86. Kurosky A, Markel DE, Peterson JW, et al: Covalent structure of the α chain of cholera enterotoxin. *J Biol Chem* 252:7257–7264, 1977
87. Lai C-Y: Determination of the primary structure of cholera toxin B subunit. *J Biol Chem* 252:7249–7256, 1977
88. Mekalanos JJ, Swartz DJ, Pearson GDN, et al: Cholera toxin genes: nucleotide sequence, deletion analysis and vaccine development. *Nature* 306:551–557, 1983

89. Betley MJ, Miller VL, Mekalanos JJ: Genetics of bacterial enterotoxins. *Ann Rev Microbiol* 40:577–605, 1986
90. Brickman TJ, Boesman-Finkelstein M, McIntosh MA: Molecular cloning and nucleotide sequence analysis of cholera toxin genes of the CtxA *Vibrio cholerae* strain Texas Star SR. *Infect Immun* 58:4142–4144, 1990
91. Marchlewicz BA, Finkelstein RA: Immunologic differences among the cholera/coli family of enterotoxins. *Diagn Microbiol Infect Dis* 1:129–138, 1983
92. Finkelstein RA, Burks MF, Zupan A, et al: Epitopes of the cholera family of enterotoxins. *Rev Infect Dis* 9:544–561, 1987
93. Lockman H, Kaper JB: Nucleotide sequence analysis of the A2 and B subunits of *Vibrio cholerae* enterotoxin. *J Biol Chem* 258:13722–13726, 1983
94. Tsuji T, Iida T, Honda T, et al: A unique amino acid sequence of the B subunit of a heat-labile enterotoxin isolated from a human enterotoxigenic *Escherichia coli*. *Microbial Pathogen* 2:381–390, 1987
95. Jacob CO, Arnon R, Finkelstein RA: Immunity towards heat labile enterotoxins of porcine and human *Eschericha coli* strains achieved with synthetic peptides. *Infect Immun* 52:562–567, 1986
96. Yamamoto T, Tamura T, Yokota T: Primary structure of a heat-labile enterotoxin produced by *Escherichia coli* pathogenic for humans. *J Biol Chem* 259:5037–5044, 1984
97. Yamamoto T, Nakazawa T, et al: Evolution and structure of two ADP-ribosylation enterotoxins, *Escherichia coli* heat-labile toxin and cholera toxin. *FEBS Lett* 169:241–246, 1984
98. Yamamoto T, Gojabori T, Yokota T: Evolutionary origin of pathogenic determinants in enterotoxigenic *Escherichia coli* and *Vibrio cholerae* 01. *J Bacteriol* 169:1352–1357, 1987
99. Vasil ML, Holmes RK, Finkelstein RA: Conjugal transfer of a chromosomal gene determining production of enterotoxin in *Vibrio cholerae*. *Science* 187:849–850, 1975
100. Holmes RK, Bramucci MG, Twiddy EM: Genetics of toxinogenesis of *Vibrio cholerae* and *Escherichia coli*. *Contr Microbiol Immunol* 6:165–177, 1979
101. Mekalanos JJ: Cholera toxin: genetic analysis, regulation and role in pathogenesis. *Curr Top Microbiol Immunol* 118:97–118, 1985
102. Guidolin A, Manning PA: Genetics of *Vibrio cholerae* and its bacteriophages. *Microbiol Rev* 51:285–298, 1987
103. Miller VL, Taylor RK, Mekalanos JJ: Cholera toxin transcriptional activator ToxR is a transmembrane DNA binding protein. *Cell* 48: 271–279, 1987
104. Gill DM: Seven toxic peptides that cross cell membranes, in Jeljaszewicz J, Wadström T (eds): *Bacterial Toxins and Cell Membranes*. London, Academic Press, 1978, pp 291–332
105. Gill DM: Cholera toxin-catalyzed ADP-ribosylation of membrane proteins, in Hayaishi O, Ueda K (eds): *ADP Ribosylation Reactions: Biology and Medicine*. New York, Academic Press Inc, 1982, pp 593–621
106. Moss J, Vaughan M: Mechanism of action of *Escherichia coli* heat-labile enterotoxin: activation of adenylate cyclase by ADP-ribosylation, in Hayaishi O, Ueda K (eds): *ADP Ribosylation Reactions: Biology and Medicine*. New York, Academic Press Inc, 1982, pp 623–636
107. Vaughan M: Choleragen, adenylate cyclase, and ADP-ribosylation, in: *The Harvey Lectures, Series 77*. New York, Academic Press Inc, 1983, pp 43–62
108. van Heyningen WE, Carpenter CCJ, Pierce NF, et al: Deactivation of cholera toxin by ganglioside. *J Infect Dis* 124:415–418, 1971
109. King CA, van Heyningen WE: Deactivation of cholera toxin by a sialidase-resistant monosialosyl ganglioside. *J Infect Dis* 127:639–647, 1973
110. Holmgren J, Svennerholm A-M: Mechanisms of disease and immunity in cholera: a review. *J Infect Dis* 136(Suppl):S105–S112, 1977
111. Eidels L, Prioa RL, Hart DA: Membrane receptors for bacterial toxins. *Microbiol Rev* 47:596–620, 1983
112. Pierce NF: Differential inhibitory effects of cholera toxoids and ganglioside on the enterotoxins of *Vibrio cholerae* and *Escherichia coli*. *J Exp Med* 137:1009–1023, 1973
113. Peterson JW, LoSpalluto JJ, Finkelstein RA: Localization of cholera toxin *in vivo*. *J Infect Dis* 126:617–628, 1972
114. Hollenberg MD, Fishman PH, Bennett V, Cuatrecasas P: Cholera toxin and cell growth: role of membrane gangliosides. *Proc Natl Acad Sci USA* 71:4224–4228, 1974
115. Moss J, Fishman PH, Mangeniello VC, et al: Functional incorporation of ganglioside into intact cells: induction of choleragen responsiveness. *Proc Natl Acad Sci USA* 73:1034–1037, 1976
116. Clements JD, Finkelstein RA: Isolation and characterization of homogeneous heat-labile enterotoxin(s) (LT(s)) with high specific activity from *Escherichia coli* cultures. *Infect Immun* 24:760–769, 1979

117. Griffiths SL, Finkelstein RA, Critchley DR: Characterization of the receptor for cholera toxin and *Escherichia coli* heat-labile toxin in rabbit intestinal brush borders. *Biochem J* 238:313–322, 1986
118. Ludwig DS, Holmes RK, Schoolnik GK: Chemical and immunochemical studies on the receptor binding domain of cholera toxin B subunit. *J Biol Chem* 260:12528–12534, 1985
119. Kazemi M, Finkelstein RA: Study of epitopes of cholera enterotoxin related enterotoxins by checkerboard immunoblotting. *Infect Immun* 58:2352–2360, 1990
120. Moss J, Richards RL, Alving CR, et al: Effect of the A and B protomers of choleragen on release of trapped glucose from liposomes containing or lacking ganglioside G_{M1} *J Biol Chem* 252:797–798, 1977
121. Tosteson MT, Tosteson DC, Rubnitz J: Cholera toxin interactions with lipid bilayers. *Acta Physiol Scand* 481(Suppl):21–25, 1980
122. Gill DM, Woolkalis M: Toxins which activate adenylate cyclase, in Evered D, Whelan J (eds): *Ciba Foundation Symposium 112: Microbial Toxins and Diarrhoeal Disease.* London, Pitman Publishing Ltd, 1985, pp 57–73
123. Fishman PH: Mechanism of action of cholera toxin: events on the cell surface, in Field M. Fordtran JS, Schultz SG (eds): *Secretory Diarrhea.* Baltimore, Waverly Press Inc, 1980, pp 85–106
124. Field M, Plotkin GR, Silen W: Effects of vasopressin, theophylline and cyclic adenosine monophosphate on short-circuit current across isolated rabbit ileal mucosa. *Nature (London)* 217:469–471, 1968
125. Field M: Intestinal secretion: effect of cyclic AMP and its role in cholera. *N Engl J Med* 284:1137–1144, 1971
126. Butcher RW, Baird CE, Sutherland EW: Effects of lipolytic and antilipolytic substances on adenosine 3′,5′-monophosphate levels in isolated fat cells. *J Biol Chem* 243:1705–1712, 1970
127. Field M, Fromm D, Wallace CK, Greenough WB III: Stimulation of active chloride secretion in small intestine by cholera exotoxin. *J Clin Invest* 486:24a(abstr), 1969
128. Vaughan M, Pierce NF, Greenough WB III: Stimulation of glycerol production in fat cells by cholera toxin. *Nature* 226:658–659, 1970
129. Greenough WB III, Pierce NF, Vaughan M: Titration of cholera enterotoxin and antitoxin in isolated fat cells. *J Infect Dis* 121(Suppl):S111–S113, 1970
130. Wolff, J, Temple R, Cook GH: Stimulation of steroid secretion in adrenal tumor cells by choleragen. *Proc Natl Acad Sci USA* 70:2741–2744, 1973
131. Donta ST, King M: Induction of steroidogenesis in tissue culture by cholera enterotoxin. *Nature* 243:246–247, 1973
132. Guerrant RL, Brunton LL, Schnaitman TC, et al: Cyclic adenosine monophosphate and alteration of Chinese hamster ovary cell morphology: a rapid, sensitive *in vitro* assay for the enterotoxins of *Vibrio cholerae* and *Escherichia coli. Infect Immun* 10:320–327, 1974
133. Field M: Mode of action of cholera toxin: stabilization of catecholamine-sensitive adenylate cyclase in turkey erythrocytes. *Proc Natl Acad Sci USA* 71:3299–3303, 1974
134. Schafer DE, Lust WD, Sircar B, et al: Elevated concentration of adenosine 3′:5′-cyclic monophosphate in intestinal mucosa after treatment with cholera toxin. *Proc Natl Acad Sci USA* 67:851–856, 1970
135. Sharp GWG, Hynie S: Stimulation of intestinal adenyl cyclase by cholera toxin. *Nature* 229:266–269, 1971
136. Chen LC, Rohde JE, Sharp GWG: Intestinal adenyl-cyclase activity in human cholera. *Lancet* i:939–941, 1971
137. Gill DM, Pappenheimer AM: Diphtheria: recent studies have clarified the molecular mechanisms involved in its pathogenesis. *Science* 182:353–358, 1973
138. Zieve PD, Pierce NF, Greenough WB III: Stimulation of glycogenolysis by purified cholera exotoxin in disrupted cells. *Johns Hopkins Med J* 129:299–303, 1971
139. Gill DM, King CA: The mechanism of action of cholera toxin in pigeon erythrocyte lysates. *J Biol Chem* 250:6424–6432, 1975
140. Gilman AG: G proteins: transducers of receptor-generated signals. *Ann Rev Biochem* 56:615–649, 1987
141. Powell CW: The role of G proteins in transmembrane signalling. *Biochem J* 272:1–13, 1990
142. Powell DW, Berschneider HM, Lawson LD, et al: Regulation of water and ion movement in intestine, in Evered D, Whelan J (eds): *Ciba Foundation Symposium 112: Microbial Toxins and Diarrheal Disease.* London, Pitman Publishing Ltd, 1985, pp 14–33
143. Peterson JW, Ochoa LG: Role of prostaglandins and CAMP in the secretory effects of cholera toxin. *Science* 245:857–859, 1989
144. Gill DM: Sequence homologies among the enzymically active portions of ADP ribosylating toxins. *Zbl Bakt Suppl* 17:315–323, 1988
145. Weiss AA, Hewlett EL: Virulence factors of *Bordetella pertussis. Ann Rev Microbiol* 40:661–686, 1986
146. O'Brien AD, Holmes RK: Shiga and shiga-like toxins. *Microbiol Rev* 51:206–220, 1987

147. Greenberg RN, Guerrant RL: *E. coli* heat-stable enterotoxin, in Dorner F, Drews J (eds): *Pharmacology of Bacterial Toxins*. Oxford, Pergamon Press, 1986, pp 115–151

148. Gorbach SL, Banwell JG, Chatterjee BD, et al: Acute undifferentiated human diarrhea in the tropics. I. Alterations in intestinal microflora. *J Clin Invest* 50:881–889, 1971

149. Sack RB, Gorbach SL, Banwell JG, et al: Enterotoxigenic *Escherichia coli* isolated from patients with severe cholera-like disease. *J Infect Dis* 123:378–385, 1971

150. Barnum DA, Glantz PJ, Moon HW: Colibacillosis, in *CIBA Veterinary Monograph Series/TWO*. Summit, NJ, CIBA Pharmaceutical Co, 1967

151. Gyles CL, Barnum DA: A heat-labile enterotoxin from strains of *Escherichia coli* enteropathogenic for pigs. *J Infect Dis* 120:419–426, 1969

152. Smith HW, Halls S: Studies on *Escherichia coli* enterotoxin. *J Path Bact* 93:531–543, 1967

153. Smith HW, Gyles CL: The relationship between two apparently different enterotoxins produced by enteropathogenic strains of *Escherichia coli* of porcine origin. *J Med Microbiol* 3:387–401, 1970

154. Gyles CL: Relationships among heat-labile enterotoxins of *Escherichia coli* and *Vibrio cholerae. J Infect Dis* 129:277–283, 1974

155. Finkelstein RA: Laboratory production and isolation of enterotoxins and isolation of a candidate live vaccine for diarrheal disease, in *Proceedings of the 43rd Nobel Symposium: Cholera and Related Diarrheas— Molecular Aspects of a Global Health Problem, Stockholm, 1978*. Basel, Switzerland, S. Karger, 1980, pp 64–79

156. Dorner F: *Escherichia coli* enterotoxin purification and partial characterization. *J Biol Chem* 250:8712–8719, 1975

157. Finkelstein RA, LaRue MK, Johnston DW, et al: Isolation and properties of heat-labile enterotoxin(s) from enterotoxigenic *Escherichia coli. J Infect Dis* 133(Suppl):S120–S137, 1976

158. Rappaport RS, Sagin JF, Pierzchala WA, et al: Activation of heat-labile *Escherichia coli* enterotoxin by trypsin. *J Infect Dis* 133(Suppl):S41–S54, 1976

159. Neill RJ, Ivins BE, Holmes RK: Synthesis and secretion of the plasmid-coded heat-labile enterotoxin of *Escherichia coli* in *Vibrio cholerae. Science* 221:289–291, 1983

160. Clements JD, Yancey RJ, Finkelstein RA: Properties of homogeneous heat-labile enterotoxin from *Escherichia coli. Infect Immun* 29:91–97, 1980

161. Kunkel SV, Robertson DC: Purification and chemical characterization of the heat-labile enterotoxin produced by enterotoxigenic *Escherichia coli. Infect Immun* 25:586–596, 1979

162. Dallas WS, Falkow S: Amino acid sequence homology between cholera toxin and *Escherichia coli* heat-labile toxin. *Nature (London)* 288:499–501, 1980

163. Leong J, Vinal AC, Dallas WS: Nucleotide sequence comparison between heat-labile toxin B-subunit cistrons from *Escherichia coli* of human and porcine origin. *Infect Immun* 48:73–77, 1985

164. Zinnaka Y, Carpenter CCJ: An enterotoxin produced by non-cholera vibrios. *Johns Hopkins Med J* 131:403–411, 1972

165. Ohashi M, Shimada T, Fukumi H: In vitro production of enterotoxin and hemorrhagic principle by *Vibrio cholerae*, NAG. *Japan J Med Sci Biol* 25:179–194, 1972

166. Yamamoto K, Takeda Y, Miwatani T, et al: Purification and some properties of a non-01 *Vibrio cholerae* enterotoxin that is identical to cholera enterotoxin. *Infect Immun* 39:1128–1135, 1983

167. Yamamoto K, Takeda Y, Miwatani T, et al: Evidence that a non-01 *Vibrio cholerae* produces enterotoxin that is similar but not identical to cholera enterotoxin. *Infect Immun* 41:896–901, 1983

168. Craig JP: The vibrio diseases in 1982, in Takeda Y, Miwatani T (eds): *Bacterial Diarrheal Diseases*. Boston, Martinus Nijhoff Publishers, 1985, pp 11–23

169. Finkelstein RA, Sobocinski PZ, Atthasampunna P, et al: Pathogenesis of experimental cholera: identification of choleragen (Procholeragen A) by disc immunoelectrophoresis and its differentiation from cholera mucinase. *J Immunol* 97:25–33, 1966

170. Vasil ML, Holmes RK, Finkelstein RA: Studies on toxinogenesis in *Vibrio cholerae*. II. An in vitro test for enterotoxin production. *Infect Immun* 9:195–197, 1974

171. Yamamoto T, Yokota T: Sequence of heat-labile enterotoxin of *Escherichia coli* pathogenic for humans. *J Bacteriol* 155:728–733, 1983

172. Tsuji T, Honda T, Miwatani T, et al: Analysis of receptor-binding site in *Escherichia coli* enterotoxin. *J Biol Chem* 260:8552–8558, 1985

173. Peterson JW: Salmonella toxin. *Pharmacol Ther* 11:719–724, 1980

174. Finkelstein RA, Marchlewicz BA, McDonald RJ, et al: Isolation and characterization of a cholera-related enterotoxin from *Salmonella typhimurium. FEMS Microbiol Lett* 17:239–241, 1983

175. Stephen J, Wallis TS, Starkey WG, et al: Salmonellosis in retrospect and prospect, in Evered D. Whelan J (eds): *Ciba Foundation Symposium 112: Microbial Toxins and Diarrheal Disease*. London, Pitman Publishing Ltd, 1985, pp 175–192

176. Peterson JW, Chopra AK, Prasad R, et al: Partial purification and characterization of cloned *Salmonella* enterotoxin, in: *Proceedings of the 23rd Joint Conference on Cholera*, US–Japan Cooperative Medical Science Program, Williamsburg VA, National Institute of Allergy and Infectious Diseases, NIH, p. 85.

177. Spira WM, Fedorka-Cray PJ: Purification of enterotoxins from *Vibrio mimicus* that appear to be identical to cholera toxin. *Infect Immun* 45:679–684, 1984

178. Shimada T, Sakazaki R, Horigome K, et al: Production of cholera-like enterotoxin by *Aeromonas hydrophila*. *Jpn J Med Sci Biol* 37:141–144, 1984

179. Potomski J, Burke V, Robinson J, et al: *Aeromonas* cytotonic enterotoxin cross reactive with cholera toxin. *J Med Micro* 23:179–186, 1987

180. Potomski J, Burke V, Watson I, et al: Purification of cytotoxic enterotoxin of *Aeromonas sobria* by use of monoclonal antibodies. *J Med Micro* 23:171–177, 1987

181. Walker RI, Caldwell MB, Lee EC, et al: Pathophysiology of *Campylobacter* enteritis. *Microbiol Rev* 50:81–94, 1986

182. Klipstein FA, Engert RF: Immunological interrelationships between cholera toxin and the heat-labile and heat-stable enterotoxins of coliform bacteria. *Infect Immun* 18:110–117, 1977

183. Holmes RK, Twiddy EM, Pickett CL: Purification and characterization of Type II heat-labile enterotoxin of *Escherichia coli. Infect Immun* 53:464–473, 1986

184. Joo I: Cholera vaccines, in Barua D, Burrows W (eds): *Cholera*. Philadelphia, WB Saunders, 1974, pp 333–355

185. Finkelstein RA: Immunology of cholera. *Curr Top Microbiol Immunol* 69:137–196, 1975

186. Finkelstein RA: Immunology of *Vibrio cholerae*, in Nahmias AJ, O'Reilly RJ (eds): *Comprehensive Immunology: Immunology of Human Infection*. New York, Plenum Publishing Corp, 1981, pp 291–315

187. Feeley JC, Gangarosa EJ: Field trial of cholera vaccine, in Ouchterlony Ö, Holmgren J (eds): *Cholera and Related Diarrheas*. Basel, S Karger, 1980, pp 204–210

188. Finkelstein RA: Vaccines (?) against the cholera-related enterotoxin family. *Microbiology* 1985:114–118, 1985

189. Finkelstein RA: Dead vaccines are "alive" but live vaccines are not dead: analysis of options for immunization against cholera, in Holmgren J. Lindberg A, Mollby R (eds): *Development of Vaccines and Drugs against Diarrhea, 11th Nobel Conference, Stockholm, 1985*. Lund, Sweden Studentlitteratur, and Kent, England, Chartwell-Bratt Ltd, 1986, pp 74–81

190. Cvjetanovic B: Economic considerations in cholera control, in Barua D, Burrows W (eds): *Cholera*. Philadelphia, WB Saunders, 1974, pp 435–445

191. Finkelstein RA, Pongpairojana S: A test of antigenicity for the selection of strains for inclusion in cholera vaccines. *Bull WHO* 39:247–259, 1968

192. Curlin G. Levine R, Aziz KMA, et al: Field trial of cholera toxoid, in: *Proceedings of the 11th Joint Conference on Cholera*, US–Japan Cooperative Medical Science Program, 1975. 1976, pp 314–329

193. Sciortino CV, Finkelstein RA: *Vibrio cholerae* express iron-regulated outer membrane proteins *in vivo. Infect Immun* 42:990–996, 1983

194. Booth BA, Sciortino CV, Finkelstein RA: Adhesins of *Vibrio cholerae*, in Mirelman D (ed): *Microbial Lectins and Agglutinins*. New York, John Wiley and Sons, 1986, pp 169–182

195. Booth BA, Dyer TJ, Finkelstein RA: Adherence of *Vibrio cholerae* to cultured human cells, in Sack RB, Zinnaka Y (eds): *Advances in Research on Cholera and Related Diarrheas*, Vol 7 *Proceedings of the 23rd Joint Conference on Cholera*, US–Japan Cooperative Medical Science Program, Williamsburg VA, 1987. KTK Scientific Publishers, Tokyo, 1990, pp 19–35

196. Kaper JB, Levine MM, Lockman HA, et al: Development and testing of a recombinant live oral cholera vaccine, in: *Vaccines 85*. Cold Spring Harbor NY, Cold Spring Harbor Laboratory, 1985, pp 107–111

197. Levine MM, Kaper JB, Morris JG, et al: Reactogenicity, colonizing capacity, and immunogenicity of further attenuated, genetically engineered *Vibrio cholerae* 01 vaccine strains, in Kuwahara S, Pierce NF (eds.): *Advances in Research on Cholera and related Diarrheas, Proceedings of the 21st Joint Conference on Cholera*, US–Japan Cooperative Medical Science Program, Bethesda MD, 1985. Tokyo, KTK Scientific Publishers, pp 225–230, 1988

198. Cash RA, Music SI, Libonati JP, et al: Response of man to infection with *Vibrio cholerae*. II. Protection from illness afforded by previous disease and vaccine. *J Infect Dis* 130:325–333, 1974

199. Owen RL, Pierce NF, Apple RT, et al: M cell transport of *Vibrio cholerae* from the intestinal lumen into

Peyer's patches: a mechanism for antigen sampling and for microbial transepithelial migration. *J Infect Dis* 153:1108–1118, 1986

200. Svennerholm A-M, Holmgren J: Synergistic protective effect in rabbits of immunization with *Vibrio cholerae* lipopolysaccharide and toxin/toxoid. *Infect Immun* 13:735–740, 1976

201. Rappaport RS, Bonde G: Development of a vaccine against experimental cholera and *Escherichia coli* diarrheal disease. *Infect Immun* 32:534–542, 1981

202. Clemens JD, Sack DA, Harris JR, et al: Field trial of oral cholera vaccines in Bangladesh. Lancet II:124–127, 1986

203. Clemens JD, Harris JR, Sack DA, et al: Field trial of oral cholera vaccines in Bangladesh: results of one year of follow-up. *J Infect Dis* 158:60–69, 1988

204. Fujita K, Finkelstein RA: Antitoxic immunity in experimental cholera: comparison of immunity induced perorally and parenterally in mice. *J Infect Dis* 125:647–655, 1972

205. Holmgren J: Experimental studies on cholera immunisation: the protective immunogenicity in rabbits of monomeric and polymeric crude exotoxin. *J Med Microbiol* 6:363–370, 1973

206. Germanier R, Fürer E, Varallyay S, et al: Preparation of a purified antigenic cholera toxoid. *Infect Immun* 13:1692–1698, 1976

207. Peterson JW: Protection against experimental cholera by oral or parenteral immunization. *Infect Immun* 26:594–598, 1979

208. Fürer E, Cryz SJ Jr, Dorner F, et al: Protection against colibacillosis in neonatal piglets by immunization of dams with procholeragenoid. *Infect Immun* 35:887–894, 1982

209. Pierce NF, Cray WC Jr, Sacci JB Jr, et al: Procholeragenoid: a safe and effective antigen for oral immunization against experimental cholera. *Infect Immun* 40:1112–1118, 1983

210. Finkelstein RA, Hollingsworth RC: Antitoxic immunity in experimental cholera: observations with purified antigens and the rat foot edema model. *Infect Immun* 1:468–473, 1970

211. Northrup RS, Fauci AS: Adjuvant effect of cholera enterotoxin on the immune response of the mouse to sheep red blood cells. *J Infect Dis* 125:672–673, 1972

212. Finkelstein RA, Sciortino CV, Rieke LC, et al: Preparation of "procoligenoids" from *Escherichia coli* heat-stable enterotoxins (LTs). *Infect Immun* 45:518–521, 1984

213. Klipstein FA, Engert RF, Houghten RA: Protection in rabbits immunized with a vaccine of *Escherichia coli* heat-stable toxin cross-linked to the heat-labile toxin B subunit. *Infect Immun* 40:888–893, 1983

214. Germanier R: Typhoid fever, in Germanier R (ed): *Bacterial Vaccines*, New York, Academic Press Inc, 1984, pp 137–165

215. Boesman-Finkelstein M, Sciortino CV, Finkelstein RA: Iron-related antibacterial activities of human milk, in Spik G, Montreuil J, Crichton JJ, Mazurier J (eds): *Proteins of Iron Storage and Transport*. Elsevier, Netherlands, Elsevier Science Publishers, 1985, pp 251–260

216. Boesman-Finkelstein M, Finkelstein RA: Antimicrobial effects of human milk: inhibitory activity on enteric pathogens. *FEMS Lett* 27:167–174, 1985

217. Dolan SA, Boesman-Finkelstein M, Finkelstein RA: Antimicrobial activity of human milk against pediatric pathogens. *J Infect Dis* 154:722–725, 1986

218. Dolan SA, Boesman-Finkelstein M, Finkelstein RA: Inhibition of enteropathogenic bacteria in human milk whey in vitro. *Pediatr Infect Dis J* 8:430–436, 1989

219. Boesman-Finkelstein M, Watson NE, Finkelstein RA: Bovine lactogenic immunity against cholera toxin-related enterotoxins and *Vibrio cholerae* outer membrane. *Infect Immun* 57:1227–1234, 1989

220. McClead RE, Gregory SA: Resistance of bovine colostral anti-cholera toxin antibody to in vitro and in vivo proteolysis. *Infect Immun* 44:474–478, 1984

221. Brüssow H, Hilpert H, Walther I, et al: Bovine milk immunoglobulins for passive immunity to infantile rotavirus gastroenteritis. *J Clin Microbiol* 25:982–986, 1987

222. Hilpert H, Brüssow H, Mietens C, et al: Use of bovine milk concentrate containing antibody to rotavirus to treat rotavirus gastroenteritis in infants. *J Infect Dis* 156:158–166, 1987

223. Tacket CO, Herrington DA, Lonsonsky G, et al: Protection by milk immunoglobulin concentrate against oral challenge with enterotoxigenic *Escherichia coli*, *N Engl J Med* 318:1240–1243, 1988

9

Colonization and Pathology

R. Bradley Sack

1. INTRODUCTION

The pathogenesis of cholera has been well characterized during the past 25 years in several animal models and cholera patients. From these studies has come an understanding of this disease which is perhaps the most complete of any infectious disease. Clearly, there are still gaps in our knowledge about many of the details of the host–parasite relationship, but the major events (inoculum size, colonization, and enterotoxin production and its physiologic effects) are known, and from this knowledge specific interventions have been devised to interfere with the establishment of the infection, aid in treating it, or hasten its termination.

Cholera is a topical infection of the small intestine with *V. cholerae* 01, in which acute diarrhea and resultant volume depletion are the sole basis of all clinical manifestations. The small bowel in humans is normally only sparsely colonized with bacteria, which are mostly of the respiratory, commensal type, i.e., gram positive cocci, such as streptococci and staphylococci. Specifically lacking are gram-negative enteric organisms, and anaerobes. The total concentration of organisms in the small bowel is less than 10^5 per ml of intestinal fluid (or per gram intestine).[1] Vibrios, therefore, have little microbial competition preventing colonization and infection of the upper small intestine.

The small bowel is also the site of the most active fluid exchanges that occur in the intestine. Normally about 10–11 liters of fluid enter the upper gut during each 24-h period, consisting of ingested fluid from the stomach, fluid secreted by the pancreas, liver, and biliary tree, and fluid secreted by the small intestine itself.[2] Nearly all of this fluid is reabsorbed in the small bowel, with only a relatively small volume reaching the large intestine, where the remainder is absorbed. Normally only about 200 ml per day are excreted in fecal material. During cholera, this finely balanced system of fluid movement is severely disrupted, and large volumes of diarrheic fluid are excreted.

Cholera, edited by Dhiman Barua and William B. Greenough III. Plenum Medical Book Company, New York, 1992.

This chapter will attempt to define our present understanding of how these events occur, at a cellular and molecular level where possible.

2. VIBRIO INGESTION

Vibrios are ingested in food and water that have been contaminated with the organisms. In nearly all cases, the vibrios have come from feces of humans infected (but not necessarily symptomatic) with the organisms. No animals have been shown to be reservoirs of the organisms, with the exception of shellfish in certain aquatic environments (see Chapter 6). Vibrios are extremely acid sensitive, being killed at a pH of <5.5. Therefore the normal gastric acid (~pH 2) is a formidable barrier in preventing these organisms from reaching the small bowel.

In volunteer experiments done in healthy young adults, the inoculum size necessary to produce clinical cholera can be decreased by 100,000 times, when the stomach acid has been neutralized by sodium bicarbonate.[3] In natural outbreaks of cholera, the risk of developing the disease is markedly increased in persons who have low gastric acidity, such as those with previous gastrectomies.[4] In patients with cholera in an endemic area, it has been determined that their gastric acid is lower than in a group of comparable persons without cholera.[5] In animal models and volunteers, gastric acid is routinely neutralized before inoculation in order to insure the highest infection rates. Clearly the presence of gastric acid markedly influences the size of the vibrio inoculum necessary to produce infection. No other factors are known to be important in determining inoculum size, although one would presume salivary enzymes, other gastric and pancreatic enzymes might also contribute to natural "resistance" to infection.

There have been no studies in which the inoculum size could be determined accurately in a field situation, although it is known that it takes about 10^{11} organisms suspended in liquid to produce a 50% attack rate in normal young volunteers with normal gastric acid.[3] Since the attack rate in an endemic area, even during an epidemic period is usually not more than 2–4 per 1000 population, it is postulated that the inoculum size may be much lower than this, perhaps in the range of 10^4 or 10^5, with the hypochloridic subjects being selected out for successful infection. Vibrios may also be protected in their journey through an acid stomach if they are within a food bolus, and if the gastric emptying time is rapid. All evidence suggests, however, that gastric acid is the major determinant of a successful inoculation of vibrios.

3. COLONIZATION OF THE SMALL BOWEL

Vibrios surviving the passage through the stomach must colonize the small bowel in order to establish infection and disease. They do this by attaching themselves to mucosal cells of the small bowel and proliferating to large concentrations, 10^7 to 10^8 vibrios per ml of small intestine.[6] While actively colonizing the mucosa, and closely approximating themselves to enterocytes, they produce the enterotoxin which is then responsible for the alterations in fluid transport of the small bowel.

Until very recently, the mechanisms whereby vibrios reach the mucosal surface and effectively colonize this area were poorly understood. A number of possible mechanisms were postulated and studied in animal models. These have included chemotactic mechanisms, motility of the vibrios through their single polar flagellum, hemagglutinins (both soluble and cell-associated), outer membrane proteins, lipopolysaccharides, enterotoxin, and fimbria. It now seems clear that fimbria are the critical factor in colonization. The possible importance of these other factors, however, will be discussed as well.

3.1. Chemotaxis and Motility

In order for vibrios to colonize the surface of enterocytes, they must overcome the normal mucous layer that covers the intestine. This mucous has been shown to be chemotactic to vibrios[7] and vibrios are known to produce proteolytic enzymes, including mucinase.[8] Although these factors may be important in allowing the vibrios to traverse the mucous layer, this has not been clearly defined.

Likewise motility has been postulated as being an important factor in facilitating vibrios in reaching the surface of enterocytes. All vibrios normally possess a single polar-sheathed flagellum. Early studies in animal models suggested that nonmotile variants of *V. cholerae* 01 were less virulent[9]; more recent studies, however, have failed to corroborate these findings.[10] Clearly, vibrios do not attach by their flagella, which can be seen protruding into the luminal space on photomicrographs (see Fig. 1). If one considers a comparable situation with enterotoxigenic *E. coli,* both naturally occurring motile and nonmotile strains cause diarrheal illness, and there is no evidence that motile strains are more virulent in animal models. The darting, rapid motility of vibrios, so impressive in the laboratory, seems not to be a critical factor in pathogenesis. This property may be of more importance to survival of these organisms in the environment, where they survive well either attached to water plants[11] or to shellfish.[12]

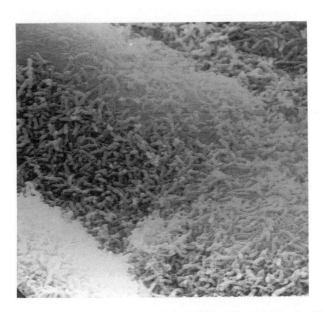

FIGURE 1. Scanning electron photomicrograph of *V. cholerae* 01 heavily colonizing the villus of the ileum of an adult rabbit. (Courtesy of Dr. Richard Finkelstein.)

3.2. Hemagglutinins

A large variety of hemagglutinins have been described in *V. cholerae* 01 which may be both soluble and cell-associated.

A summary of this extensive body of information has recently been published.[8] The cell-associated, mannose-sensitive hemagglutinin, which can be used to differentiate classical and El Tor strains of *V. cholerae* 01 was postulated as being important in the epidemiologic behavior of El Tor strains, where asymptomatic infection is more widespread.[13] It is now clear, however, that all strains of *V. cholerae* 01 produce cell-associated hemagglutinins[8] and that these are not essential for virulence.[14] The gene controlling one of these cell-associated hemagglutinins has been cloned and sequenced[15]; this will allow more detailed studies of the function of these proteins.

A soluble hemagglutinin has also been characterized that is also a proteolytic enzyme, which digests mucin and fibronectin, as well as nicking the A subunit of the cholera enterotoxin.[16] Although there are interesting theoretical possibilities for the importance of this protein, such as allowing detachment of the vibrios after initial colonization, or of activating the cholera enterotoxin, none have yet been clearly defined.

In a recent study in which a large number of *V. cholerae* 01 strains were surveyed, there was considerable variation in the presence of hemagglutinins, and no clear correlation with virulence.[14]

Slime layers have also been described in some vibrio strains, which are hemagglutinins, but again there is no clear evidence that these are virulence factors.[17]

3.3. Outer Membrane Proteins and Lipopolysaccharides

The outer membrane of vibrios contains several major proteins, some of which are strongly antigenic.[18,19] Some studies have suggested that the flagellar sheath is a continuation of the outer membrane.[20] No studies have clearly implicated these outer membrane proteins as virulence factors, however. One study[21] has suggested that an iron-regulated outer membrane protein may be important in the colonization process.

The lipopolysaccharide (LPS) of *V. cholerae* 01, though a clear virulence factor (since only 01 strains are capable of causing epidemic cholera) and an important protective antigen, has not been clearly defined as an adhesive factor. Purified LPS has been found to cause hemagglutination, and monoclonal antibodies directed against LPS inhibit this hemagglutination.[8] Antibodies against LPS are highly protective in animal models, and part of this protection may be in interference with colonization, either directly or indirectly. The genes controlling O antigen synthesis have now been cloned into *E. coli*,[22] and it may be possible to specifically isolate its role in pathogenesis.

3.4. Fimbria

Fimbria have long been suspected of being important in vibrio adherence, particularly since they are well characterized as virulence factors in enterotoxigenic *E. coli*. Although fimbria were occasionally visualized in preparations of vibrios, they were not convincingly demonstrated until the past 4–5 years. Using specially designed bacteriologic media,[23] these protein appendages have been clearly identified, and their genetic control characterized (Fig.

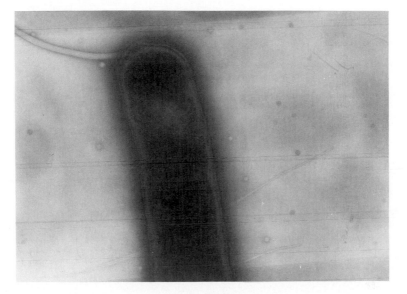

FIGURE 2. Photomicrograph of *V. cholerae* 01 with its attached fimbria and polar flagellum. (Courtesy of Dr. John Mekalanos.)

2), The major subunit of the pilus (fimbria) is encoded by the gene *tcpA*, which is found uniformly in all clinical isolates of *V. cholerae* 01.[24] This TCP pilus is expressed coordinately with cholera enterotoxin under a wide variety of culture conditions; this effect appears to be dependent on regulation by the ToxR gene,[25] which also plays a role in regulating other potential virulence factors, such as outer membrane proteins.[26] The *tcpA* gene has been sequenced and the amino acid sequence of the pili deduced[25]; amino acid homology with pili of other pathogenic bacteria has been observed. In volunteer studies[27] mutant strains which did not produce the pili failed to colonize the intestine and failed to produce an effective immune response. Thus, TCP pili seem to be the elusive "colonization factor" of *V. cholerae* 01, analogous to the colonization factors of ETEC. Unlike ETEC, however, to date, all strains of *V. cholerae* 01 have produced a pilus of the same antigenic type. This is not unexpected because of the known cross-protection afforded by killed whole cell cholera vaccines. The receptors for the pili have not yet been identified.

The presence of the conjugative plasmid P has been shown to suppress virulence of some strains of *V. cholerae* 01, possibly through interfering with the production of TCP pili.[28]

V. cholerae 01 have also been shown to produce other pili, which have hemagglutinating activity, but have no role in colonization.[29] Likewise *V. cholerae* non-01 have been shown to produce pili which are closely related to the TCP pili, but which have no role in colonization.[30]

4. PATHOLOGY

The colonization of the small bowel and the action of the enterotoxin on the mucosal cells leads to marked biochemical and physiological changes in small bowel function. The integrity of the mucosa, however, remains intact, and there are few histologic changes that

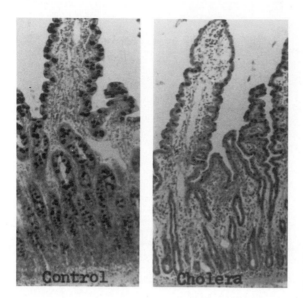

FIGURE 3. Histologic section of dog jejunum before and during experimentally induced clinical cholera. (Courtesy of Dr. Charles Carpenter, *J Infect Dis* 126:551–564, 1972.)

can be demonstrated. These are best demonstrated in animal models of cholera, particularly the dog, where the same section of bowel can be biopsied before and during the acute infection.[31] This is shown in Fig. 3. During cholera, the goblet cells have discharged their mucus, there is some edema in the interstitial spaces, and there are a few inflammatory cells present in the lamina propria. The fluid lost through this mucosa has only a low concentration of protein, also confirming the integrity of the mucosal layer.

Studies of small bowel biopsies during cholera in patients in endemic areas showed evidence of chronic inflammation, originally thought to be part of the "lesion" of cholera. When adequate control biopsies were done, however, this chronic lesion was found to be present in all biopsies, whether or not they were from patients with cholera[32] (Fig. 4). This biopsy appearance has been termed "tropical enteropathy" by some, and is an exaggeration of the "normal" physiologic inflammation present in the intestine, as compared to the germ-free state.[33] Early studies of intestinal tissues obtained at autopsy of patients dying of cholera

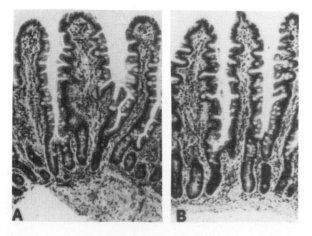

FIGURE 4. (A) Histologic section of human upper small bowel during cholera from patient in Pakistan. (B) Histologic section, for comparison, of a normal Pakistani subject. (Courtesy of H. Thomas Norris in *Cholera*, Barua D, Barrow PA (eds.), Philadelphia, W.B. Saunders Co, 1974.)

often revealed degenerative changes, which we now recognize as being due to post-mortem autolysis.

5. ANIMAL MODELS FOR THE STUDY OF PATHOGENESIS

Natural infection with *V. cholerae* 01 does not occur in animals, although other serotypes of *V. cholerae* can be recovered in animal feces; therefore all animal models are unnatural hosts. In spite of that limitation, much information obtained from these models has been found to apply closely to human disease.

A large number of animals have been used to study *V. cholerae* infection since the early studies of Koch.[34] Both parenterally injected and enterically administered vibrios were used in these models. None were developed that mimicked the clinical disease of cholera until about 35 years ago when rabbit models were successfully developed.

The first two reproducible animal models were developed in India; the ligated intestinal loop of adult rabbits,[35] and the infant rabbit.[36] Both continue to be used to study certain aspects of pathogenesis, in particular, colonization and the physiologic effects of cholera enterotoxin.

There are only two adult intact animal models, in which lethal watery diarrhea can be predictably produced: the dog[37] and the rabbit (the RITARD model, Removable Intestinal Tie Adult Rabbit Diarrhea).[38] Both of these have been used extensively to study both pathogenesis and protective immunity. Both have limitations, including cost and the high inoculum needed to produce clinical cholera.

Intact infant animal models have also been used in studies of pathogenesis: the rabbit and the mouse. Both of these models have limitations of age; the animals are susceptible only during a relatively short period after birth.

A large number of animals have been used in the ligated intestinal loop model; these include rats, mice, and chickens, as well as rabbits and dogs.

A detailed summary of the animal models used in the study of cholera and other diarrheal diseases has recently been published.[39]

REFERENCES

1. Drasar BS, Barrow PA: *Intestinal Microbiology*. American Society for Microbiology, Washington, D.C., 1985
2. Phillips SF: Diarrhea: a current review of the pathophysiology. *Gastroenterology* 63:1495, 1972
3. Hornick RB, Music SI, Wenzel R, et al: The Broad Street pump revisited: Response of volunteers to ingested cholera vibrios. *Bull NY Acad Med* 47:1192–1203, 1971
4. Gitelson S: Gastrectomy, achlorhydria and cholera. *Israel J Med Sci* 7:663–667, 1971
5. Sack Jr GH, Pierce NF, Hennessey KN: Gastric acidity in cholera and noncholera diarrhoea. *Bull WHO* 47:31–36, 1972
6. Gorbach SL, Banwell JG, Jacobs B: Intestinal microflora in Asiatic cholera II, the small bowel. *J Infect Dis* 121:38–45, 1970
7. Freter R, Allweiss B, O'Brien PCM: The role of chemotaxis in the virulence of cholera *Vibrios*. in: *Proceedings of the 13th Joint Conference on Cholera*. US–Japan Cooperative Medical Science Program (NIH, Bethesda, MD). Department of Health, Education, and Welfare Pub. No. 78-1590, 1978, pp 152–181
8. Booth BA, Sciortino CV, Finkelstein RA: Adhesins of Vibrio cholerae, in Mirelman D (ed): *Microbial Lectins and Agglutinins*, New York, John Wiley & Sons, 1986, pp 169–182
9. Guentzel MN, Berry LJ: Motility as a virulence factor for *Vibrio cholera. Infect Immun* 11:890–897, 1975
10. Teppema JS, Guinee PAM, Ibrahim AA, et al: *In vivo* adherence and colonization of Vibrio cholerae strains that differ in hemagglutinating activity and motility. *Infect Immun* 55:2093–2102, 1987

11. Spira WM: Environmental factors in diarrhea transmission: the ecology of *Vibrio cholerae* 01 and cholera, in Holme T, Holmgren J, Merson MH, et al (eds): *Acute Enteric Infections in Children. New Prospects for Treatment and Prevention.* Elsevier/North-Holland Biomedical Press, Amsterdam, 1981, p 273

12. Morris Jr JG, Black RE: Cholera and other vibrioses in the United States. *N Engl J Med* 312:343–349, 1985

13. Woodward WE, Mosley WH: The spectrum of cholera in rural Bangladesh. 2. Comparison of El Tor Ogawa and classical Inaba infection. *Am J Epidemiol* 96:342–35, 1972

14. Booth BA, Finkelstein RA: Presence of hemagglutinin/protease and other potential virulence factors in 01 and non-01 Vibrio cholerae. *J Infect Dis* 154:183–186, 1986

15. Franzon VL, Manning PA: Molecular cloning and expression in Escherichia coli K-12 of the gene for a hemagglutinin from Vibrio cholerae. *Infect Immun* 52:279, 1986

16. Booth BA, Boesman-Finkelstein M, Finkelstein RA: Vibrio cholerae hemagglutinin/protease nicks cholera enterotoxin. *Infect Immun* 45:559, 1984

17. Attridge SR, Rowley D: The specificity of Vibrio cholerae adherence and the significance of the slime agglutinin as a second mediator of *in vitro* attachment. *J Infect Dis* 147:873, 1983

18. Kabir S: Composition, and immunochemical properties of outer membrane proteins of Vibrio cholerae. *J Bacteriol* 144:382, 1980

19. Sengupta D, Datta-Roy K, Banerjee K, et al: Identification of some antigenically related outer-membrane proteins of strains of *Vibrio cholerae* 01 and non-01 serovars involved in intestinal adhesion and the protective role of antibodies to them. *J Med Microb* 29:33, 1989

20. Richardson K, Parker CD: Identification and occurrence of *Vibrio cholerae* flagellar core proteins in isolated outer membrane. *Infect Immun* 47:674, 1985

21. Goldberg MB, DiRita VJ, and Calderwood SB, Identification of an iron-regulated virulence determinant in *Vibrio cholerae,* using TnphoA mutagenesis. *Infect Immun* 58:55, 1990.

22. Manning PA, Heuzenroeder MW, Yeadon J, et al: Molecular cloning and expression in *Escherichia coli* K-12 of the O-antigens of the Inaba and Ogawa serotypes of the *Vibrio cholerae* 01 lipopolysaccharides and their potential for vaccine development. *Infect Immun* 53:272, 1986

23. Ehara M, Ishibashi M, Ichinose Y, et al: Fimbriae of *Vibrio cholerae* 01: observation of fimbriae during colonization of the upper small intestine and a new medium to facilitate fimbriae production. Presented at the 22nd Joint Conference US–Japan Cooperative Medical Science Program Cholera Panel, Toyama, Japan, July 20–23, 1986

24. Taylor R, Spears P, Mekalanos JJ: Applications of the TCP in cholera vaccine development. Presented at the 23rd Joint Conference on Cholera, US–Japan Cooperative Medical Science Program, Williamsburg, VA, November 10–12, 1987

25. Taylor RK, Miller VL, Furlong DB, et al: Use of phoA gene fusions to identify a pilus colonization factor coordinately regulated with cholera toxin. *Proc Natl Acad Sci* 84:2822–2837, 1987

26. Miller VL, Mekalanos JJ: A novel suicide vector and its use in construction of insertion mutations: osmoregulation of outer membrane proteins and virulence determinants in *Vibrio cholerae* requires toxR. *J Bact* 170:2575, 1988

27. Harrington DA, Hall RKH, Losonsky G, et al: Toxin, toxin-coregulated pili, and the toxR regulon are essential for *Vibrio cholerae* pathogenesis in humans. *J Exper Med* 168:1487, 1988

28. Bartowsky EJ, Attridge SR, Thomas CJ, et al: Role of the P plasmid in attenuation of *Vibrio cholerae* 01. *Infect Immun* 58:3129, 1990

29. Iwanaga M, Nakasone N, and Ehara M: Pili of *Vibrio cholerae* 01 Biotype El Tor: a comparative study of adhesive and non-adhesive strains. *Microb Immunol* 33:1, 1989

30. Nakasone N, Iwanaga M: Pili of *Vibrio cholerae* non-01. *Infect Immun* 58:1640, 1990.

31. Elliott HL, Carpenter CCJ, Sack RB, et al: Small bowel morphology in experimental canine cholera: a light and electron microscopic study. *Lab Invest* 22:112–120, 1970

32. Sprinz H, Sribhibhadh R, Gangarosa EJ, et al: Biopsy of small bowel of Thai people with special reference to recovery from Asiatic cholera and to an intestinal malabsorption syndrome. *Am J Clin Pathol* 38:43–51, 1962

33. Dubos RJ: *Man Adapting,* in Hepsa Ely Silliman Memorial Lectures, New Haven, Yale University Press, 1980, p 538

34. Pollitzer R: *Cholera,* in Monograph Series No. 43, Geneva, World Health Organization, 1959

35. De SN, Chatterjee DN: An experimental study of the mechanism of action of *Vibrio cholerae* on the intestinal mucous membranes. *J Pathol Bacteriol* 66:559–562, 1953

36. Dutta NK, Habbu MK: Experimental cholera in infant rabbits: a method for chemotherapeutic investigation. *Br J Pharmacol* 10:153–159, 1955

37. Sack RB, Carpenter CCJ: Experimental canine cholera. I. Development of the model. *J Infect Dis* 119:138–149, 1969
38. Spira WM, Sack RB, Froehlich JL: Simple adult rabbit model for *Vibrio cholerae* and enterotoxigenic *Escherichia coli* diarrhea. *Infect Immun* 32:739–747, 1981
39. Sack RB, Spira WM: Animal models of acute diarrheal diseases of bacterial etiology, in Zak O (ed.): *Experimental Models in Antimicrobial Chemotherapy*, Vol. 2, London, Academic Press Inc., Basel, Switzerland, 1986, p 43

10

Pathogenesis

Jan Holmgren

The pathogenesis of cholera is intimately associated with the production and action of the enterotoxin molecule known as cholera toxin (in earlier work sometimes called choleragen or permeability factor) by the cholera vibrios. It is now 20 years since experimental evidence first clearly suggested that cholera is a toxin-mediated disease. Robert Koch, who identified *V. cholerae* as the causative agent of cholera, had already proposed in 1884 that the disease was toxin-mediated[1] but it was not until 1959 that the Indian scientists De[2] and Dutta[3] and their co-workers convincingly demonstrated the existence of the cholera toxin. Today, cholera is recognized as the prototype of a large group of diarrheal diseases that are also mediated by enterotoxins, some of which are structurally and functionally related to the cholera enterotoxin. Collectively, these other "enterotoxic enteropathies"[4] are more important than cholera as causes of morbidity and mortality in most parts of the world. Still, however, the main information about the pathogenesis of this whole group of diseases was derived from basic research about the pathogenesis of cholera and to a large extent to specific studies of the cholera toxin molecule and its mode of action.

During a cholera infection, the cholera toxin molecule is produced and released by the cholera vibrios during their colonization and multiplication in the small intestine. The toxin binds to specific receptors on the mucosal cells and stimulates intestinal adenylate cyclase activity. This results in the formation of excessive amounts of cyclic AMP in the epithelial cells, and through not yet fully understood mechanisms, this, in its turn, leads to a net secretion of electrolytes and water from the body into the gut lumen giving rise to severe diarrhea and fluid loss, and in severe cases to dehydration, metabolic acidosis and often death. These events are summarized in Fig. 1 and discussed more fully below, together with other aspects of cholera toxin relevant to the pathogenesis of cholera; for additional and broader aspects of the cholera toxin molecule the reader is also referred to pertinent reviews.[5-7]

Cholera, edited by Dhiman Barua and William B. Greenough III. Plenum Medical Book Company, New York, 1992.

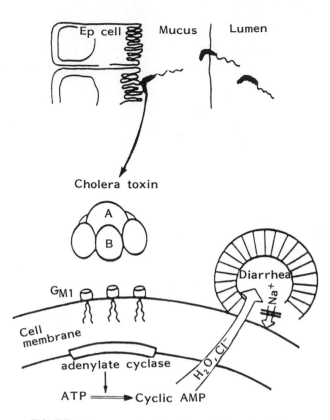

FIGURE 1. Summary of pathogenic mechanisms in cholera.

1. SYNTHESIS, ASSEMBLY, AND SECRETION OF CHOLERA TOXIN

1.1. Subunit Structure and Function

Cholera toxin is a protein built from two types of subunits: a single "heavy" A subunit of molecular weight 28,000 which is noncovalently attached to a 58,000-molecular weight aggregate of five "light" B subunits, each with a molecular weight of 11,600.[5-7]

The B subunits are aggregated in a ring by tight noncovalent bonds; the A subunit is linked to and partially inserted in the B ring through weaker noncovalent interactions. The A subunit, although synthesized as a single polypeptide chain (one gene) is usually "nicked" between its two cystein residues (see below) and thus splits into fragments A_1 (molecular weight ~22,500) and A2 (molecular weight ~5500) when treated with thiol-reducing agents. Reduction of whole toxin releases the A_1 fragment from the A_2-5B complex, indicating that A is attached to the B ring by its A_2 portion.[8]

The different role of the two types of subunits for the intoxication process became evident when it was found[9] that choleragenoid, a protein which is immunologically related to cholera toxin and able to bind to intestinal epithelium without having toxic activity, contains the same light subunits as the toxin but lacks the heavy subunit. This finding strongly suggested that the light subunits are responsible for cell binding (B subunit) and the heavy subunit for the direct toxic activity (A subunit). Experiments with toxin subunit fractions, prepared by gel filtration in acidic buffer and dialyzed to allow renaturation and reassociation of subunits, confirmed that the B subunits bound strongly both to intact cells and to the isolated cell receptors (see below), but were nontoxic. Purified A subunit neither bound to nor was toxic for intact cells; however, A reassociated with B subunits had both binding and toxic activity in various whole cell systems.[9,10]

The requirement for membrane binding by the B subunits can in experimental systems be circumvented by using disrupted cells; in these conditions purified A subunit can activate adenylate cyclase.[11] Furthermore, the characteristic lag period of 10–90 min observed in intact cells before any effect of cholera toxin on adenylate cyclase is seen, essentially disappears in the broken cells. Reduction of the disulphide bond between the A_1 and A_2 regions seems to be necessary for the activity of A on adenylate cyclase.

1.2. Genetics

Cholera toxin is encoded by chromosomal structural genes for the A and B subunits, respectively. These genes have been cloned, and their nucleotide sequences have been determined. The genes for the A and B subunits of cholera toxin are arranged in a single transcriptional unit with the A cistron (ctxA) preceding the B cistron (ctxB). Studies on the organization of cholera toxin genes in classical and El Tor biotypes showed that there are two copies of cholera toxin genes in classical biotype strains while there is only one copy in most El Tor strains.[12]

The synthesis of cholera toxin is positively regulated by a gene, toxR that increases ctx expression by more than 100-fold.[13] The toxR acts at the transcriptional level, and is present in strains of either classical or El Tor biotypes. ToxR probably increases ctx transcription by encoding a regulatory protein that interacts positively with the ctx promoter region.

In addition to its role in cholera toxin gene expression, toxR is required for production of a pilus colonization factor and for expression of an outer membrane protein of V. cholerae.[14] The toxR gene product therefore seems to play a central role in the coordinate transcription regulation of multiple virulence determinants of V. cholerae. Recent data indicate that the toxR product is a 32.5-kDa protein, the amino acid composition of which is consistent with a transmembrane membrane structure. The transmembrane nature of the toxR protein may then explain how this protein can transduce environmental signals across the cell envelope of V. cholerae.

1.3. Toxin Assembly and Secretion

Studies on heat-labile enterotoxin in E. coli (the subunit structure and function of which is closely similar to cholera toxin) have shown that the A and B subunits are initially synthesized as precursors.[15] These are rapidly processed and translocated across the inner membrane into the periplasm, where unassembled monomeric B subunits have been shown to assemble relatively slowly with a half-time of 1–2 min. Most likely these events are very similar for cholera toxin subunits in V. cholerae.[16,17] However, in E. coli the assembled holotoxin remains within the periplasm and is not secreted through the outer membrane. This contrasts with V. cholerae which completely secretes its enterotoxin into the surrounding milieu.[16,17]

Such a secretion pathway in *V. cholerae* poses certain fundamental questions because of the structural complexity of the toxins involved. For example, are the component A and B subunits secreted independently or are they assembled at some stage during the secretion process? At what location does this occur and which toxin structure domains are important for secretion?

These questions have recently been addressed in this laboratory using pulse–chase experiments. The results indicate that: (1) the A and B subunits transiently enter the periplasm as they traverse the envelope[17]; (2) Oligomerization of the toxin subunits occurs in the periplasm prior to their secretion across the outer membrane[18]; (3) The pathway of toxin assembly proceeds via A subunit association with B monomers or small oligomers, e.g., dimers[19]; and (4) B subunits contain structural domains important for toxin translocation across the *V. cholerae* outer membrane.[16]

It therefore seems that the events of toxin secretion are remarkably well-coordinated in ensuring the formation of a functional toxin that is successfully delivered across the bacterial cell-envelope. In fact, the data suggest that the periplasm of *V. cholerae* is an ideal location for toxin assembly because it ensures a high concentration of monomers.[18]

2. TOXIN BINDING AND ACTIVATION OF ADENYLATE CYCLASE IN EPITHELIAL CELLS

2.1. Receptors

The first event in the action of cholera toxin on cells is rapid, tight binding to receptors on the cell surface. Studies with isotope-labeled toxin have shown that binding occurs almost instantaneously, has a high affinity, and is initially reversible.[10,20] The number of binding sites per cell varies widely with the cell type but the affinity of binding varies very little ($K_A \sim 1 \times 10^9$ mol/liter) indicating that the receptor is the same for various cell types.[21]

It is now well established that the membrane receptor for cholera toxin is a specific ganglioside called GM1 (for review see ref. 5). van Heyningen *et al.*[22] observed that a crude ganglioside mixture inactivated cholera toxin. Holmgren *et al.*,[23] Cuatrecasas,[24] and King and van Heyningen[25] showed that this inactivation resulted from the specific binding between the toxin and a single ganglioside GM1. Studies of various cell types, including small intestinal mucosal cells of different species, demonstrated that there existed a direct relationship between the cell content of GM1 and the number of toxin molecules that the cells could bind.[21] Furthermore, exogenous GM1 ganglioside could be incorporated into the membrane of various cells and then served as functional receptors for cholera toxin both in cell lines and *in vivo* in the intestine of rabbits.[21,24]

Many strains of *V. cholerae* produce sialidase, an enzyme which can increase the GM1 content of cell membranes by hydrolyzing sialic acid from more complex gangliosides (di-, tri-, tetrasialogangliosides, etc.) of the GM1-series (in contrast the sialic acid residue in GM1 itself is resistant to sialidase treatment).[23,25] Although incubation of nonintestinal tissues or cells with *V. cholerae* sialidase usually increased the number of toxin-binding sites and the cellular susceptibility to the toxin, these effects, however, could not be reproduced on intestinal tissue. Thus, *V. cholerae* sialidase failed to increase the number of receptors for cholera toxin in intestinal epithelium and also did not enhance the intestinal sensitivity to the toxin.[21] The role of *V. cholerae* sialidase in the pathogenesis of cholera therefore remains unclear and it may, if at all existing, not be related to toxin receptor density.

2.2. Effects on Adenylate Cyclase

Even though the binding of cholera toxin to cell membrane receptors is almost instantaneous, there is a substantial lag period, 20–90 min, before this results in any detectable effects on cell metabolism. This lag period partly reflects the kinetics of cyclic AMP accumulation and subsequent "second messenger"-induced events in the cholera toxin action, but also (approx. 15–30 min) the time it takes for the cholera toxin A subunit to penetrate the cell membrane to initiate activation of adenylate cyclase.[5] Once such penetration has occurred, however, the generation of the A1 fragment and the subsequent action on adenylate cyclase occur within 1 min.[11] The cell penetration process is poorly understood. The time it takes is markedly influenced by incubation temperature and the composition of the cell membrane. Lateral diffusion of the toxin in the cell membrane to allow for the initial uni- or bivalent toxin binding to GM1 receptors to become pentavalent is important and this may take longer in cells with relatively little GM1 than in cells with more receptors (see ref. 5). Also, capping and uptake of cholera toxin in vesicles have been observed. It has been speculated that such events, in analogy with the situation for, e.g., diphtheria toxin or Shiga toxin, might be important for enabling the A subunit of cholera toxin to penetrate into the cytosol, but this hypothesis has not convincingly been supported experimentally.[26]

The biochemical intracellular events that lead to activation of adenylate cyclase are mainly known. Gill and King[11] showed that, in broken cell preparations, activation depends on NAD, undefined cellular cytosol factors, and ATP, in addition to the A1 fragment of cholera toxin and cell membrane. Moss et al.[27] identified that cholera toxin, like diphtheria toxin, has ADP–ribosyltransferase activity and catalyzes the reaction: NAD + acceptor protein → ADP-ribose-acceptor protein + nicotinamide + H^+.

The protein that is ADP ribosylated by cholera toxin has been identified as the guanylnucleotide-binding component (the N_s protein) of the membrane-bound adenylate cyclase.[28] This observation fitted nicely with the previous one by Cassel and Sellinger[29] that cholera toxin blocks the inherent GTPase action of the N_s protein. Adenylate cyclase is active while GTP is bound to the GTP-binding component but becomes inactive when GTP is being hydrolyzed to GDP; thus cholera toxin stabilizes adenylate cyclase in an active conformation.

3. EFFECTS ON FLUID TRANSPORT MECHANISMS

3.1. Physiology

Diarrhea results from a disturbance in the normal balance between absorption and secretion in intestine. Absorption predominates in the normal situation. However, diarrhea may occur when the balance is shifted towards secretion either by inhibition of absorption or by stimulation of secretion. We will therefore briefly review the main absorptive and secretory processes in the intestine, before discussing the specific disturbances that are characteristic of cholera (for more comprehensive reviews see 30–32).

In the jejunum, absorption of salt and water is stimulated by the absorption of nutrients, and is largely a passive process. In the ileum and colon, on the other hand, active transport of Na and Cl ions is mainly responsible for dehydrating the luminal contents. Impaired absorption leading to diarrhea may occur because of the presence of non-absorbed solutes in the lumen (osmotic diarrhea), reduced jejunal permeability, impaired active transport processes, or increased intestinal motility. Diarrhea may also be produced when intestinal secretion is stimulated. Secretion results from an increase in apical membrane permeability for Cl ions and occurs when one or more of three intracellular "second messengers" are generated in increased amounts. These are cAMP, cGMP, and free calcium. Each of these may be increased by a number of secretagogues, including bacterial toxins, mediators of inflammatory responses, and various neuropeptides.

3.2. Pathophysiology

The main, though probably not exclusive, site of action for cholera toxin is the small intestine and especially the duodenum and jejunum.[33,34] This site reflects the large number of cholera vibrios and, thus, the comparatively large amounts of cholera toxin released there, as well as a decreasing secretory response to cholera toxin from the proximal towards the distal part of the intestine.[35] However, there are substantial numbers of cholera vibrios also in the ileum and in the colon. Therefore, in severe cholera, there is a substantial contribution of ileal dysfunction, and effects by cholera toxin on colonic (absorptive) function may also contribute to disease.

Cholera is regarded a the archtypal cAMP-mediated intestinal secretory process. The early studies by Field et al., [36] and subsequent confirmatory experiments by many others (see refs. 5–7), showed that cholera toxin could concomitantly stimulate cyclic AMP formation and electrolyte and fluid secretion in isolated intestinal epithelium, stripped from its muscle layer, and mounted for electrolyte transport analyses in an Ussing chamber system. The net fluid secretion induced by cholera toxin depended on two separate effects, active chloride (and bicarbonate) secretion from the serosal to the mucosal side, and inhibition of active coupled NaCl absorption from the mucosal to the serosal side (see ref. 30). Furthermore, other agents which induced cyclic AMP formation or prevented cyclic AMP degradation, as well as added cyclic AMP itself, had similar effects as cholera toxin on intestinal electrolyte and water transport both as studied using isolated epithelium in Ussing chambers and on using ligated intestinal loops in vivo. The current view is that the normal absorption of NaCl (and water) that is inhibited by cholera toxin is a property residing in mature villus cells, whereas the secretion of chloride and bicarbonate with the associated transport of water that is increased by the toxin takes place in the less differentiated crypt cells.

The activation of adenylate cyclase and generation of cAMP in the intestinal epithelium, resulting from the action of cholera toxin, are described above and known in considerable detail. The precise biochemical mechanisms by which cholera toxin and cAMP inhibit active NaCl absorption and cause active chloride and bicarbonate secretion are less well known. The intracellular cAMP activates a protein kinase, which in its turn promotes phosphorylation of a number of proteins. Among the proteins phosphorylated, one or more may be directly concerned with regulating chloride permeability of the apical membrane, the increase in which is the direct cause of the secretory process. These aspects have recently been discussed in detail.[37]

3.3. Other Secretory Mechanisms?

As described above cholera toxin is assumed to induce net fluid secretion by its direct effects on the cAMP metabolism of the intestinal epithelial cells. This picture to a large extent was derived from the results of Ussing chamber experiments.

While these experiments convincingly showed that cholera toxin could induce intestinal secretion and cyclic AMP accumulation in intestinal epithelium without a need for blood flow, they are, however, less conclusive than initially thought in defining the action of cholera toxin as directly on the intestinal epithelial cells. In addition to the epithelial cells, the intestinal wall has a prominent muscular layer, and an enteric nervous system which can function independently of the central nervous system. The intestine also contains various cells that can produce hormones and neuropeptides with effects on intestinal secretion [e.g., the enterochromaffin cells producing serotonin (5-HT)]. There is also a number of immuno- logically active cells, including mast cells, located both dispersed among the polar epithelial cells and underneath the epithelial cells in the lamina propria. All of these cells probably respond with cAMP formation when exposed to cholera toxin. It is therefore conceivable that cholera toxin could stimulate secretion indirectly by first acting on a "receptor cell" and, only indirectly via factors released from the primary cells, affect the fluid transport processes of the epithelial cells.

It is therefore important that intestinal epithelial cell lines have now become available, which are sufficiently differentiated to allow electrolyte transport studies. For instance, the T_{84} human intestinal epithelial cell line, which forms tight junctions, shows polarity, and develops a resistance, has been extensively examined in recent years in Ussing chamber experiments (38). Strikingly, the results in this defined unicellular system have almost com- pletely confirmed those previously obtained using intact tissue. Thus, the T_{84} cell line responds with chloride and water secretion when exposed to each of the three previously proposed intracellular mediators of intestinal secretion, i.e., cAMP, cGMP, and calcium or to agents that induce increases in these substances. The T_{84} cell lines has receptors for cholera toxin, and it characteristically responds to cholera toxin with adenylate cyclase activation and cAMP formation as well as active chloride secretion.[38]

Lundgren and co-workers have proposed an important role for the enteric nervous system in the pathophysiology of enterotoxin-induced secretory states including cholera.[39] According to their hypothesis the toxin first adheres to a receptor cell and then triggers the release of amines and/or peptides. These, in turn, stimulate intramural nervous reflexes by activation of dendrites adjacent to the receptor cells. The stimulated reflex(es) contain(s) at least one cholinergic synapse, and it is being proposed that vasoactive intestinal polypeptide (VIP), a known intestinal secretion-inducing neurotransmitter, is the final mediator signal on the polar epithelial cells to start the electrolyte and fluid secretion in response to cholera toxin and other enterotoxins. Lundgren et al. have provided two main observations to support their hypothesis: (1) enterotoxin-induced secretion is markedly inhibited by tetrodotoxin (a so- dium-gate blocker in nerve membranes), by hexamethonium (a cholinergic nicotinic receptor antagonist), and by lidocain (a local anaesthetic agent) placed on the mucosal or serosal side in the intestine; and (2) cholera secretion is accompanied by an increased release of VIP from the small intestinal gut (and cholera patients also show increased levels of VIP in blood). Each of the ganglionic or neuro-transmittor blockers used, however, has multiple effects including a potential direct effect on mucosal epithelial cell function. Also, it is possible that these agents merely block a normal "background" nervous stimulation on the intestinal epithelium rather than interrupting a specific enterotoxin signal. Clearly, further work is required to define the role of nerves and neurotransmitters in cholera secretion, an area of research that might also give new clues to pharmalogical intervention of secretory diar- rheas.[31]

This conclusion also applies to the need to better define the importance of cholera toxin–induced increased motility as a contributing factor to cholera diarrhea. Mathias et al.[40] found that both live V. cholerae organisms and purified cholera enterotoxin evoked strong intestinal myoelectric activity in rabbit ileum, and proposed that this motility-promoting activity might be of pathogenic significance in cholera. Thus, in addition to its direct secretion-stimulating effects on intestinal enterocytes, cholera toxin might also affect some other target cells in the intestinal mucosa and this may be a contributing factor to cholera diarrhea.

4. ADDITIONAL TOXINS?

Before 1983, it was strongly believed that cholera toxin was the sole mediator of fluid secretion and diarrhea in cholera. It was therefore a great surprise when Kaper *et al.*,[41] who, by well-defined genetical methods, had deleted the genes for both A subunit and B subunit production in a *V. cholerae* strain, found that this mutant, JBK70, still gave rise to diarrhea in many volunteers who were fed this organism. Furthermore, this strain seemed to produce a heat-labile toxic factor that could stimulate fluid secretion in ligated intestinal loops of rabbits. The nature and significance of a second toxin for the pathogenesis of cholera remains obscure. Several second toxin candidates have been considered, e.g., the hemolysin produced by especially *V. cholerae* 01 organisms of the El Tor biotype[42]; the Shiga-like toxin described by O'Brien[43]; the soluble hemagglutinin/protease produced in different quantities by most *V. cholerae* organisms[44]; LT-like toxin not binding to GM1 ganglioside (not yet found in *V. cholerae* organisms); or simply nonspecific "metabolic products" of the bacteria which, for example, might change the pH of the microclimate. One or more of these factors may play a role in explaining the diarrhea caused by non–cholera toxin producing *V. cholerae* 01 mutants. However, their role is clearly at most secondary to that of cholera toxin, since really severe cholera has, to date, never been observed in volunteers fed cholera toxin-negative mutants.

REFERENCES

1. Koch R: An address on cholera and its bacillus. *Br Med J* (August 30): 403–407; 453–459, 1884
2. De SN: Enterotoxicity of bacteria-free culture-filtrate of *Vibrio cholerae. Nature (London)* 183:1533–1534, 1959
3. Dutta NK, Panse MV, Kulkarni DR: Role of cholera toxin in experimental cholera. *J Bact* 78:594–595, 1959
4. Craig JP: A survey of the enterotoxic enteropathies, in Ouchterlony Ö, Holmgren J, (eds): *Cholera and Related Diarrheas*. 43rd Nobel Symposium, Stockholm 1978. Basel, Karger, 1980, p 15
5. Holmgren J: Actions of cholera toxin and the prevention and treatment of cholera. *Nature* 292:413–417, 1981
6. Lai C-Y: The chemistry and biology of cholera toxin. *CRC Crit Rev Biochem.* 9:171–206, 1980
7. Moss J, Vaughan M: Activation of adenylate cyclase by choleragen. *A Rev Biochem* 48:581–600, 1979
8. Gill DM: The arrangement of subunits in cholera toxin. *Biochemistry NY* 15:1242–1248, 1976
9. Lönnroth I, Holmgren J: Subunit structure of cholera toxin. *J Gen Microbiol* 76:417–427, 1973
10. Holmgren J, Lindholm L, Lönnroth I: Interaction of cholera toxin and toxin derivatives with lymphocytes. I. Binding properties and interference with lectin-induced cellular stimulation. *J Exp Med* 139:801–819, 1974
11. Gill DM, King CA: The mechanism of action of cholera toxin in pigeon erythrocyte lysates. *J Biol Chem* 424–432, 1975
12. Mekalanos JJ, Swartz DJ, Pearson GDN, Harford N, Groyne F, DeWilde M: Cholera toxin gene: nucleotide sequence, deletion analysis and vaccine development. *Nature (London)* 306:551–557, 1983
13. Miller VL, Mekalanos JJ: Synthesis of cholera toxin is positively regulated at the transcriptional level by *toxR. Proc Natl Acad Sci USA* 81:3471–3475, 1984
14. Taylor RK, Miller VL, Furlong DB, Mekalanos JJ: The use of *PhoA* gene fusions to identify pilus colonization factor coordinately regulated with cholera toxin. *Proc Natl Acad Sci USA,* 84:2833–2837, 1987

15. Palva ET, Hirst TR, Hardy SJS, Holmgren J, Randall, L: Synthesis of precursors to the B subunit of heat-labile enterotoxin in *Escherichia coli. J Bacteriol* 146:325–339, 1981

16. Hirst TR, Sanchez J, Kaper JB, Hardy SJS, Holmgren J: Mechanisms of toxin secretion by *Vibrio cholerae* investigated in strains harboring plasmids that encode heat-labile enterotoxins of *Escherichia coli. Proc Natl Acad Sci USA* 81:7752–7756, 1984

17. Hirst TR, Holmgren J: Transient entry of enterotoxin subunits into the periplasm during their secretion from *Vibrio cholerae. J Bacteriol* 169:1037–1045, 1987

18. Hirst TR, Holmgren J: Conformation and protein secreted across bacterial outer membranes: A study of enterotoxin translocation from *Vibrio cholerae. Proc Natl Acad Sci USA* 84:7418–7422, 1987

19. Hardy SJS, Holmgren J, Johansson S, Sanchez J & Hirst TR: Coordinated assembly of multisubunit proteins: Oligomerization of bacterial enterotoxins in vivo and in vitro. *Proc Natl Acad Sci USA* 85:7109–7113, 1988

20. Cuatrecasas P: Interaction of *Vibrio cholerae* enterotoxin with cell membranes. *Biochemistry NY* 12:3547–3558, 1973

21. Holmgren J, Lönnroth I, Månsson JE, Svennerholm L: Interaction of cholera toxin and membrane GM1 ganglioside of small intestine. *Proc Natl Acad Sci USA* 72:2520–2524, 1975

22. Heyningen WE van, Carpenter CCJ, Pierce NF, Greenough WB: Deactivation of cholera toxin by ganglioside GM1. *Science* 183:656–657, 1974

23. Holmgren J, Lönnroth I, Svennerholm L: Tissue receptor for cholera exotoxin: postulated structure studies with GM1 ganglioside and related glycolipids. *Infect Immun* 8:208–214, 1973

24. Cuatrecasas P: Gangliosides and membrane receptors for cholera toxin. *Biochemistry NY* 12:3558–3566, 1973

25. King CA, van Heyningen WE: Deactivation of cholera toxin by a sialidase-resistant monosialosylganglioside. *J Infect Dis* 127:639–647, 1973

26. Fishman PH: Internalization and degradation of cholera toxin by cultured cells: relationship to toxin action. *J Cell Biol* 93:860–865, 1982

27. Moss J, Vaughan M: Mechanism of action of choleragen. Evidence for ADP-ribosyl transferase activity with arginine as an acceptor. *J Biol Chem* 252:2455–2457, 1977

28. Pfeuffer T, Cassel D: Mechanism of cholera action: covalent modification of the guanyl nucleotide-binding protein of the adenylate cyclase system. *Proc Natl Acad Sci USA* 75:2669–2673, 1978

29. Cassel D, Selinger Z: Mechanisms of adenylate cyclase activation by cholera toxin: inhibition of GTP hydrolysis at the regulatory site. *Proc Natl Acad Sci USA* 74:3307–3311, 1977

30. Field M: Regulation of small intestine ion transport by cyclic nucleotides and calcium, in Field M, Fordtran JS, Schultz SG, (eds): *Secretory Diarrhea.* Bethesda, MD, American Physiology Society, 1980, p 21

31. Powell DW, Berschneider HM, Lawson LD, Marens H: Regulation of water and ion movement in intestine, in *Microbial Toxins and Diarrheal Disease,* London, Pitman, (CIBA Foundation Symposium 112), 1985 p 14

32. Turnberg LA: Mechanisms of intestinal absorption and secretion of electrolytes and water, in Holmgren J, Lindberg A, Möllby R (eds): *Development of Vaccines and Drugs against Diarrhea.* 11th Nobel Conference Stockholm 1985. Lund, Sweden, Studentlitteratur, 1986, p 231

33. Carpenter CCJ, Sack RB, Feeley JC, Steenberg RW: Site and characteristics of electrolyte loss and effect of intraluminal glucose in experimental canine cholera. *J Clin Invest* 47:1210–1220, 1968

34. Banwell JG, Pierce NF, Mitra RC, Brigham K, Caranasos GJ, Keimowitz RI, Redson DS, Thomas J, Gorbach SL, Sack RB, Mondal A: Intestinal fluid and electrolyte transport in human cholera. *J Clin Invest* 49:183–195, 1970

35. Carpenter CCJ, Greenough WB III: Response of the canine duodenum to intraluminal challenge with cholera exotoxin. *J Clin Invest* 47:2600–2607, 1968

36. Field M, Fromm D, Wallace CK, Greenough WB: Stimulation of active chloride secretion in small intestine by cholera exotoxin. *J Clin Invest.* 48:24a, 1969

37. De Jonge HR, Lohmann SM: Mechanisms by which cyclic nucleotides and other intracellular mediators regulate secretion, in *Microbial Toxins and Diarrheal Disease,* London, Pitman, (CIBA Foundation Symposium 112), p 116, 1985

38. Dharmaathaphorn K, McRoberts JA, Mandal KG, Tisdale LO, Masui H: A human colonic tumor cell line that maintains vectorial electrolyte transport. *Am J Physiol* 246:G204–G208, 1984

39. Jodal M, Lundgren O: Enterotoxin-induced fluid secretion and the enteric nervous system, in Holmgren J, Lindberg A, Möllby R (eds), *Development of Vaccines and Drugs against Diarrhea.* 11th Nobel Conference, Stockholm 1985. Lund, Sweden, Studentlitteratur, 1986, p 278

40. Mathias JR, Carlson GM, DiMarino AJ, Bertiger G, Morton HE, Cohen S: Intestinal myoelectric activity in response to live *Vibrio cholerae* and cholera enterotoxin. *J Clin Invest* 58:91–96, 1976

41. Kaper JB, Lockman H, Baldini MM, Levine MM: Recombinant nontoxinogenic *Vibrio cholerae* strains as attenuated cholera vaccine candidates. *Nature (London)* 308:655–658, 1984

42. Honda T, Finkelstein RA: Purification and characterization of the hemolysin produced by *Vibrio cholerae* biotype El Tor: Another toxic substance produced by cholera vibrios. *Infect Immun* 26:1020–1027, 1979

43. O'Brien AD, Chen MI, Holmes RK, Kaper J, Levine MM: Environmental and human isolates of *Vibrio cholerae* and *Vibrio parahemolyticus* produce a *Shigella dysenteriae* 1 (Shiga)-like cytotoxin. *Lancet* i:77–78, 1984

44. Svennerholm A-M, Strömberg Jonson G, Holmgren J: *Vibrio cholerae* soluble hemagglutinin: purification and development of ELISA methods for antigen and antibody quantitations. *Infect Immun* 41:237–243, 1983

11

Pathophysiology and Clinical Aspects of Cholera

G. H. Rabbani and William B. Greenough III

1. INTRODUCTION

Cholera may have been prevalent as an epidemic disease since antiquity (see Chapter 1), but only in the 1960s did research illuminate the mechanism of this disease. Before the discovery that a bacteria caused cholera, John Snow showed remarkable insight into the pathophysiology of the disease. For almost 80 years after Robert Koch's isolation of *Vibrio cholerae*, the causative organism of epidemic cholera, however, a false idea of pathophysiology was propagated from teachings of Virchow.[1] In 1959, SN De[2] in India demonstrated that *Vibrio cholerae* produces a diarrheagenic toxin (cholera toxin). Over the next 30 years the toxin was fully characterized as were the mechanisms of toxin-induced diarrhea.[3] In cholera patients, the origin and characteristics of diarrheal fluids were determined, the molecular basis of the action of cholera toxin (CT) was demonstrated, and its clinical consequences were established. Effective, low-cost therapeutic interventions were designed. This chapter will examine the progressive development of knowledge concerning the pathophysiologic and clinical aspects of cholera.

> The stools and vomited matter in cholera consist of water, containing a small quantity of the salts of the blood, and a very little albuminous substance. It would seem that the cholera poison, when reproduced in sufficient quantity, acts as an irritant on the surface of the stomach and intestines, or, what is still more probable, it withdraws fluid from the blood circulating in the capillaries, by a power analogous to that by which epithelial cells of the various organs abstract the different secretions of the healthy body.
>
> The change in the blood is precisely that which the loss by the alimentary canal ought to produce. . . The loss of water from the blood causes it to assume a thick tarry appearance. . . The diminished volume of the blood causes many of the symptoms of a true haemorrhage, as debility,

Cholera, edited by Dhiman Barua and William B. Greenough III. Plenum Medical Book Company, New York, 1992.

faintness, and the coldness. . . all the symptoms attending cholera, except those connected with the alimentary canal, depend simply on the physical alteration of the blood.

. . . the whole quantity of fluid that requires to be effused into the stomach and bowels, in order to reduce the blood of a healthy adult individual to the condition in which it is met with in the collapse of cholera is, on the average, 100 ounces, or 5 imperial pints. This calculation may be useful. . .

. . . the effects of a weak saline solution injected into the veins in the stage of collapse. . . : The shrunken skin becomes filled out, and loses its coldness and lividity; the countenance assumes a natural aspect; the patient is able to sit up, and for a time seems well. If the symptoms were caused by a poison circulating in the blood, and depressing the action of the heart, it is impossible that they should be thus suspended by an injection of warm water, holding a carbonate of soda in solution. (Snow, J., *On the mode of Communication of cholera,* 2nd ed. John Churchill, London, 1855.)

2. PATHOGENESIS OF CHOLERA

Cholera is caused by infection of the small intestine of man by a gram-negative toxigenic bacteria called *Vibrio cholerae* 01.[4] The illness is characterized by the sudden onset of watery diarrhea, vomiting, dehydration often leading to death. The route of entry of the organisms into the human body is through the mouth. There is ample evidence in the epidemiologic literature that in most outbreaks, *V. cholerae* infections have been traced to drinking of contaminated water[5] (see Chapter 7). Once the viable organisms are swallowed, the establishment of a small intestinal infection depends on several factors related to man, the host, and the parasite. These are briefly discussed below.

2.1. Gastric Acid

The importance of gastric acid as a nonspecific defense mechanism against enteric infections is well recognized. Studies in human volunteers[6] have shown that the number of *V. cholerae* cells required to infect half of the volunteers was large (10^6) relative to that required for other enteric pathogens such as *Shigellae* (10^2) and *S. typhimurium* (10^4). In experimental animals, attack rates never reach 100% no matter how large the infecting dose of *V. cholerae* is. It has been shown in human volunteers[7,8] that neutralization of stomach acid with sodium bicarbonate reduces the infecting dose of *V. cholerae* from 10^{11} to 10^6. During epidemics of cholera in Israel and Italy, attack rates were significantly higher in subjects with hypochlorhydria due to the surgical resection of the stomach or chronic ingestion of antacids.[9,10] These findings are consistent with the observation that in areas where cholera is endemic, an inverse relationship exists between the basal levels of gastric acid and the development of clinical cholera. A recent study has shown that gastric colonization with gram-negative organisms including *V. cholerae* were frequently associated with hypochlorhydria in a group of malnourished Bangladeshi children.[11]

2.2. Intestinal Colonization by *V. cholerae*

Successful colonization of the small intestine by *V. cholerae* depends on the adhesion of vibrios to the intestinal mucosal surface. *V. cholerae* strains which are unable to colonize the gut are also unable to cause disease. Adhesion secures the bacteria against the effect of intestinal motility and facilitates the delivery of enterotoxin that is produced. Much is yet to be learned about the mechanism of adhesion of *V. cholerae* to the mucosal surface of human intestine.

The intestinal tract offers an elegant array of defences against the pathogenic organisms. Intestinal motility, phagocytosis, chemotaxis, mucous secretion, and microbial interaction are just a few of these host defense mechanisms. However, pathogenic bacteria likewise vary greatly in their ability to overcome these host factors. It has been shown that the glycoprotein component of mucus may contain a variety of carbohydrate molecules which can act as specific receptors for bacteria. *V. cholerae*[12] and *E. coli*[13] have both been shown to possess carbohydrate-mediated attachment to intestinal cells. Walker *et al.*[14] has demonstrated that proteolytic activity of the pancreatic enzymes interferes with the ability of enterotoxins and bacterial antigens to attach to and penetrate the microvillous membrane.

2.3. Bacterial Pili and Mucus Coat

Toxigenic *E. coli* possess fine, filamentous surface appendages called "pili" which have been shown to facilitate adhesion to specific mucosal receptors of the microvillous membrane.[15] Although similar structures have not yet been identified with *V. cholerae*, it has been suggested that the flagellum of the motile strains possesses an adhesive component which facilitates its attachment to intestinal mucosa.[16] It has been shown that *V. cholerae* motility and *in vitro* production of hemolysin are associated with the adherence capacity of the organism. Recent *in vivo* electron microscopic studies, however, have shown that certain human *V. cholerae* strains adhere to and colonize the small intestinal epithelium, despite the absence of haemagglutinating activity and motility.[17]

The process of *V. cholerae* colonization of the human intestine appears to be complex, involving factors like proteolytic enzymes, hemagglutinins, colonization pili, along with a coordinated expression of chemotatic and motility functions. The importance of bacterial pili in the colonization process has only recently been recognized. Taylor *et al.*[18] characterized a pilus, designated as toxin coregulated pili (TcpA) elaborated by *V. cholerae* 01 of Classical and El Tor biotypes that is required for colonization in mouse and in humans. Herrington *et al.*[19] subsequently showed that an isogenic mutant of *V. cholerae* lacking TcpA was unable to colonize volunteers. Expression of TcpA, CT, and other proteins is coordinately regulated by a transmembrane DNA-binding regulatory protein called ToxR. Thus, ToxR-regulated surface and secreted proteins (TcpA and toxin B subunit) may provide potential immunogens for future cholera vaccines.

One recent report by Yamamoto[20] suggested the importance of mucus lining of the microvillous membrane in the colonization process. The authors demonstrated that *V. cholerae* 01, irrespective of the biotype or serotype, adheres to the mucus coat of the human small intestine and that adherence to the mucus coat is more extensive than adherence to the villous surface of the human intestine.

2.4. Cell Membrane Interaction and Bacterial Binding

Changes in the composition of the intestinal cell membrane may also interfere with the binding properties of the bacterial cell or its toxins. Studies in animals have shown that more CT molecules bind to the microvillous membrane of the newborn rabbit as compared with adults.[21] This effect may be related to a decreased ratio of protein to phospholipids, commonly found in the immature mucous membranes of newborn animals. This may partly explain why children are more susceptible to enteric pathogens than are adults.

The interaction of *V. cholerae* with other organisms in the gut appears to be important in the pathogenesis of cholera but is poorly understood. There is indirect evidence that nontoxigenic *E. coli* are able to subsequently exclude toxigenic *E. coli* from the small intestine, probably due to competition for intestinal receptor sites.[22] Similar findings with *V. cholerae* have not yet been reported. The clinical implications of such bacterial interactions are speculative at present.

More recently Finkelstein[23] has described a protein made by *V. cholerae*. This protein also called "cholera lectin" has a molecular weight of 32,000 and is a hemagglutinin, a mucinase, and a protease that appears to be involved in the attachment of *V. cholerae* to the mucosal cells, probably by altering mucin, fibronectin, or lactoferrin. This protein alone is not diarrheagenic, but may be involved in splitting the A1 subunit from the complete cholera toxin molecule or from "choleragen."

2.5. Enterotoxin Production and the Clinical Disease

Scientists have now established that the intestinal secretion in cholera is due to the action of a toxin (CT) produced by all strains of *V. cholerae* 01. This toxin has been purified, characterized, and its diarrheagenic properties are well studied. CT has been discussed in detail elsewhere in this book and will not be repeated here. In brief, the toxin is a 84-kDa protein consisting of an active A subunit (with A1 and A2 peptides) and a cluster of 5 B subunits which bind the toxin molecule to the mucosal GM1 ganglioside receptors. The active A subunit enters the cell and increases cAMP concentrations by activating the enzyme, adenyl cyclase. cAMP then stimulates secretion of water and electrolytes resulting in massive secretory diarrhea.

2.6. Role of Prostaglandins in Cholera

It has been suggested that the effects of cholera toxin may be mediated through intracellular messengers other than cAMP. These include prostaglandins, serotonin (5-hydroxytryptamine), and neurotransmitters. That the prostaglandins are involved in the pathogenesis of cholera is shown by the observation that CT-induced intestinal secretion can be prevented by drugs which inhibit prostaglandin synthesis. These drugs, including aspirin and indomethacin, have been shown to inhibit secretory effects of cholera toxin in experimental animals.[24,25] A recent study using intestinal perfusion technics in cholera patients showed that during active disease the jejunal prostaglandin E2 concentrations were significantly elevated (172–1435 pg/ml) as compared to early convalescent stage (60–270 pg/ml, $P < 0.001$).[26] The prostaglandin E2 concentrations were negatively correlated ($r = 0.71$, $P < 0.05$) with the time after the onset of the disease. Patients with higher jejunal prostaglandin E2 concentrations also have high stool output ($r = 0.84$, $P < 0.01$). However, when cholera patients are treated with conventional doses of aspirin and indomethacin, there are no antisecretory effects. The reason these drugs do not reduce intestinal fluid loss is not known. It is possible that local intestinal prostaglandin E2 production in severe cholera results in mucosal prostaglandin E2 concentrations above those required for maximal secretory response. An alternate hypothesis is that cholera toxin maximally stimulates the secretory system and any increases of prostaglandin E2 cannot enhance it further.

TABLE 1
Electrolyte Composition of Small Intestinal Fluids in Patients with Acute Cholera

	Na^+ (mmol/liter)	K^+ (mmol/liter)	Cl^- (mmol/liter)	HCO_3^- (mmol/liter)	Osmolality (mOsm/kg)
Jejunum	147 ± 6	5.6 ± 0.7	138 ± 5	15 ± 4	292 ± 8
Ileum	140 ± 6	5.7 ± 0.9	122 ± 8	41 ± 5	290 ± 12
Stool	133 ± 21	20.1 ± 7.7	100 ± 7	41 ± 9	301 ± 9
Dhaka Solution (cholera saline)	133	14	99	48[a]	294

[a]As acetate, which in the body is metabolically converted to bicarbonate (Table adapted from ref. 30 and 36). Values are given as mean ±sd

2.7. Toxin-Induced Intestinal Secretion of Salt and Water

Diarrhea in cholera results from the stimulation of small intestinal secretion due to the enterotoxin. It has been shown in animals that after a 5–10 min exposure to the enterotoxin, the small intestinal epithelium secretes isotonic fluid for a period of 12–24 h.[27] The enterotoxin stimulates secretion by activating an intracellular biochemical process and there are no changes in the integrity of the intestinal mucosa.[28] However, histologic lesions in the mucosa, including epithelial sloughing, vacuolation, edema, and necrosis of renal tubules have been described in the past. These changes were subsequently found to be postmortem artifacts.[28] There has been no evidence in the literature that the enterotoxin enters the systemic circulation or the organisms penetrate the intestinal epithelium.

Studies in man and animal show that fluid loss occurs from all segments of the small intestine, mostly from the upper part and there appears to be little contribution from the salivary glands and gastric mucosa. The contribution of the pancreas and the liver has not been fully assessed.[29,30] Experimental evidence indicates that in canine cholera, as well as in human, the diarrheal fluid loss is highest in the duodenum and least in the ileum.[30]

The electrolyte composition of intestinal fluids in cholera varies significantly at different segments of the small intestine and is given in Table 1. Intestinal perfusion studies in man and animals have shown that in the duodenum, the bicarbonate concentration is less than that of plasma, whereas in the ileum it is 2–3 times higher.[32,33] The electrolyte patterns of the fluid produced by the duodenum, jejunum, and ileum in cholera are similar to the electrolyte patterns reached when the respective bowel segments are perfused with isotonic saline solutions.

2.8. Colonic Potassium Secretion and Reduced Water Absorption

Our understanding of the small intestinal function is more complete when compared to that of the colon in cholera. Although the transport functions of the large intestine are in many ways similar to that of the small bowel, there are many differences that make the large intestine an important determinant in the development of diarrhea. Unlike the small intestine, the large intestine does not actively absorb glucose and amino acid, nor there is any glucose- and amino acid-stimulated sodium absorption, except in neonatal period.[37,38] The colon possesses significantly greater capabilities than small intestine in absorbing sodium against considerable sodium concentration gradients. In healthy adults, colon can absorb a maximum of 0.5 liters of water in 24 h with a ileocecal flow of approximately 2 liters per 24 h.[39,40] Several factors, including the volume, composition, and the rate of flow of luminal fluids, determine colonic fluid absorption. Because of the great absorptive power of the colon, diarrhea does not occur so long as the ileocecal flow rate remains within the limits of the colonic absorptive capacity. In contrast, a small alteration in colonic absorption due to any disease would result in significant diarrhea in the face of normal small intestinal function and ileocecal flow rate.[41] In health, human colon absorbs water, sodium, and chloride, and secretes potassium and bicarbonate. During cholera diarrhea, alteration of colonic function certainly occurs, but is poorly understood. The only study that has assessed the colonic function during acute cholera was that by Speelman and co-workers.[42] These authors carefully conducted colonoscopic perfusion studies in patients with active diarrhea and during convalescence. The results showed that during acute cholera the colon is in a state of dysfunction characterized by diminished water absorption and increased potassium secretion (Table 2 and Fig. 1). The net water transport was approximately zero. These results showed that the colon contributes to the clinical expression of cholera by failing to absorb normally and by secreting potassium at a higher rate. There is conflicting evidence in the literature, however, about the effects of cholera toxin in the colon. Studies in animals indicate that there is no alteration of colonic water and electrolyte transport due to cholera toxin.[43,44] In contrast, more definitive studies by Donowitz and Binder[45] showed that CT stimulates cAMP production and net fluid secretion in the rat cecum. The mechanism of colonic dysfunction in human cholera can be considered to be the result of cholera toxin causing an elevation of cAMP in the colonic mucosa. On the other hand Shultz[46] pointed out that sodium absorption in the rabbit descending colon occurs in a manner different from that in the small bowel, that is, by simple diffusion through sodium-specific channels. Unlike sodium absorption in the small bowel, the sodium absorption in the colon can be blocked by the diuretic amiloride[47] and is enhanced by aldosterone.[48] The colon also possesses a mechanism to absorb chloride by secreting bicarbonate in the exchange process.[49] These differences

TABLE 2
Net Colonic Ion Absorption (+) or Secreton (−) in Patients with Acute
Cholera Measured by Colonoscopic Perfusion[a]

Patient no.	Sodium	Potassium	Chloride	Bicarbonate
1	−378	−78	−441	−285
2	−26	−50	+46	−115
3	−241	−33	−17	−242
4	+279	−24	+409	−52
5	+652	−34	+461	−85
6	+260	−36	+244	−81
7	−67	−38	−5	−82
8	−126	−52	−20	−222
9	−98	−38	−76	−95
10	+480	−71	+433	−6
11	+335	−51	+335	−58
12	+132	−1	+160	−17
Mean	+100	−42	+127	−112
SD[b]	308	21	265	90

[a]Table from ref. 42.
[b]SD, standard deviation. Values are given in microequivalents per min.

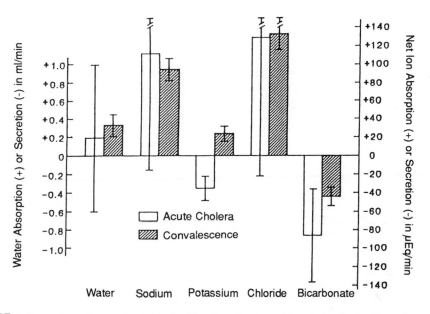

FIGURE 1. Comparison of rates of net colonic absorption of water and ions in 5 patients with cholera who were studied both during their acute illness and during convalescence. Bars show the mean values and the brackets the SEM. The mean secretion of potassium was significantly greater in acute cholera than during convalescence ($p <$ 0.05 by paired t-test). Figure from ref. 42.

between the handling of electrolyte by the small intestine and the colon and the known action of elevated cAMP in the small intestine to inhibit the neutral cotransport of sodium chloride into epithelial cells[50] suggest that the mechanism of CT action on the colon should be distinct from that in the small intestine. Observations of Speelman et al.[42] show that sodium and chloride absorption are intact in most patients with cholera. These findings agree with the isotopic flux studies of Love et al.,[51] who found that in cholera the colon is in a state of net absorption of sodium of about 80 µl per min.

The increased potassium secretion by the colon during acute cholera may also be explained by the action of CT on the colonic epithelium. Direct administration of dibutyryl cAMP to the rat proximal colon has been shown by Foster et al.[52] to stimulate potassium secretion. An alternative explanation for the enhanced potassium secretion by the colon in acute cholera is that aldosterone is exerting an effect on the colon. Patients with acute cholera are hypovolemic and are expected to have elevated blood aldosterone levels. Johnson et al.[53] showed that the mineralocorticoid deoxycorticosterone acetate causes a marked increase in the concentrations of potassium in the intestinal fluid of canine ileal loops exposed to CT. It has been suggested accordingly that aldosterone can act on the colon in acute cholera to augment potassium secretion.[54] It is possible that an aldosterone response in cholera moderates the severity of disease by antagonizing the effects of CT on the colon, which are to cause secretion of water, sodium, and chloride.[55] The colonic dysfunction in cholera may also be attributable to nonspecific factors. These include high flow rates of intestinal contents in the colon that occur naturally in patients with active cholera and during experimental perfusion. Another factor may be the alteration of normal colonic bacterial flora leading to reduced production of volatile fatty acids which are shown to promote sodium absorption in the colonic mucosa.[56]

TABLE 3
Assessment of Dehydration and Fluid Deficit in Cholera[a]

Signs and symptoms	Mild dehydration	Moderate dehydration	Severe dehydration
General appearance	Alert, thirsty, and restless	Thirsty, restless, irritable, giddiness with postural changes	Drowsy, cold and sweaty extremities, wrinkled, muscle cramps
Radial pulse	Normal rate and volume	Rapid and weak	Feeble, may not be palpable
Respiration	Normal	Deep, may be rapid	Deep and rapid
Anterior fontanelle	Normal	Sunken	Very sunken
Systolic blood pressure	Normal	Low	Very low, many be unrecordable
Skin elasticity	Retracts	Retracts slowly	Retracts very slowly (>2 sec)
Eyes	Normal	Sunken	Very sunken
Voice	Normal	Hoarse	Not audible
Loss of fluid	4–5% of body weight	6–9% of body weight	10% or more of body weight

[a]Table from ref. 102.

3. CLINICAL MANIFESTATIONS OF CHOLERA

Studies of naturally occurring cholera suggest that the incubation period may be only a few hours or as long as 5 days, usually 2–3 days.[6,57] In human volunteer studies, the incubation period varies inversely with the number of viable *V. cholerae* fed by mouth, being shortest when the greatest challenge dose was given.[6,57] The clinical manifestations of infection with *V. cholerae* vary from asyptomatic infection to severe diarrhea. Many cases are mild and cannot be distinguished from other milder forms of diarrhea; such patients rarely seek therapy. Clinical manifestations are given in Table 3.

3.1. The Mild Disease

The ratio of individuals with mild disease to those requiring hospital care is about 1 : 1 in infections due to classical *V. cholerae* and about 7 : 1 in infections due to El Tor biotype.[58] In most mild cases there are no prodromal symptoms. There may be few bouts of loose stools without mucus and blood. Clinically significant nausea and vomiting are usually uncommon. In adults the stool volume is usually less than a liter per day[57] and clinically significant fluid deficit does not develop, they do not require fluid replacement to maintain normal hydration. Patients are well ambulatory, feeling little if any disability and there is little risk of complications. The diagnosis can only be established by bacteriologic studies of stool. The watery diarrhea usually stops by the end of a week and there is usually no prolonged fecal excretion of vibrios.

3.2. The Typical Disease

In most cases, the illness is characterized by the onset of vomiting, voluminous watery stools, with severity of dehydration depending entirely on total losses. In its most severe form, cholera is a frightening and rapidly fatal disease. If salt and water are not adequately replaced, severely ill patients develop hypovolemic shock, acidosis, and may die in less than 24 h. Death rates may be as high as 70% in untreated patients.[59] Diarrhea is painless and may begin slowly or abruptly and is commonly associated with vomiting of clear, watery alkaline fluid from the small intestine. There is little nausea and usually no blood or bile in the vomit. In the first few stools, there may be some fecal materials, but later the fluid is clear and is characteristically known as "rice-water" stools (i.e., water in which uncooked rice has been washed). The "rice-water" has a characteristic "fishy" odor and may contain flecks of mucus and occasional polymorphonuclear leucocytes but no red blood cells.

The diarrhea is most severe during the first 48 h of the onset; the fluid loss may equal 1 liter per h in the severely ill adult but usually the loss is less than 500 ml per h. After 48 h, the rate of stool output declines slowly, diarrhea terminating in 4 to 6 days in individuals given adequate intravenous or oral replacement of fluid and electrolytes but no antibiotics.[60-62] The total volume of fluid lost during an average illness by a 40-kg Bengali adult male is 25 to 30 liters[3] but volumes as high as 80 liters have been reported.[34]

3.3. Pathogenesis and Clinical Manifestations of Dehydration

So long as the loss of fluid by vomiting and diarrhea is balanced by the amount of oral intake, there is no dehydration. As the disease progresses, however, if the loss exceeds the intake, symptoms and signs of isotonic dehydration soon appear. The clinical manifestations of cholera and other dehydrating diarrheas result from the underlying deficit due to loss of large quantities of extracellular fluid in diarrheal stool. The magnitude of this loss of fluids and electrolytes is the major determinant of the severity of the clinical condition of patients with cholera.

Thirst: The first symptom that appears as a result of dehydration is thirst, which starts manifesting when the fluid loss is 2 to 3 percent of the patient's body weight. The patient may have mild dehydration and drinking of adequate amount of properly constituted oral rehydration fluid at this stage may prevent development of severe dehydration. The patient continues to pass watery stools. He or she is uneasy but alert. The radial pulse may be a little fast and there is little sign of dehydration.

Loss of skin turgor: The immediate sign of fluid deficit appears in the skin due to loss of water from the subcutaneous tissues. A 5 to 10 percent loss of body weight due to fluid loss results in moderate dehydration: the skin loses its elasticity, a fold of skin picked up by fingers does not fall quickly back when released. In healthy individuals this sign is elicited on the skin over the abdomen, but in undernourished children with loose skin due to little subcutaneous fat, and in the elderly the sign may not be a reliable indicator of dehydration.

Hypovolemia and shock: With increasing loss of fluid and electrolytes in the diarrheal stool, signs of fully developed hypovolemia and shock appear. Fluid loss may be more than 10 percent of the body weight resulting in a serious fall in the amount of fluid in the extracellular compartment and also in the volume of circulating blood. The systolic blood pressure is usually low and sometimes undetectable; the pulse rate may exceed 100 per min. The radial pulse volume is low, thready, and sometimes undetectable. However the femoral and carotid pulses are usually present. The body is cold peripherally in the arms and legs. In most patients the rectal temperature is slightly elevated. The fingers are shrivelled and wrinkled ("washer women's hand"), the tips of tongue and lips may be blue, the mouth is dry and the eyes are sunk into their sockets. The voice is hoarse, there are pain and cramps in the limbs and sometimes in the muscles of the abdomen. The respiratory rate and volume are increased, about 35 per min, often with deep gasps. The abdomen is nontender and looks scaphoid in appearance; the bowel sounds may be active or diminished in frequency and in intensity. Adults with severe cholera are usually conscious, but occasionally stuporous or rarely in frank coma.

4. COMPLICATIONS OF CHOLERA

In cholera, complications that are not directly related to fluid loss are rare. Such complications include, pneumonia, sepsis, renal failure, hypoglycemia, corneal ulceration, electrolyte abnormalities, and cardiac abnormalities. Complications commonly occur as a result of prolonged shock in patients with severe cholera who are not properly treated with fluid and electrolytes.

4.1. Metabolic Acidosis

The acidosis of cholera has been shown to be a base-deficit acidosis due to loss of bicarbonate ions in the stool.[34,35,62] However, more definitive studies have shown that acidosis results from a combination of several factors including lactic acidemia, hyperphosphatemia, hyperproteinemia, and transient renal failure (Table 4).[63] These metabolic features can be explained by the action of cholera toxin in promoting secretion by the small intestinal mucosal cells of a bicarbonate-rich, protein-free isotonic fluid from the extracellular body water. Thus, hyperproteinemia results from hemoconcentration of serum protein after the loss of plasma water. Lactic acidemia results from decreased perfusion of

TABLE 4
Serum Electrolytes, Anion Gaps, and other Biochemical Parameters before Rehydration, after Rehydration, and during Early Convalescence in Adult Patients with Severe Cholera[a]

Parameter	Before hydration	After hydration	Convalescence	P-value[b]
Sodium (mmol/l)	134.8 ± 3.5	139.5 ± 2.2	138.6 ± 2.6	<0.001
Potassium (mmol/l)	4.6 ± 0.6	4.7 ± 1.2	4.0 ± 0.6	<0.01
Chloride (mmol/l)	103.2 ± 4.4	107.1 ± 1.9	104.6 ± 3.1	NS
Bicarbonate (mmol/l)	11.4 ± 4.0	17.8 ± 2.8[c]	22.6 ± 4.0[c]	<0.001
Anion Gap[d] (mmol/l)	20.2 ± 3.4.8	14.6 ± 2.8[e]	11.4 ± 3.0[e]	<0.001
Protein (g/dl)	10.8 ± 1.3	6.6 ± 0.8	6.5 ± 0.6	<0.001
Lactate (mmol/l)	4.05 ± 1.96	—	1.61 ± 0.90	<0.001
Phosphate (mmol/l)	4.4 ± 1.3	2.0 ± 0.8	1.9 ± 0.5	<0.001
Creatinine (mg/dl)	2.48 ± 1.01	1.7 ± 0.81	1.02 ± 0.92	<0.001
Calcium (mg/dl)	11.6 ± 1.0	8.5 ± 0.6	9.1 ± 0.5	<0.001
Magnesium (mg/dl)	3.1 ± 0.5	2.0 ± 0.4	2.1 ± 0.3	<0.001

[a]Table from Ref. 63.
[b]P-values by paired student's t-test comparing mean values on admission and during convalescence.
[c]Mean bicarbonate values are significantly higher after rehydration than on admission (before rehydration) and are higher during convalescence than after rehydration (P<0.001).
[d]Anion gap = sodium - (chloride + bicarbonate); normal range 8 to 12 mmol/liter.
[e]Mean anion gaps are significantly lower after rehydration than on admission (P<0.01) and are lower during convalescence than after rehydration (P<0.001).

tissues during hypovolemic shock. Hyperphosphatemia probably results from a combination of hydrolysis of cellular phosphate esters during acidosis, a shift of this inorganic phosphate into the extracellular fluid, and failure of the kidney to excrete this added phosphate load. Vomiting, which occurs in most cholera patients, would be expected to ameliorate the metabolic acidosis through the loss of hydrogen ions. Thus, it appears that severe cholera causes acidosis with relatively little change in serum chloride but an increased serum anion gap. The acidosis is more profound than would be expected on the basis of stool losses of bicarbonate, because of superimposed lactic acidemia and renal failure.

Patients with severe acidosis develop increased rate of respiration, 35 or more breaths per min in adults and 40 or more in children are commonly seen.[31,64] In patients with untreated acidosis, deep Kussmaul-type breathing develops, which slowly disappears after correcting acidosis. In extreme and neglected cases pulmonary edema ensues and can be a direct cause of death.[65] Abnormalities of serum electrolyte concentrations are also common. During hypokalemic acidosis with lower concentrations of potassium ions and higher concentrations of hydrogen ions in the extracellular fluid, potassium ions move from the intracellular to the extracellular fluid compartment in exchange for a movement of hydrogen ions into the cells ($K^+ - H^+$ exchange). This results in normal or elevated plasma potassium concentrations before treatment. With the correction of acidosis, however, net potassium movement into the cell occurs and serum potassium concentrations fall to hypokalemic levels if no potassium is concurrently administered.[60,64]

4.2. Renal Failure

The renal failure in cholera has been described as a consequence of hypovolemic shock which induces acute tubular necrosis.[60,66] The renal failure is usually mild, the serum creatitine concentration is 2.48 mg per dl and is promptly improved by providing adequate amounts of isotonic intravenous fluid.[63] Carpenter et al.[67] noted that azotemia is mild at the time of admission for acute cholera; blood urea nitrogen values were 21 to 26 mg per dl (7.5 to 9.3 mmol per liter) and rose during hospitalization only if rehydration therapy was given in inadequate volumes. The correction of renal failure was not immediate, however; the elevated creatinine concentration persisted throughout the initial rehydration period and did not become normal until convalescence. The high phosphate concentration, on the other hand, fell to normal immediately after rehydration. Thus, the hyperphosphatemia appears to depend on the acidic pH of blood as well as on the renal failure, allowing more rapid correction of the serum phosphate levels than of the creatinine level after an improvement in acidosis. This rapid normalization of the serum phosphate level suggests that extracellular phosphate shifted into cells during correction of acidosis.[68] In mild cases there is oliguria and if the fluid deficit is not corrected it may lead to anuria, uremia, and death. With proper replacement of fluid and electrolytes, there is little kidney damage and urine flow returns quickly.

4.3. Hypoglycemia

Hypoglycemia has been recognized as an important complication of many diarrheal diseases, including cholera.[69-71] In some reports,[71] 50% of the children with cholera develop clinically significant hypoglycemia, the blood glucose concentration ranging between 1 to

2 mmol per dl or lower. Patients are usually severely dehydrated when first seen; they may be acidotic, comatose, or have neurologic findings including motor seizures, spasticity, generalized convulsion, and sometimes hemiplegia. Deaths occur in about 40% of hypoglycemic children even after treatment with intravenous glucose.[69] In one recent study 14.3% of the children with cholera and hypoglycemia died compared to 0.7% children who died without hypoglycemia.[70] It has been observed that the relative risk of death from hypoglycemia is 6.4 in a group of Bangladeshi children with diarrhea.[41] The mechanism of hypoglycemia in cholera and in other diarrheal diseases is not known. However the possible contributions of hyperinsulinism, hypoxia, fasting, undernutrition, ketosis, failure of gluconeogenesis, and failure of counterregulatory mechanisms have been suggested. Hypoglycemic individuals with cholera were found to have normal or low plasma insulin concentrations and hyperinsulinemia has not been considered responsible for hypoglycemia. The failure of counterregulatory mechanisms is not an important cause because the major counterregulatory hormones, epinephrine and glucagon concentrations are not diminished.[71,72] More definitive studies indicate that defective gluconeogenesis due to altered enzyme pathways and transport systems is the cause of hypoglycemia.[72] It has been shown that failure of gluconeogenesis is due to reduced store and oxidation of fats, reduced plasma concentrations of alanine (the major protein for gluconeogenesis), and presence of sepsis and endotoxemia, which are known to impair enzyme activities necessary for gluconeogenesis.[73–75] Patients with hypoglycemia need special clinical care during management. During diarrhea, it is of special importance that they should continue feeding, which may prevent weight loss as well as fatal hypoglycemia. An effective way of treating patients with hypoglycemic diarrhea requiring parenteral fluids would be to routinely administer intravenous fluid containing glucose; this may be life-saving in many instances.

4.4. Cardiac Abnormalities

Individuals with moderately severe cholera rarely have cardiac abnormalities. However, cardiac arrhythmias may sometimes occur in severely ill patients due to excess loss of potassium and bicarbonate ions in the stool resulting in hypokalemia and acidosis.[76] In acutely ill patients, electrocardiographic changes may be present, these include; giant P and T waves, T-wave inversion, and ST segment depression.[67,76,77] Sinus tachycardia is occasionally present. Sometimes hypokalemic arrhythmia and focal myocarditis may develop and lead to sudden death during dehydration. Children with severe uncorrected hypoglycemia and acidosis may develop fatal cardiac arrhythmias. Timely administration of adequate amount of proper fluids and electrolytes can prevent all these cardiac abnormalities in patients with severe cholera.

4.5. Paralytic Ileus

If increasing losses of potassium ions in the stool are not quantitatively replaced, signs of paralytic ileus and abdominal distension may appear. This is more commonly seen in children. Paralytic ileus is rarely seen in adults (even without treatment) or in patients receiving proper fluid and electrolytes.[65,78] With adequate treatment abdominal distension gradually improves and no residual effects have been observed.

4.6. Seizures

Seizures of grand mal type may occur in children with cholera before or during therapy. Seizures rarely occur in adults. The cause of these seizures is not known. In a majority of cases the seizure is associated with hypoglycemia and is treated with intravenous glucose administration and low doses of diazepam or phenobarbitone.[59,60,78] Seizures are a poor prognostic sign, sometimes leading to coma and death.

4.7. Cholera in Pregnancy

Pregnant mothers with cholera carry a 50% risk of fetal death during third trimester.[79] Most fetal deaths occur within 24 h of the disease. The cause of fetal death is not known. It has been suggested that placental ischemia and hypoxia resulting from poor visceral perfusion may play an important role. Retention of placenta after abortion is also a complication of severe cholera during pregnancy.

4.8. Pulmonary Edema

Acute pulmonary edema is sometimes associated with cholera and severe acidosis. The pathogenesis of pulmonary edema is not clear. However, it has been observed that acidotic children who are treated with solutions not containing base (bicarbonate) frequently develop pulmonary edema.[65,80] Untreated metabolic acidosis and sometimes overhydration may also cause pulmonary hypertension and edema. In most children these complications can be prevented by proper treatment with rehydration fluids containing adequate amounts of electrolytes.

4.9. Changes in Biochemical Parameters in Blood

Abnormalities of serum electrolytes, blood pH, and other biochemical parameters in blood result from metabolic defects due to isotonic fluid loss, acidosis, and their consequences. The changes in common laboratory findings are given in Table 5.

Isotonic fluid loss produces hypovolemia and hemoconcentration. This is manifested by a rise in blood hematocrit and serum specific gravity values.[60,64,67] Increases in plasma protein concentrations result from the loss of fluid from the extracellular compartment. Changes in the hematocrit, plasma protein, and serum specific gravity values are useful clinical indicators of dehydration during treatment. Loss of bicarbonate in the stool together with lactic acidemia and renal failure results in a drop of pH of arterial blood as well as arterial pCO_2 concentrations due to ventilatory compensation.[82] Most patients have lower than normal serum sodium concentrations when first seen before treatment. In some instances, hypernatremia (serum sodium concentration > 160 mmol per liter) has been observed, particularly in children receiving improperly constituted oral rehydration fluids with excessive sugar and salt before coming to the hospital.[31] In untreated patients, serum calcium concentrations are usually elevated and return to normal after rehydration. In these patients, there is no justification to administer calcium in the form of calcium gluconate during

TABLE 5
Mean Arterial Blood or Plasma Values in Severe Untreated Cholera[a]

	Adult	Children
pH	7.19	7.18
pCO_2 (mmHg)	28	—
Bicarbonate (mmol/liter)	9	12
Sodium (mmol/liter)	141	138
Potassium (mmol/liter)	4.5	4
Chloride (mmol/liter)	107	110
Glucose (mg/dl)	180	165
Osmolality (mOsm/kg)	326	293
Urea nitrogen (mg/dl)	26	—
SGOT (Unit/ml)	40	—
Alkaline phosphatase (Unit/ml)	5.1	—
Magnesium (mmol/liter)	—	2.6
Calcium (mmol/liter)	—	7.3
Lactate (mmol/liter)	—	2.4
Total protein (g/dl)	10.1	9.5
Plasma (sp. gr.)	1.040	1.033
Hematocrit (%)	47	47
White blood cells/mm³	23,000	—

[a]Adapted from ref 81.

treatment. Many children present with clinical signs of severe hypoglycemia, their blood glucose concentrations varying between 1 mmol to 2.2 mmol per dl on admission. Serum osmolality and serum chloride concentrations are usually within normal limits. In some cases minimal elevations of serum alkaline phosphatase[82] and serum glutamic oxaloacetic transaminase activities have been observed.[83] Serum creatinine concentrations are slightly elevated but return to normal after rehydration. Mild leukocytosis has been observed. However, it is most likely that the leukocytosis is due to hemoconcentration.

5. CHOLERA IN CHILDREN

It has been convincingly shown that more children than adults are susceptible to infectious diarrheas. Epidemiologic studies in endemic areas like Bangladesh show that case–fatality rates of cholera in children 1 to 5 years old is ten times higher than that in adults.[84] However, the mechanism(s) for the increased susceptibility of the children to enterotoxin-induced diarrhea is unknown. It may be related to several factors, including increased exposure to infectious agents, impaired host immunity, and/or increased sensitivity to the elaborated toxin. It has been shown that in young animals (14- and 21-day-old rats) E. coli heat-stable toxin (ST) causes significantly greater secretion than in adult rats.[85] Although similar findings have not yet been reported with CT, it suggests that the increased number of jejunal receptors in the immature rat may, in part explain the increased sensitivity and secretory response to E. coli ST observed in vivo. Cholera in children presents an especially alarming clinical situation which can rapidly lead to death. Symptoms such as fever, lethargy, seizures, altered consciousness, and hypoglycemia are seen more commonly in children than in adults; the last two are important risk factors for death.[10,64] This underlines the extreme urgency of early rehydration therapy and feeding in children during cholera epidemics.

Children, more commonly than adults, develop hyponatremia and hypokalemia because of the proportionately greater loss of sodium and potassium in the stool.[64,86] The nutritional status of the child also appears to be an important determination of the clinical severity of the disease. It has been reported that malnourished children are more prone to develop severe dehydration and prolonged diarrhea in spite of antibiotic therapy.[64,71] Because of the increased risk of death in children, special attention by the clinician is needed. Metabolic studies of malnourished children indicate that the prompt introduction of a full diet during illness will hasten nutritional recovery. However, the effect of cholera on long-term nutritional status of children has not yet been adequately studied.

5.1. Characteristics of Diarrheal Stool in Children

Most children with cholera who seek treatment are brought to the hospital within 24 h of onset of watery diarrhea and vomiting.[87–89] It is difficult to determine the volume of diarrheal stool lost before coming to hospital and the clinician has to estimate the loss by clinical findings. It has been observed that the water and electrolyte deficit at the time of admission results primarily from the stool losses with smaller contributions from vomiting and evaporation from the skin. Children with cholera may lose water from the skin as much as 2.9 ml/kg to 3.6 ml/kg per h.[64,86] Other factors, however, also are important; these include volume and electrolyte contents of urine, evaporative loss from the lungs, nutritional status, and the volume and composition of rehydration fluid given before coming to hospital. There is a wide variation in clinical severity and in the total volume of diarrheal stool among children with cholera. In some instances the child may stop having diarrhea in a few days and in others, the illness may be prolonged for more than a week.

The electrolyte composition of ileal and jejunal fluids in children with acute cholera are similar to that of adults and are given in Table 6. Unlike adults, however, the small intestinal fluid of children contains more sodium and less potassium than those in the stool. These differences in the electrolyte composition of stool probably occur in the colon. The normal human colon absorbs sodium and secretes potassium and bicarbonate. It has been observed that the colonic mucosa exchanges potassium for sodium more efficiently in children than in adults.[64,90] In childhood cholera, the stool potassium is increased almost two-fold and sodium content is lower than that found in adults. The stool osmolality in childhood cholera

TABLE 6
Small Bowel Fluid Composition in Children and Adults with Cholera[a]

	Na$^+$ (mEq/liter)	K$^+$ (mEq/liter)	HCO$_3^-$ (mEq/liter)	Cl$^-$ (mEq/liter)	pH	Osmolality (mOsm/kg)
Children						
Jejunum	140.6 ± 13.9	4.6 ± 1.6	7.8 ± 4.8	129.6 ± 16.8	7.28 ± 0.42	281 ± 10
Ileum	140.9 ± 5.0	4.4 ± 1.0	27.8 ± 9.5	115.1 ± 14.5	7.94 ± 0.27	279 ± 5
Adults						
Jejunum	147.5 ± 5	5.6 ± 0.7	14.8 ± 4.3	137.8 ± 5	—	292 ± 8
Ileum	145.8 ± 4.0	5.7 ± 0.9	42.0 ± 4.0	129.9 ± 7.6	—	285
Children stool	101	28	32	92	—	—
Adults stool	140	13	44	104	—	300

[a]Adapted from ref. 101.

is similar to that of adults.[35] The stool CO_2 content is lower in childhood cholera than that in adults.[64,91] It has been observed that both in children and adults, as the rate of purging declines, sodium content of stool decreases while stool potassium content increases.[35,64] Changes in blood chemistry depend on the severity of dehydration and duration of illness. On admission serum osmolality is usually normal, indicating isotonic dehydration (135–293 mmol/liter). Normal plasma sodium concentrations (135–140 mmol/liter) are usual but low sodium concentrations (below 130 mmol/liter) are also common. There is significant hypo-kalemia, serum potassium concentrations as low as 1.2 mmol/liter are not infrequent. Hypo-kalemia is usually associated with low arterial pH (7.18) and marked acidosis characterized by lactic acidemia (mean ± sd serum lactate, 4.05 ± 1.96 mmol/liter) and low serum bicarbonate concentrations (10 mmol/liter).[63] Plasma specific gravity is increased due to loss of isotonic fluid from the extracellular fluid compartment. In children with severe cholera the plasma specific gravity values may range from 1.035 to 1.040 before rehydration.[64] Higher values of plasma specific gravity are usually common in adults with similar status of de-hydration,[92,93] probably because of smaller extracellular fluid compartment per unit body mass in adults. The blood urea nitrogen and the serum creatinine concentrations are within normal limits when first seen in the hospital.[94] This indicates that the duration of circulatory insufficiency is too brief to cause a measurable change in renal function. Changes in other biochemical parameters associated with acidosis and hypoglycemia are described in the relevant sections of this chapter.

6. NUTRITION IN CHOLERA

Nutritional consequences of cholera are important, especially in the children of the tropics where preexisting undernutrition is common.[95,96] During cholera normal feeding is usually interrupted either because of intense vomiting or because of the common tradition of withholding food in some communities. These may lead to a negative nitrogen balance and retardation of normal growth in children. In malnourished children whose nutritional reserve is marginal, a 24-h period of starvation may lead to depletion of liver glycogen stores and precipitate hypoglycemia. It has been shown that undernourished children with cholera suffer prolonged illness when compared to those with better nutrition.[59] Metabolic balance studies in children indicate that nitrogen retention during recovery does not depend on the severity of the disease; nitrogen balance becomes quickly positive within 2 days of diarrhea when a moderate amount of milk is given.[64] It has been observed that normal food given during active disease accelerates clinical recovery.

Diarrhea affects child nutrition by reducing food intake due to anorexia or the withhold-ing of food, and reduced food absorption. It has been observed that in children with acute cholera there is a reduction of calorie and protein intake of 20% to 40%.[97,98] Interestingly, however, calorie intake from breast milk does not decrease in these children compared to that of healthy breast-fed children. It has been observed that in children with cholera, food and calorie intake improved every day during the course of the illness, reaching an intake of 100 kcal/kg per day on the fourth day of cholera.[99] The intake is even higher than the recom-mended allowances (120 kcal/kg per day) on the seventh day, and it remains the same after recovery. Metabolic balance studies have indicated that carbohydrates are well absorbed (80% to 85%) during acute attacks of cholera but absorption of proteins and fats is reduced; protein and fat malabsorption may last for several weeks after recovery.[99] Nutritional status of children does not make any difference in nutrient absorption during cholera; both undernourished and well-nourished children absorb carbohydrates equally well.[97,100] In these children, however, absorption of proteins and fats is reduced during acute illness and returns to normal during the convalescence. The cause of transient reduction of protein and fat malabsorption is not known, but may be related to inadequate pancreatic enzymes or their dilution by voluminous small intestinal secretion that occurs in cholera. Interference with the formation of micellar fat in the intestine may also be responsible for poor fat absorption. Anorexia frequently accompanies diarrheal diseases, including cholera, and interferes with the food intake. It has been observed, however, that if offered, there is substantial intake of food and calories by children suffering from acute cholera.[101] However, it is clear that despite some malabsorption, feeding during cholera is beneficial for nutritional purposes and may decrease diarrheal stool volume and duration of diarrhea.

REFERENCES

1. Carpenter CCJ: Treatment of cholera—Tradition and authority versus science, reason, and humanity. *Johns Hopkins Med J* 139:153–162, 1976
2. De SN: Enterotoxicity of bacteria free culture filtrate of *Vibrio cholerae. Nature* 183:1533, 1959
3. Rabbani GH: Cholera. *Clin Gastroenterol* 15:507–528, 1986
4. Baumann P, Furniss Al, Lee JV: Vibrio, in Kreig NR, Holt JG (eds): *Bergey's Manual of Systematic Bacteriology,* Vol 1. Baltimore, Wiliams and Wilkins, 1984, pp 518–538
5. Christie AB: Cholera, in Christie AB (ed): *Infectious Diseases: Epidemiology and Clinical Practice.* Churchill Livingston, Edinburgh, 1987, pp 193–230
6. Hornick RB, Music SI, Wenzel R, et al: The Broad Street pump revisited: response of volunteers to ingested cholera vibrios. *Bull NY Acad Med* 47:1181–1191, 1971
7. Cahs R, Music S, Libonate J, et al: Response of man to infection with *V. cholerae.* 1. Clinical, serologic, and bacteriologic response to a known inoculum. *J Infect Dis* 129:45, 1974
8. Carpenter CCJ: Pathogenesis and pathophysiology of cholera. *Pub Hlth Pap* 40:53, 1970
9. Gitelson S: Gastrectomy, achlorhydria and cholera. *Israel J Med Sci* 7:633–637, 1971
10. Bain WB, Zampieri A, Mazzotti M, et al: Epidemilogy of cholera in Italy in 1973. *Lancet* ii:1370–1374, 1974
11. Gilman RH, Partanen R, Brown KH, Spira WM, Khanam S, Greenberg B, Bloom SR, Ali A: Decreased gastric acid secretion and bacterial colonization of the stomach in severely malnourished Bangladeshi children. *Gastroenterol* 94:1308–1314, 1988
12. Jones GW, Freter R: Adhesive properties of *Vibrio cholerae:* nature of the interaction with isolated rabbit brush border membranes and human erythrocytes. *Infect Immun* 14:240–245, 1976
13. Boedeker EC: Enterocyte adherence of *Escherichia coli:* its relation to diarrheal disease. *Gastroenterol* 83:489–492, 1982
14. Walker WA, Wu M, Isselbacher KJ, Block KJ: Intestinal uptake of macromolecules. IV. The effect of pancreatic duct ligation on the breakdown of antigen and antigen–antibody complexes on the intestinal surface. *Gastroenterol* 69:1223–1229, 1975
15. Evans DG, Silver RP, Evans DJ Jr, Chase DG, Gorbach SL: Plasmid controlled colonization factor associated with virulence in *Escherichia coli* enterotoxigenic for humans. *Infect Immun* 12:656–667, 1975
16. Holt SC: Bacterial adhesion in pathogenesis: an introductory statement, in: Schlessinger D (ed.): *Microbiology, 1982.* Washington DC, American Society for Microbiology, 1982, pp 261–265
17. Teppema JS, Guinee PAM, Ibrahim AA, Paques M, Ruitenberg EJ: In vivo adherence and colonization of *Vibrio cholerae* strains that differ in hemagglutinating activity and motility. *Infect Immun* 55:2093–2102, 1987
18. Taylor RK, Miller VL, Furlong DB, Mekalanos JJ: Use of phoA gene fusion to identify a pilus colonization factor coordinately regulated with cholera toxin. *Proc Natl Acad Sci USA* 84:2833–2837, 1987
19. Herrington DA, Hall RA, Losnosky G, Mekalanos JJ, Taylor RK, Levine MM: Toxin, toxin-coregulated pili, and the toxR regulation are essential for *Vibrio cholerae* pathogenesis in human. *J Exp Med* 168:1487–1492, 1988
20. Yamamoto T, Takeshi Y: Electron microscopic study of *Vibrio cholerae* 01 adherence to the mucus coat and villous surface in the human small intestine. *Infect Immun* 56:2753–2759, 1988
21. Bresson JL, Pang KY, Walker WA: Microvillous membrane differentiations: quantitative difference in cholera toxin binding to the intestinal surface of new born and adult rabbits. *Paediatr Research* 18:984–987, 1984

22. Davidson JN, Hirschhorn DC: Use of the K88 antigen for in vivo bacterial competition with porcine strains of enteropathogenic *Escherchia coli*. *Infect Immun* 12:134–136, 1975
23. Finkelstein RA, Boesman-Finkelstein M, Holt P: *Vibrio cholerae* hemagglutination (lectin) protease hydrolyses fibronectin and ovomucin. *Proc Natl Acd Sci USA* 80:1092–1095, 1983
24. Wald A, Gotterer, GS, Rajendra GR, Turjjman NA, Hendrix TR: Effect of indomethacin on cholera-induced fluid movement, unidirectional sodium fluxes, and intestinal cAMP. *Gastroenterol* 72:106–110, 1977
25. Jacoby HI, Marshall CH: Antagonism of cholera enterotoxin by antiinflammatory agents in the rat. *Nature* 235:163–165, 1972
26. Speelman P, Rabbani GH, Bukhave K, Rask-Madesn K: Increased jejunal prostaglandin E2 concentrations in patients with acute cholera. *Gut* 26:188–193, 1985
27. Pierce NF, Greenough WB III, Carpenter CCJ: *Vibrio cholerae* enterotoxin and its mode of action. *Bactreriol Rev* 35:1–12, 1971
28. Gangarosa EJ, Beisel WR, Benyajati C, et al: The nature of the gastrointestinal lesion in Asiatic cholera and its relation to pathogenesis: A biopsy study. *Am J Trop Med* 9:125–135, 1960
29. Greenough WB III: Pancreatic and hepatic hypersecretion in cholera. *Lancet* ii:991–993, 1965
30. Banwell JG, Pierce NF, Mitra RC, Brigham KL, Caranasos GJ, Keimowitz RI, Fedson DS, Thomas J, Gorbach SL, Sack RB, Mondal A: Intestinal fluid and electrolyte transport in human cholera. *J Clin Invest* 49:183–195, 1970
31. Pierce NF, Sack RB, Mitra RC, Banwell JG, Brigham KL, Fedson DS, Mondal A: Replacement of water and electrolyte losses in cholera by an oral glucose electrolyte solution. *Ann Int Med* 70:1173–1181, 1969
32. Carpenter CCJ, Sack RB, Feeley JC, Steenberg RW: Site and characteristics of electrolyte loss and effect of intraluminal glucose in experimental canine cholera. *J Clin Invest* 47:1210–1220, 1968
33. Carpenter CCJ, Greenough WB III: Response of canine duodenum to intraluminal challenge with cholera toxin. *J Clin Invest* 47:2600–2608, 1968
34. Carpenter CCJ, Mondal A, Sack RB, Mitra PP, Dans PE, Wells SA, Hinman EJ, Chaudhury RN: Clinical studies in Asiatic cholera. *Bull Johns Hopkins Hosp* 118:174–196, 1966
35. Watten RH, Morgan RM, Songkhla YN, Vanikiati V, Phillips RA: Water and electrolyte studies in cholera. *J Clin Invest* 38:1879–1889, 1959
36. Greenough WB III, Rosenberg IS, Gordon RS, Davies BI: Tetracycline in the treatment of cholera. *Lancet* i:355–357, 1964
37. Batt ER, Schacter D: Developmental pattern of some intestinal transport mechanisms in new born rats and mice. *Am J Physiol* 261:1064–1068, 1969
38. Binder HJ: Amino acid absorption from the mammalian colon. *Biochem Biophys Acta* 219:503–506, 1970
39. Debongnie JC, Phillips SF: Capacity of the human colon to absorb fluid. *Gastroenterol* 74:698–703, 1978
40. Phillips SF, Giller J: The contribution of colon to electrolytes and water conservation in man. *J Lab Clin Med* 81:733–746, 1973
41. Read NW: Diarrhea: the failure of colonic salvage. *Lancet* ii:481–483, 1982
42. Speelman P, Butler T, Kabir I, Ali A, Banwell J: Colonic dysfunction during cholera infection. *Gastroenterol* 91:1164–1170, 1986
43. Sack RB, Carpenter CCJ, Steenberg RW, Pierce NF: Experimental cholera: a canine model. *Lancet* ii:206–207, 1966
44. Swab EA, Hynes ZA, Donowitz M: Elevated intramural pressure alters rabbit small intestinal transport in vivo. *Am J Physiol* 242:G58–G64, 1982
45. Donowitz M, Binder HJ: Effect of enterotoxins of *Vibrio cholerae, Escherichia coli,* and *Shigella dysentariae* type 1 on fluid and electrolyte transport in the colon. *J Infect Dis* 134:135–143, 1976
46. Schultz SG: Sodium and chloride absorption by small and large intestine: an overview, in: Janowitz HD, Sachar DB (eds): *Frontiers of Knowledge in the Diarrheal Diseases.* Upper Montclair, NJ, Projects in Health, Inc, 1979
47. Schultz SG, Frizzel RA, Nellans HN: Sodium transport and the electrophysiology of rabbit colon. *J Membr Biol* 33:351–384, 1977
48. Frizzel RA, Schultz SG: Effects of aldosterone on ion transport by rabbit colon in vitro. *J Membr Biol* 39:1–26, 1978
49. Phillips SF, Schmalz PF: Bicarbonate secretion by the rat colon: effect of intraluminal chloride and acetazolamide. *Proc Soc Exp Biol Med* 135:116–122, 1970
50. Field M: Intestinal secretion. *Gastroenterol* 66:1063–1084, 1974
51. Love AHG, Phillips RA, Rhode JE, Veall N: Sodium ion movement across intestinal mucosa in cholera patients. *Lancet* ii:151–153, 1972

52. Foster ES, Sandle GI, Hayslett JP, Binder HJ: Cyclic adenosine monophosphate stimulates active potassium secretion in the rat colon. *Gastroenterol* 84:324–330, 1983

53. Johnson J, Casper AGT, Carpenter CCJ: Effects of desoxycorticosterone on potassium concentration in enterotoxin-stimulated small intestinal secretions. *Johns Hopkins Med J* 133:201–206, 1973

54. Carpenter CCJ, Mondal A, Sack RB, et al: Clinical studies in Asiatic cholera. II. Development of 2:1 saline lactate regimen. *Johns Hopkins Med J* 118:174–196, 1966

55. Levitn R, Ingelfinger FI: Effect of *d*-aldosterone on salt and water absorption from the intact human colon. *J Clin Invest* 44:801–808, 1965

56. Argenzio RA: Short chain fatty acids and the colon. *Dig Dis Sci* 26:97–99, 1981

57. Oseasohn R, Ahmad S, Islam MA, Rahaman ASMM: Clinical and bacteriological findings among families of cholera patients. *Lancet* i:340–342, 1966

58. Bart KJ, Huq Z, Khan M, Mosley WH: Seroepidemiologic studies during a simultaneous epidemic of infection with *El Tor* Ogawa and classical Inaba *Vibrio cholerae*. *J Infect Dis* 121(suppl.):S17–S24, 1970

59. Lindenbaum J, Greenough WB III, Islam MR: Antibiotic therapy of cholera. *Bull WHO* 36:871–833, 1967

60. Carpenter CCJ, Barua D, Wallace CK, Mitra P, Sack RB, Khanra SR, Wells SA, Dans PE, Chaudhury RN: Clinical studies in Asiatic cholera. IV. Antibiotic therapy in cholera. *Bull Johns Hopkins Hosp* 118:216–229, 1966

61. Hirschhorn N, Kinzie JL, Sachar DB, Northrup RS, Taylor JO, Ahmed SZ, Phillips RA: Decrease in net stool output in children during intestinal perfusion with glucose-containing solutions. *N Eng J Med* 279:176–181, 1968

62. Pierce NF, Banwell JG, Mitra RC, Caranasos GJ, Keimowitz RI, Thomas J, Mondal A: A controlled comparison of tetracycline and furazolidone in cholera. *Brit Med J* 3:277–280, 1968

63. Wang F, Butler T, Rabbani GH, Jones PK: The acidosis of cholera: contributions of hyperproteinemia, lactic acidemia, and hyperphosphatemia to an increased serum anion gap. *N Eng J Med* 315:1591–1595, 1986

64. Mahalanabis D, Wallace CK, Kallen RJ, Mondal A, Pierce NF: Water and electrolyte losses due to cholera in infants and small children: A recovery balance study. *Pediatrics* 45:374–385, 1970

65. Greenough WB III, Hirschhorn N, Gordon RS Jr, Linderbaum J, Ally KM: Pulmonary edema associated with acidosis in patients with cholera. *Trop Geogr Med* 28:86–90, 1976

66. Benyajati C, Keoplug M, Beisel WR, Gangarosa EJ, Sprinz H, Sitprija V: Acute renal failure in Asiatic cholera: clinicopathologic correlations with acute tubular necrosis and hypokalemic nephropathy. *Ann Int Med* 52:960–975, 1960

67. Carpenter CCJ, Mitra RP, Sack RB: Clinical studies in Asiatic cholera. I. Preliminary observations, November, 1962–March, 1963. *Bull Johns Hopkins Hosp* 118:165–173, 1966

68. Knochel JP: Biochemical, electrolyte, and acid-base disturbance in acute renal failure, in, Brenner BM, Lazarus JM (eds): *Acute Renal Failure*. Philadelphia, WB Saunders, 1983, pp 568–585

69. Molla AM, Hossain M, Islam R, Bardhan PK, Sarkar SA: Hypoglycemia: a complication of diarrhea in childhood. *Indian Pediatr* 18:181–185, 1981

70. Jones RG: Hypoglycemia in children with acute diarrhea. *Lancet* ii:643, 1966

71. Hirschhorn N, Lindenbaum J, Greenough III WB, Alam SM: Hypoglycemia in children with acute diarrhea. *Lancet* ii:128–132, 1966

72. Bennish ML, Azad Ak, Rahman O, Phillips RE: Hypoglycemia during diarrhea in childhood: Prevalence, pathophysiology, and outcome. *N Eng J Med* 322:1357–1363, 1990

73. Senior B, Sadeghi-Nejad A: Hypoglycemia: a pathophysiologic approach. *Acta Ped Scand* (suppl)352, 1989

74. McCallum RE, Seale TW, Stith RD: Influence of endotoxin treatment on dexamethasone induction of hepatic phosphoenolpyruvate carboxylase. *Infect Immun* 39:213–239, 1983

75. Knowles RG, McCabe JP, Beevers SJ, Pogson CI: The characteristics and sign of inhibition of gluconeogenesis in rat liver cells by bacterial endotoxin. *Biochem J* 242:721–728, 1987

76. Carpenter CCJ, Biern RO, Mitra PP, Sack RB, Dans PE, Wells SA, Khanra SS: Electrocardiogram in Asiatic cholera. Seperated studies of effects of hypovolemia, acidosis, and potassium loss. *Brit Heart J* 29:103–111, 1967

77. Ally KM, Greenough WB III: Electrocardiographic changes during shock due to cholera and other causes. *East Pakistan Med J* 10:1–8, 1966

78. Mahalanabis D, Brayton JB, Mondal A, Pierce NF: The use of Ringer's lactate in the treatment of children with cholera and acute noncholera diarrhea. *Bull WHO* 46:311–319, 1972

79. Hirschhorn N, Chaudhury AKMA, Lindenbaum J: Cholera in pregnant women. *Lancet* i:1230–1232, 1969

80. Harvey RM, Enson Y, Lewis ML, Greenough III WB, Ally KM, Panno RA: Hemodynamic studies on cholera. Effect of hypovolemia and acidosis. *Circulation* 37:709–728, 1968

81. Pierce NF, Mondal A: Clinical features of cholera, in Barua D, Burrows W (eds): *Cholera*. Philadelphia, WB Saunders, 1974, p 216

82. Pierce NF, Graybill JR, Kaplan MM, Bauwman DL: Systemic effects of parenteral cholera enterotoxin in dogs. *J Lab Clin Med* 79:145–156, 1972

83. Iwert ME, Deb BD, Srivastava DL, Burrows W: Cholera toxins: Increased levels of serum glutamic-ox-alloacetic transaminase in human cholera. *J Infect Dis* 118:422–426, 1968

84. Mosley WH, Benenson AS, Barui KR: A serological survey of cholera antobodies in rural East Pakistan. 1. The distribution of area and the relation of antibody titer to the pattern of endemic cholera. *Bull WHO* 38:327–334, 1968

85. Cohen MB, Moyer S, Lutterell M, Gianella RA: The immature rat small intestine exhibits an increased sensitivity and response to *Escherichia coli* heat-stable enterotoxin. *Pediatr Res* 20:555–560, 1986

86. Griffith LSC, Fresh JW, Watten RH, Willaroman MP: Electrolyte replacement in pediatric cholera. *Lancet* i:1197–1199, 1967

87. Rabbani GH, Islam MR, Butler T, Shahriar M, Alam K: Single-dose treatment of cholera with furazolidone or tetracycline in a double-blind randomized trial. *Antimicrob Agents Chemother* 33:1447–1450, 1989

88. Rabbani GH, Greenough III WB, Holmgren J, Kirkwood B: Controlled trial of chlorpromazine as antisecretory agent in patients with cholera hydrated intravenously. *Brit Med J* 284:1361–1364, 1982

89. Koch SW, Metcoff J: Physiologic considerations in fluid and electrolyte therapy with particular reference to diarrheal dehydration in children. *J Pediatr* 62:107–131, 1963

90. Beisel WR, Watten RH, Blackwell RQ, Benyajati C, Phillips RA: The role of bicarbonate pathophysiology and therapy in Asiatic cholera. *Am J Med* 35:58–66, 1963

91. Friis-Hansen B: Body water compartments in children: changes during growth and related changes in the body composition. *Pediatr* 28:169–181, 1961

92. Cheek DB: Extracellular volume, its structure and measurement and the influence of age and disease. *J Pediatr* 58:103–125, 1961

93. Carpenter CCJ: Clinical and pathophysiologic features of diarrhea caused by *Vibrio cholerae* and *Escherichia coli*, in Field M, Fordtran JS, Schultz SG (eds): *Secretory Diarrhea*. Bethesda, MD, American Physiological Society, 1980, pp 67–83

94. Scrimshaw NS, Taylor CE, Gordon JE: Interactions of nutrition and infection. World Health Organization Monograph Series no. 57. Geneva World Health Organization, 1968

95. Rowland MG, Cole TJ, Whitehead RG: A quantitative study into the role of infection in determining nutritional status in Gambian village children. *Brit J Nutr* 37:441–450, 1977

96. Hoyle B, Yunus M, Chen LC: Breast feeding and food intake among children with acute diarrheal disease. *Am J Clin Nutr* 33:2365–2367, 1980

97. Molla AM, Molla A, Sarker SA, Rahaman MM: Food intake during and after recovery from diarrhea in children, in Chen LC, Scrimshaw S (eds): *Diarrhea and Malnutrition*. New York, Plenum Press, 1983, pp 113–123

98. Molla AM, Molla A, Khatun M: Does oral rehydration therapy alter food consumption and absorption of nutrients in children with cholera. *J Trop Med Hyg* 89:113–117, 1986

99. Martorell R, Yarbrough C, Yarbrough S, Klein RE: The impact of ordinary illness on the dietary intakes of malnourished children. *Am J Clin Nutr* 33:345–357, 1980

100. Hirschhorn N, Molla A: Reversible jejunal disaccharidase deficiency in cholera and other acute diarrheal diseases. *Johns Hopkins Med J* 125:291–293, 1969

101. Mahalanabis D, Watten R, Wallace CK: Clinical aspects and management of pediatric cholera, in: Barua D, Burrows W (eds): *Cholera*. Philadelphia, WB Saunders, 1974, pp 223–227

102. Molla AM: Cholera, in: Rakel ED (ed): *Conn's Current Therapy*, Philadelphia, WB Saunders, 1989, pp. 48–51

12

Laboratory Diagnosis

Sudhir Chandra Pal

1. INTRODUCTION

Laboratory diagnosis of acute untreated cholera is fairly simple and straight forward as large number of cholera vibrios are present in the stools of such cases. The number of vibrios may vary from about 10^6 to 10^9 per ml of fecal material with relatively fewer organisms of the normal intestinal flora.[1-3] Therefore, it may be possible for a trained laboratory worker to isolate and identify the pathogen, using inexpensive media and reagents in a minimally equipped laboratory.

With the wide clinical spectrum of El Tor cholera, it is almost impossible to establish the diagnosis without the help of a laboratory and a prompt diagnosis is extremely important for instituting early control measures in the face of an epidemic. Laboratory examination of each and every case, however, may not be required once the cause of the epidemic has been established.

2. COLLECTION OF SPECIMENS

The key to the success in laboratory diagnosis is the proper collection of the sample. Improperly collected material is more likely to yield erroneous results in the laboratory; therefore, the practical importance of sample collection cannot be overemphasized. The stool samples should be collected as early as possible following the onset of clinical symptoms and prior to administration of any antimicrobial drugs. Samples should never be collected directly from the bedpans, as the pan may be contaminated by previous use and thus give false-positive results. On the other hand, the presence of disinfectants in the pan might result in a false-negative report.

Cholera, edited by Dhiman Barua and William B. Greenough III. Plenum Medical Book Company, New York, 1992.

2.1. Stool

A specimen of liquid stool is best collected by introducing a No. 26 or 28 soft rubber catheter lubricated with sterile paraffin into the rectum for a distance of about 8 to 10 cm and allowing the stool to flow into a sterile screwcapped bottle or test tube. Approximately 2 to 3 ml of stool may be sufficient for laboratory examination.

2.2. Rectal Swab

A rectal swab is often used where a catheter specimen cannot be obtained. The swab should be wrapped well with good-quality absorbent cotton wool that will absorb about 0.1 to 0.2 ml of liquid feces. It is important to ensure that the swab is introduced properly for at least 2 to 4 cm beyond the anus and that the fecal matter is collected. Contamination from the perinium should be avoided as far as possible. Rectal swabs are good for very-young babies and for collecting specimens from convalescents who no longer have any watery diarrhea. For ease of introduction, the swab may be moistened with the transport medium and the excess fluid removed by pressing the swab against the side of the tube. A rectal swab has been found to be more convenient in the field situation though possibly less rewarding than a catheter specimen.

2.3. Labeling

All specimens should be labeled properly with the name and age of the patient and the date and time of collection of the samples. A properly filled proforma giving the relevant epidemiological informations and clinical history of the patient should be sent along with the specimens.

3. TRANSPORTATION OF THE SPECIMENS

If the specimens of stool cannot be processed within 2h or are required to be transported to a distant laboratory, they have to be preserved at about 4°C or placed in holding medium and kept at room temperature. They should never be kept under direct sun. A number of holding or transport media have been found to be most useful for the purpose.

3.1. Venkatraman–Ramakrishnan Medium

Venkatraman and Ramakrishnan's[4] buffered sea-salt (V–R medium) is a simple and inexpensive medium and has been extensively used in the Indian subcontinent. The medium can be prepared by dissolving 12.405 g boric acid (H_3BO_3) and 14.902 g potassium chloride (KCl) in 800 ml of hot distilled water. The solution is cooled and then made up to 1 liter. Two hundred fifty ml of this stock solution is mixed with 133.5 ml of 0.20 M NaOH and then made up to 1 liter to which 20 g of sea salt or common salt is added. The pH should be adjusted to 9.2. The solution is filtered through paper and distributed in 10-ml volumes in 1-oz screwcapped fairly wide mouth vials and then autoclaved.

About 1 to 2 ml of feces should be inoculated in 10 ml of V–R medium which may be kept at the room temperature. *V. cholerae* has been found to survive from 6 weeks to 6 months[5] in this medium even at room temperature. A simple modification of the V–R medium by using 20 g of crude sea salt and 5 g peptone in 1 liter of distilled water (pH 8.6) has been found to be useful.[6] V–R fluid in its original or modified form is not much used at present.

3.2. Cary–Blair Medium

Cary and Blair[7] developed a semisolid medium for the preservation of specimens for the isolation of Salmonella, Shigella, *E. coli,* and Pasteurella. This medium has also been found to be useful for isolation of *V. cholerae* and provides comparable results with that of V–R medium.[6,8] The medium contains: sodium thioglycolate, 1.5 g; dibasic sodium phosphate, 1.1. g; sodium chloride, 5.0 g; agar–agar, 5.0 g; and distilled water, 991.0 ml. The medium can be prepared by dissolving the constituents in a flask by heating and then adding 9 ml of 1.0% $CaCl_2$ solution when the solution is cooled to about 50°C. The pH is adjusted to 8.4. The medium should be dispensed in 7.5-ml volumes in 9-ml screwcapped vials, leaving a small air space, and sterilized by steaming for 15 min. The main advantage of the medium is that it can be used for other intestinal pathogens and transported easily due to its semisolid consistency. The Cary–Blair medium has been extensively used by various workers with satisfactory results.[9–11]

3.3. Alkaline Peptone Water

Alkaline peptone water (APW) is by far the simplest and most extensively used medium for holding as well as for enrichment. It can be prepared easily by dissolving 10.0 g peptone and 10.0 g of sodium chloride in 1 liter of distilled water. The pH is adjusted to 8.4. The medium is dispensed in 8- to 10-ml amounts either in screwcapped vials or in test tubes and autoclaved.

The rectal swab or a small amount of fecal matter may be inoculated into the medium and transported to the laboratory. The only disadvantage of the medium is that when the specimen is kept for a long period at ambient temperature other organisms such as *Pseudomonas* and non-01 *V. cholerae* may overgrow the *V. cholerae* 01. The medium was extensively used by the Cholera Research Centre, Calcutta in their different field studies.[12–15]

3.4. Monsur's Transport Medium

A fluid medium developed by Monsur[16] has been found to be suitable for both holding and enrichment for *V. cholerae*. It contains 1.0% each of trypticase and sodium chloride with pH adjusted to 8.4 to 9.2. About 25 ml of the medium is dispensed in 2-oz screwcapped vials and autoclaved. Potassium tellurite is added to the medium to a concentration of 1 in 200,000 or 1 in 100,000 just before inoculation. The main disadvantages of the medium are wide variations in the quality of potassium tellurite available in market and the solution needs to be freshly prepared before use. Monsur's medium has been used extensively in Bangladesh.[17–19]

3.5. Blotting Paper Strip

A strip of filter paper soaked in liquid stool was successfully used for transporting stool for laboratory diagnosis for typhoid fever and shigellosis.[20,21] It was found that thick blotting paper strips are better than filter paper for *V. cholerae* as they retain moisture for a long period when kept in sealed plastic bags. *V. cholerae* was found to survive up to 5 weeks in such strips.[22] The efficacy of the blotting paper strips method was compared with Cary–Blair transport medium for transportation of cholera stools. A significantly higher isolation rate was observed from the specimens transported in blotting paper strips (93.7 percent) than that in Cary–Blair medium (83.4 percent), even after 14 days of collection.[23]

3.6. International Postal Regulations

When the specimens are required to be sent by mail, these should be packed in double containers: the inner container must be leakproof, and the outer container must protect against breakage.

4. ISOLATION/DETECTION OF *V. CHOLERAE* FROM STOOL

4.1. Rapid Laboratory Diagnosis

Prompt laboratory diagnosis of cholera is often advantageous not only for early isolation of the patient and initiation of control measures but also for conducting certain clinical and epidemiological studies. A number of such rapid laboratory diagnostic methods have been used.

4.1.1. Bandi's[24] Agglutination Method

Cholera stool is incubated in 5 ml of alkaline peptone water containing adequate amount of specific cholera antiserum. In positive cases, clumps of *V. cholerae* could be seen after 2–7 h at the bottom and along the side of the tubes. Satisfactory results were also obtained by Cossery[25] by keeping the final dilution of the agglutinating serum at 1 : 100. However, 38% more positive results were obtained by cultural method than Bandi's method.[26]

A modification of Bandi's method has been described[27] where a biphasic medium was used for inoculation of diluted cholera stool and a drop of antiserum was added after 2–4 h of incubation. Agglutinated particles were seen after 1 h with the help of a hand lens. As all the above methods based on agglutination require the supply of large amount of anticholera serum, none of them gained popularity among the laboratory workers.

4.1.2. Dark-Field Microscopy[28]

This consists of detection by dark-field or phase contrast microscopy of characteristic motility (shooting stars) of *V. cholerae* in liquid stools that can be inhibited by addition of specific antiserum. This diagnosis can be made with 2–5 min in about 50% of the cases.[29] The antisera used for this purpose should not contain any antibacterial preservative but these are not readily available from commercial sources. Again, the presence of about 10^5 vibrios per ml of stool may be needed for detection by this method.

4.1.3. Fluorescent-Tagged Antibody (F.A.) Technique

This technique that demonstrates *V. cholerae* 01 in artificially contaminated stool[30] as well as in the feces of acute cases of cholera after initial enrichment in alkaline peptone water[31] was found to be useful for early diagnosis of cholera. Applying the same principle on direct smears prepared from stool of cholera patients, Sack and Barua[32] found about 90% correlation with cultural method and that the results could be available within 2 h. However, the F.A. technique did not gain popularity among the laboratory workers as it needs costly apparatus, good quality conjugated sera, and special skill for operation, besides requiring the presence of large number of organisms (10^6 to 10^7 per ml) for the success of the technique.[33]

4.1.4. Oblique Light Illumination Technique

Colonies of *V. cholerae* can be located on a noninhibitory nutrient agar (pH 8.6) plate with the help of a stereomicroscope as described elsewhere.[31,34] This method was modified and applied for rapid diagnosis by Barua[35] as the growth on predried agar plate (after 4 to 5 h incubation at 37°C) is sufficient for the colonies of *V. cholerae* to be spotted by this technique. It consisted of directing a beam of light at an angle of 30–40° from a 100-watt microscope lamp from a distance of 4 to 6 in onto a concave mirror placed on the table in front of the stereoscopic microscope used for examining the plates. With this technique, it is possible to scan the plates using 10× or 20× magnification and detect typical flat, gray, homogenous, translucent colonies or confluent growth of *V. cholerae*. The growth can then be used for slide agglutination with specific antisera for confirmation.

4.1.5. Coagglutination Technique

Early detection by coagglutination of *V. cholerae* in stools has also been described.[36] The reagent is prepared by sensitizing a 10% suspension of *Staphylococcus aureaus,* Cowan 1 strain with specific *V. cholerae* 01 antisera. One drop of the reagent is mixed with an equal volume of liquid stool on a slide with rings and the clumping of the organisms can be observed within 2 min. A clearer positive result has been claimed to be obtained using growth after 4 h of enrichment in peptone water. The results correlated favorably (93.6 %) with that of cultural method. While a complete correlation between coagglutination test and the conventional methods for identification of growth from culture plates has recently been reported[37] several other workers have found it difficult to get reproducible results with different antisera for sensitizing *S. aureus.*

4.2. Cultural Methods

4.2.1. Enrichment for *V. cholerae*

The tolerance of *V. cholerae* to higher pH 9.2 to 9.4 and its highly aerophilic nature have been utilized by the laboratory workers to give selective growth advantage to the vibrios over other intestinal bacteria. This technique of selective enrichment of *V. cholerae* has been found to be very useful for laboratory diagnosis of cholera especially when the number of organisms in the stool was low. There is hardly any need for enrichment of stool specimens collected from acute untreated cholera patients. Direct plating on selective media often yielded better results than enrichment followed by plating in these cases as there is a chance of over growth by non-01 *V. cholerae* or *Pseudomonas species*. However, as instances of growth only after enrichment are also known, both direct streaking and enrichment should be routinely performed in a diagnostic laboratory.[38,39] The following media for enrichment are commonly used.

4.2.1.1. Alkaline Peptone Water (APW)

This medium has been most widely used for the purpose of enrichment for *V. cholerae*. The medium is simple, inexpensive, and can be prepared in any laboratory with minimum facilities. *V. cholerae* can multiply in a fairly wide range of pH varying from 6.0 to 9.2. Generally, the media with pH of 8.4 to 8.6 are preferred but a pH up to 9.2 can be used to achieve better inhibition of other intestinal organisms.

One or several loopfuls of stool from a case of cholera may be inoculated in 8 to 10 ml of APW and incubated at 37°C for 6 to 8 h. As highly aerophilic vibrios tend to grow on the surface of the liquid medium, sometimes in the form of a thin film, it is advisable to use the growth from the surface for plating on a solid medium. Incubation in APW for more than 8 h may result in overgrowth by other organisms. Alkaline peptone water with potassium tellurite (1 : 200,000) has been found to yield better isolation than APW, probably by inhibiting *Pseudomonas*.[40]

4.2.1.2. Monsur's[16] Trypticase–Tellurite Tourocholate Broth (TTB)

This has also been used extensively by several workers for transportation of specimen as well as for enrichment of *V. cholerae*. This medium, though more complex than APW in composition, may give better isolation due to inhibition of *Pseudomonas*. However, alkaline peptone water with tellurite (PWT) has been found to be as good as TTB.[40]

4.2.2. Plating Media for the Isolation of *V. cholerae*

Media such as MacConkey, DCA, SS Agar, and Bismuth Sulphite Agar, which are routinely used for isolation of the enteric pathogens, are not suitable for isolation of *V. cholerae*. Therefore, a large number of selective media have been developed from time-to-time to obtain better isolation of *V. cholerae*. Earlier, these media have been reviewed at length.[41−43] Some of these media were too complex to be prepared in the routine laboratory and did not find favor among the laboratory workers. Dieudonne's blood alkali agar and the Aronson's medium were used by many laboratories with varying degrees of success but were given up ultimately in favor of some of the simplified and more efficient media in current use.

The solid media that are being extensively used can be broadly classified into two groups: (1) poorly selective and nonselective; (2) selective or selective and differentiating media.

4.2.2.1. Poorly Selective and Nonselective Media

4.2.2.1a. Bile-Salt Agar (BSA). This is a nutrient agar containing 0.5% sodium taurocholate or sodium desoxycholate with pH adjusted to about 8.2, and has been extensively used in India for the last several decades.[41] It is a simple, poorly selective medium that can be prepared in any laboratory with rudimentary facilities.

On a freshly prepared medium the colonies look very clear, distinctly translucent with a clear, round margin and a flat top which can be easily distinguished from the opaque grayish white colonies with elevated center of *E. coli* and other enteric bacteria. Even without much experience, it is difficult to miss these colonies, which are so transparent that they take the color of the medium. The bile-salts not only inhibit the growth of certain aerobic gram-positive organisms present in stool but also add to the translucency of the colonies. Oblique light illumination is often helpful in spotting the colonies when they are few in number.[44] The preliminary enrichment in alkaline peptone water followed by plating in BSA are extensively used by Indian workers.

4.2.2.1b. Meat Extract Agar (MEA). This agar consists of 0.3% beef extract, 1% peptone, 0.5% NaCl, 1.5 to 2% agar, has been successfully used for the laboratory diagnosis of acute cases of cholera.[31] On a freshly prepared medium, the colonies of V. *cholerae* appear as large, translucent, grayish, and can easily be differentiated from the opaque colonies of other enteric bacteria with the naked eye or by using the oblique light illumination technique.

4.2.2.2. Selective Media

4.2.2.2a. Thiosulphate Citrate Bile Salt Agar (TCBS). This culture medium was developed by Kobayashi *et al.*,[45] has been most extensively used for the laboratory diagnosis of cholera cases and carriers as well as for isolation from environmental specimens.[2,13,73,96,99] The medium has been made commercially available in dehydrated form by Eiken, Difco, BBL and Oxoid with the following composition per liter: yeast extract, 5 g; peptone, 10 g; sodium citrate, 10 g; sodium thiosulfate, 10 g; oxgall, 5 g; sodium cholate, 3 g; saccharose, 20 g; sodium chloride, 10 g; ferric citrate, 1 g; bromothymol blue, 0.04 g; thymol blue, 0.04 g; Agar, 15 g; pH, 8.6.

The sucrose-fermenting colonies of V. *cholerae* can be detected easily; they appear as large, yellow, smooth and round against the bluish-green background of the medium, whereas the colonies of sucrose nonfermenting organisms like V. *parahaemolyticus* appear bluish in color. It is a highly selective medium and the growth of most of the enteric bacteria, except occasionally Proteus and fecal streptococcus, is inhibited. However, the medium prepared in the laboratory with the ingredients available from local sources often do not give as satisfactory results as those available from commercial sources. The major constraint for the laboratories in developing countries where the actual problem of cholera exists, is the difficulty of importing the dehydrated media from abroad. The other difficulty is the stickiness of colonies, which makes it unsuitable for direct slide agglutination. The colonies need to be subcultured on a nonselective media for the purpose; Therefore, the result can be obtained only on the following day. The quality of medium may vary from brand to brand and also between different batches of the same brand.

4.2.2.2b. Tellurite Taurocholate Gelatin Agar (TTGA). This medium developed by Monsur[16] is another highly selective medium used extensively by the cholera workers in Bangladesh. The composition of the medium is: trypticase, 10 g; sodium chloride, 10 g; sodium taurocholate, 5 g; sodium carbonate, 1 g; gelatin (Difco), 30 g; agar, 15 g in 1 liter of distilled water; pH adjusted to 8.5.

The medium is sterilized by autoclave, after which potassium tellurite is added to a final concentration of 1 in 200,000 to 1 in 100,000. The plates should be used within 5 days. After overnight incubation colonies appear as small and opaque with a zone of cloudiness around them. After 48 h incubation colonies become larger (3 to 4 mm) with typical black centers and well-defined haloes. The medium is highly inhibitory to enteric bacteria except *Proteus*.

The efficacy of the medium primarily depends on the quality of tellurite and gelatin available locally as well as the experience of the laboratory workers in preparing the media and identifying the colonies properly. It is not commercially available.

4.2.2.2c. Vibrio Agar. This medium, modified by Tamura *et al.*,[46] was used to a limited extent by the Cholera Research Centre, Calcutta. The medium provided better isolation than bile-salt agar but was less selective than TCBS. Vibrio colonies are bluish gray, translucent and sticky and are larger than the sucrose-fermenting colonies of *Proteus* and *Aeromonas*. However, the medium has not been used much outside Japan.

4.2.2.2d. *Vibrio parahaemolyticus* Agar (V.P. Agar). This is a modified TCBS agar medium developed by De *et al.*[47] with locally available ingredients primarily for the isolation of *V. parahaemolyticus* but was also found suitable for *V. cholerae*. The composition of the medium is as follows: yeast extract, 5 g; peptone, 10 g; sodium taurocholate, 5 g; sodium thiosulfate, 10 g; sodium chloride, 20 g; sodium lauryl sulfate, 0.2 g; sodium citrate, 10 g; sucrose, 20 g; bromothymol blue, 0.04 g; thymol blue, 0.04 g; agar, 20 g; and distilled water, 1 liter; pH is adjusted to 8.5.

V. cholerae colonies were more or less similar to those seen in TCBS. However, the colonies could be readily emulsified for the slide agglutination test. Samples of stool from 1632 patients and 3636 of the family contacts were tested both in TCBS and V.P. agar. V.P. agar was found to be slightly less selective than TCBS for the isolation of *V. cholerae* but the rate of isolation of *V. parahaemolyticus* was identical. The V.P. agar, being less expensive and easy to prepare, is currently in use in a number of laboratories in India.

In spite of the development of more efficient selective media during the last two decades, most of the laboratories in developing countries are continuing to use nonselective media, which can be prepared with the locally available ingredients. Imported dehydrated medium like TCBS or potassium tellurite of dependable quality for the preparation of TTGA is still beyond the reach of most of these laboratories.

4.2.2.2e. Polymixin Mannose Tellurite Agar. A new selective and differential medium for differentiation of *V. cholerae* 01 from the *V. cholerae* non 01 has been developed.[107] This differentiation is based on mannose fermentation. The colonies of *V. cholerae* 01 on this medium are agglutinated with 01 antiserum much more easily than those on thiosulphate–citrate bile salt sucrose (TCBS) agar. The composition of the medium in gms/liter is as follows: Lab. lamco, 5 g; polypeptone (BBL), 10 g; sodium chloride, 10 g; mannose, 20 g; sodium dodecylsulphate, 0.2 g; polymixin B, 180,000 U; cresol red, 0.04 g; bromothymol blue, 0.04 g; agar, 15 g; and distilled water, 1 liter. The pH is adjusted to 8.4.

5. IDENTIFICATION AND CHARACTERIZATION OF *V. CHOLERAE* 01

5.1. Species Identification

The flow chart of identification and characterization of *V. cholerae* is shown in Fig. 1. Typical colonies of *V. cholerae*, preferably from a nonselective medium, can be tested for agglutination with *V. cholerae* 01 antiserum. If positive, a provisional diagnosis of *V. cholerae* 01 can be made. This provisional identification should be sufficient for all practical purposes and can be made in a peripheral laboratory with limited facilities.[35]

For final identification a part of the agglutinable colony or a colony from a highly selective medium like TCBS or others may be transferred to nutrient agar slant and Kligler iron agar (KIA) and incubated overnight at 37°C. If there is only acid production and no gas or H_2S in KIA, i.e., K/A reaction, the identity can be confirmed by slide agglutination tests with polyvalent 01 and type-specific Inaba and Ogawa antisera. A clear-cut slide agglutination within 30 sec, with an adequate saline control will clinch the final diagnosis.

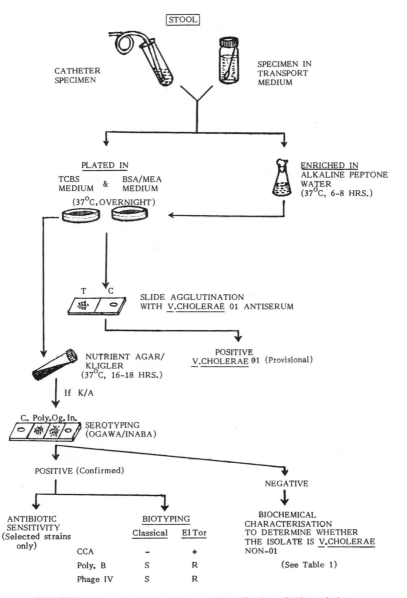

FIGURE 1. Flow chart for isolation and identification of *Vibrio cholerae*

The importance of good quality agglutinating antisera in the laboratory diagnosis of *V. cholerae* 01 cannot be overemphasized. These antisera should preferably be obtained from a reputed commercial firm or production unit and should be tested at frequent intervals with known positive and negative strains in the laboratory. Diagnostic anticholera sera can also be prepared in any well-equipped laboratory but should be left to the reference laboratory in a country.

In case of doubtful or nonagglutination with *V. cholerae* 01 antiserum, it is imperative

TABLE 1
Differentiation of *V. cholerae* from Related Organisms

Tests	*Vibrio cholerae* (01 & Non-01)	*Aeromonas hydrophila*[a]	*Plesiomonas shigelloides*	*Enterobacteriaceae*[a]
Oxidase	+	+	+	−
String	+	−+	−	−
Mannitol fermentation	+	+	−	+−
Sucrose fermentation	+	+	−	+−
Lysine decarboxylase	+	−	+	+−
Arginine dihydrolase	−	+	+	+
Ornithine decarboxylase	+	−	+	+−

[a]−+ or +− indicates variable results.

to perform some of the tests mentioned in Table 1 to confirm whether the isolate is *V. cholerae* non-01 and differentiate it from the related organisms.

5.2. Biotyping of *V. cholerae* 01

V. cholerae 01 can be differentiated into classical and El Tor biotypes on the basis of certain biological tests, namely, direct hemagglutination tests with chicken or sheep RBC, polymycin B sensitivity, and sensitivity to classical *V. cholerae* phage Group IV. However, biotyping may not be required routinely as it is not necessary for treatment or for institution of control measures. Again, El Tor biotype has a worldwide distribution in comparison to classical strains, which are encountered only in Bangladesh at the moment. Therefore, it may be of interest to biotype only some of the selected isolates for the purpose of surveillance.

5.2.1. Direct Hemagglutination Test

Finkelstein and Mukherjee[48] and Barua and Mukherjee[49] independently observed that the hemagglutinative property of El Tor vibrios towards chicken and sheep RBC is of great practical value for its differentiation from classical *V. cholerae*. Erythrocytes from other species such as goat and human cells were also found to be satisfactory[50] but guinea pig red cells were found to be unsuitable.[51] The test is performed on a clean glass slide which is divided into several columns with a glass-marking pencil for different strains to be tested. A 3-mm loopful of 2.5% suspension of thrice-washed red cells is placed in each column. A small portion of the growth from an agar or KIA slant (not from a fluid medium) is added to the red cells with a needle or loop and mixed well. Clumping of the red cells occurs within 30–60 sec in positive cases. Known positive and negative strains should be used as controls for each new suspension of red cells. Strains of classical *V. cholerae* 01 which has undergone repeated passage in the laboratory may give false positive results.[50,52] Rizvi *et al.*[53] also had an exceptional experience of isolating eight hemagglutinating strains of classical *V. cholerae* 01 from the routine isolates in Dhaka. However, other workers[47,54,55] did not encounter even a single aberrant strain.

The direct hemagglutination test has been extensively used by several workers during the last decade and has been found to be very reliable and usually runs parallel with polymyxin B sensitivity and susceptibility of *V. cholerae* phage group IV tests. Some irregular results, however, are being noted particularly among the environmental isolates.

5.2.2. Polymyxin B Sensitivity Test

Gan and Tjia[56] were the first to report that classical *V. cholerae* can be differentiated from the El Tor biotype by its sensitivity to 50 μg disc of polymyxin B. This has been further confirmed as a reliable test by several cholera workers. A 50-unit sensitivity disc of polymyxin B is placed on a bacterial lawn prepared on nutrient agar (NA), meat extract agar (MEA), or Muellar Hinton agar plates (pH 7.6) from a 2- to 4-h-old growth in nutrient broth. Several strains can be tested on the same plate by making separate lawns on zones marked on the back of the plate. Known strains of classical and El Tor biotypes should always be included as controls. The discs should be gently pressed onto the medium and the plates kept at 4°C for about 1 h before incubating overnight. A clear zone of inhibition around the disc suggests sensitivity of classical *V. cholerae* 01 whereas El Tor vibrios are resistant to this concentration.

A plate method where 15 μg/ml of polymyxin B is added to nutrient agar medium as an alternative to the disc method has also been developed.[57] Thirty to forty strains can be tested on each plate by spotting a 2- to 4-h-old nutrient broth culture on marked zones along with known sensitive and resistant strains as controls. It was observed that the pH of the nutrient agar should be kept between 7.0 and 7.6.[58] It was suggested that highly selective media such as TCBS and TTGA should not be used for this purpose as the test in these media often shows false zones of inhibition.[39] The authors also felt that this test may have a lasting differential value as there is evidence that the genetic control for the resistance property is located in the chromosome. However, polymyxin B–sensitive variants among the colonies in primary culture of El Tor vibrios were reported.[59,60]

5.2.3. Susceptibility to Cholera-Phage Group IV

Mukherjee[61] observed that the strains of classical *V. cholerae* 01 are uniformly susceptible to classical cholera-phage group IV whereas the strains of El Tor vibrios are resistant to it and recommended that the test be used as a valuable tool for differentiation between El Tor and classical *V. cholerae* 01. Classical cholera-phage group IV at its routine test dilution (RTD) should be applied with a 2-mm loop on a bacterial lawn on nutrient agar plate prepared with a 2-h growth of the test strain in nutrient broth. The results may be read after overnight incubation at 37°C.

During the last two decades the cholera-phage group IV sensitivity test has been used extensively at the WHO Collaborating Centre for Reference and Research on Vibrios in Calcutta for testing large numbers of *V. cholerae* 01 strain, received from far and wide, and has been found to be the most useful test for characterization of El Tor strains of *V. cholerae* 01, although a few phage IV–resistant strains of classical *V. cholerae* 01 have been reported.[62,63]

As it may not be possible for the small laboratories with limited facilities to maintain the phage in a pure state and to make the correct dilution, the central laboratory in the country should take the responsibility for performing the differentiation tests, including phage susceptibility.

5.2.4. Hemolysis Test

Originally, the El Tor vibrios were differentiated from the classical *V. cholerae* by their ability to produce heat-labile hemolysin and the production of acetylmethylcarbinol in Voges–Proskauer reaction. At the beginning of the Seventh pandemic, *V. cholerae* biotype El Tor, invading Hong Kong and the Philippines in 1961, were also found to be hemolytic.[48,61,64] However, the number of such hemolytic strains in the Philippines gradually decreased in subsequent years to about 1% but about 85% of these strains were found to produce hemolysin when grown in heart infusion broth with 1% glycerol.[58] El Tor strains reached Delhi in 1965, during the first year 29.1% and in the second year 1.5% of the strains were hemolytic, but during the subsequent years all the strains were found to be non-hemolytic by the conventional test.[5] The El Tor strains isolated currently in different countries are mostly nonhemolytic and, therefore, the hemolysis test is no longer useful for differentiation between El Tor and classical cholera vibrios. It is useful, however, for characterization of strains from environmental sources like water in cholerafree areas and from cases in areas like Louisiana, USA, and Queensland, Australia, which appear to be old endemic areas of El Tor infection.

The more sensitive test[58] can be performed by mixing 0.5 ml of a 24-h culture in heart infusion broth (HIB) or in HIB with 1% glycerol grown at 37°C in a tube containing 10 ml of medium with 0.5 ml of 1% suspension of thrice-washed sheep RBC. The mixture is mixed well and incubated for 2 h at 37°C and then held overnight at 4°C. The tubes are read without shaking for the presence of hemolysis. Known positive and negative strains should always be included as controls.

6. SEROLOGICAL TESTS FOR RETROSPECTIVE DIAGNOSIS OF CHOLERA

Since the very early days, attempts have been made to develop serological tests for retrospective diagnosis of cholera. Some of the techniques developed earlier were reviewed by Pollitzer and Burrows.[65] The following tests, however, have been used during the recent years.

6.1. Agglutination Test

Clinical serology has expanded considerably since Goodner *et al.*[66] reaffirmed and demonstrated the usefulness and superiority of live vibrio suspensions as antigens in the agglutination test. They also showed that a complete correlation exists between the serological and bacteriological diagnosis, and that the serotype of infection cannot be inferred from such serological examination. Barua and Sack[67] also used live antigen prepared from a log phase culture of a *V. cholerae* Inaba strain grown in peptone water for 3 h. The growing organism was agglutinated rapidly by antiserum and a preliminary reading of the results could be made after 1 h of incubation at 37°C. However, overnight refrigeration facilitated the reading of the results. The clumps of agglutinated bacteria were fine and granular in appearance, typical of the O-type agglutination. H-agglutinogen in *V. cholerae* appears to be a very weak antigen. It was found necessary to give 20 or 25 injections of large doses of 0.01% merthiolated antigen to rabbits to produce H-antisera and crude flageller preparation was more appropriate for the production of H-antiserum.[68] Demonstration of the presence of anti-H antibody in serum is not always possible. This is because *V. cholerae* possesses only a single flagellum, which is covered by a sheath, thereby making access to the H-antigenic sites rather difficult. Removal of the sheath component may be achieved by aging of the cultures[69] or by the treatment with phenol, formalin,[70] or a detergent.[71]

Bacterial agglutination tests carried out in test tubes have been adopted for a micro-technique requiring 0.025 ml of serum or plasma,[72] the test being performed in U-well microtiter plates. They used pretested suitable strains as antigen grown in broth, which was adjusted for a transmission of 74 to 80% at a wavelength of 515 nm in a Coleman Junior spectrophotometer. The agglutination test by the microtechnique with certain modifications was used by others.[73] These studies would indicate that there is, as yet, no uniformity in the method of preparing the antigen although they all used live antigen for the O-agglutination test and the strain used as antigen was selected carefully in many cases. It is generally believed that heat-killed antigen gives 2 to 4 times lower titers than those of live antigen.

6.2. Vibriocidal Test

Finkelstein[74] developed a complement-dependent vibriocidal test of great sensitivity. He diluted his sera in 10-fold serial dilutions in 1 : 20 lyophilized guinea pig complement reconstituted in phosphate buffer in 0.5 ml volumes; to each tube were added equal volumes of the vibrio suspension containing 2 to 4 × 10^3 viable cells/ml. The tubes were maintained in an ice-water bath during the above operations, after which they were incubated at 37°C for 1 h, placed once again in the ice bath and plated by the technique of Miles *et al.*[75] for a viable count. After overnight incubation, the colony counts were compared with those in the controls. The titer was determined as the dilution of the serum causing 50% inhibition of the bacterial growth.

McIntyre and Feeley[76] titrated the vibriocidal antibody by mixing two-fold serial dilutions of sera in 0.5-ml amounts, 0.25 ml of 1.5 nonvibriocidal guinea pig complement and 0.25 ml of one opacity unit suspension of a suitable strain of *V. cholerae*. After incubation at 37°C for 1 h, 3 ml of brain–heart infusion broth were added to each tube to support the growth of the surviving vibrios. The tubes were incubated until the tube containing the complement, saline, and organism reached an opacity density of 0.15 at 580 mμ. By comparing it with the turbidity of the complement control tube by the naked eye, the turbidity in the tubes with test-sera dilutions could be graded from 0 to +4. The titer was determined as the highest dilution of the serum showing a +2 turbidity (i.e., approximately 50% killing of the culture).

The technique of Finkelstein[74] was later used by various investigators in cholera serology in its original or modified form.[67,77,78] A microtechnique using the Microtiter kits (Cooke Engineering Co., Alexandria, VA, USA) and nondisposable plastic microtiter plates with "U" cups was also developed.[79] The plates were prepared with 0.025 ml of serial two-fold saline dilutions (1 : 10 to 1 : 1280) of the test sera or plasma. The latter could be obtained as supernatant after collecting 0.025 or 0.05 ml of finger-tip blood with a calibrated capillary pipette and adding the blood to 0.475 or 0.45 ml of sterile saline giving 1 : 20 or 1 : 10 dilutions of the whole blood. For technical details the interested worker is referred to the original paper.

In spite of the fact that the microtiter-based technique is less sensitive than the tube dilution (plate count) technique, the test has been widely used by many laboratories because of its obvious advantages in handling of large numbers of samples.[80–82]

A close and highly significant agreement was found between the bacterial agglutination and vibriocidal tests[67,77,78,83] and the vibriocidal titer was found to be uniformly higher than the corresponding agglutinin titer.

6.3. Indirect Bacterial Hemagglutination Test

An indirect hemagglutination (IHA) test was developed by Barua and Sack,[67] who incubated equal volumes (0.5 ml) of a 5% sensitized sheep red cell suspension and serial two-fold dilutions of serum in round-bottomed test tubes at 37°C for 1 h. Sheep red cells were previously sensitized by incubation for 2 h at 37°C with the supernatant of a thick *V. cholerae* suspension (heated at 100°C for 1½ h). Following incubation, the serum-sensitized red cell mixture was refrigerated overnight and results were recorded the next day by observing the hemagglutination patterns. However, the test was found to be less sensitive than the live bacterial agglutination test.

In another indirect hemagglutination technique[78] human group O erythrocytes were sensitized with *V. cholerae* lipopolysaccharide. For this, 200 μg of *V. cholerae* 569B Inaba LPS was used to sensitize each ml of a 2% erythrocyte suspension. Indirect hemagglutination test was carried out in microtiter plates using serially double-diluted serum. Anti-LPS IHA titers showed highly significant correlation ($P < 0.001$) to both vibrio agglutination and vibriocidal titers.

6.4. Enzyme-Linked Immunosorbent Assay

In recent years, enzyme-linked immunosorbent assay (ELISA)[84] has been widely used in the serology of cholera.[78,80,81,85–87] The technique offers several advantages as it is quite sensitive and can be adopted to disposable microtitration plates (Micro-ELISA). Further, it is possible to determine immunoglobulin class-specific serum antibody titers to defined *V. cholerae* antigens.

Holmgren and Svennerholm[85] used the method to determine class-specific serum antibody titers to *V. cholerae* endotoxin (LPS) and exotoxin (enterotoxin). They used 1 ml of antigen solutions (100 μg/ml for LPS or 10 μg/ml for cholera toxin) made in phosphate-buffered saline (PBS) to coat disposable polystyrene tubes (Nunc, Denmark) by mere incubation at 37°C. After removal of nonattached antigen by washing, the tubes were incubated with 1 ml of antiserum dilutions at room temperature. Non–antigen bound material was washed off and anti-immunoglobulin–enzyme conjugate (1 ml) at an appropriate dilution was then allowed to react with antigen-bound antibodies. After washing of the tubes, 1 ml of *p*-nitrophenyl-phosphate (1 mg/ml) was added as substrate. The yellow color that developed was registered spectrophotometrically at 400 nm after arresting the reaction by 1 N NaOH. Majumdar *et al.*[78] used the micro-ELISA technique to determine class-specific anti-LPS and anti-cholera toxin (CT) titers in the sera of convalescent cholera patients. Disposable Micro-ELISA plates (Dynatech Laboratories Inc., Alexandria, VA) were sensitized by the addition of 20 μg of LPS or 2 μg of CT in 100 μl of a coating buffer in each well, followed by overnight incubation at 4°C. Wells were washed with PBS containing 0.05% Tween-20.

Next, the wells were filled with 100 μl of test serum serially double diluted with PBS-Tween containing 1% fetal calf serum, the initial dilution being 1 : 25. Plates were incubated for 1 h, washed, and an appropriate dilution of enzyme-labeled anti-serum IgM/IgG or IgA was added. After further incubation for 1 h, the wells were washed, substrate solution added, and color development was recorded. Titer was expressed as the highest dilution of the test serum giving comparable color as the negative controls.

More recently, test sera were diluted to an appropriate single dilution and assayed in blind fashion by micro-ELISA.[82,87,88] The dilution was so chosen to minimize the non-specific reactivity of the control serum. The optical densities of the diluted test and control sera were measured by an automatic ELISA reader and the results are expressed in terms of increment of O.D. values.[85]

A highly sensitive sandwich enzyme-linked immunosorbent assay using polystyrene beads to detect cholera and other enterotoxins has been developed recently.[108] The sensitivity of this bead-ELISA was found to be quite high with various bacterial toxins such as those of *V. parahaemolyticus, E. coli,* and cholera enterotoxin. In a recent study conducted at Calcutta[109] this bead-ELISA was found to be very sensitive in the detection of cholera enterotoxin in stools of cases from whom no cholera vibrios could be isolated by conventional cultural techniques.

In the determination of the pandemic potentiality of *V. cholerae* 01, one must demonstrate both the presence of the 01 antigen and the production of enterotoxin (CT). A latex agglutination assay kit developed commercially (VET-RPLA kit, Oxoid, USA) has been recently evaluated.[110] The kit was found to be highly appropriate for the rapid detection of CT in situations involving smaller numbers of specimens and compared favorably with that of the ELISA assay technique.

6.5. Toxin Neutralization Tests

Benenson *et al.*[89] developed a test for the detection of toxin-neutralizing antibody in the sera of patients. In this method, a volume of 0.2 ml of serial three-fold dilutions of sera is mixed with an equal volume of cholera toxin diluted to contain a standard dose of 0.05 ml. These mixtures, together with a control mixture of toxin diluted in the same way with saline, are incubated in a 37°C water bath for 30 min and 0.1 ml is injected intradermally in duplicate into shaven skin of a guinea pig. After 18 h the sites of injection are examined for size of induration and 0.12 ml of a 5% solution of pontomine sky blue 6XB in 0.5 N saline per 100 g of body weight is injected intravenously. After about 1 to 1½ h, the intensity of bluing is registered as +1 to +4 and the diameter is recorded in millimeters. The titer of the sera is considered to be the dilution at which the mean diameter was reduced to one-half or less than that of the control sites. A nine-fold rise, which was considered significant was found in 73% of 111 bacteriologically confirmed cholera cases and 2.5% of bacteriologically negative cases.

Pierce *et al.*[90] determined serum antitoxin titers by performing neutralization tests in ligated loops of the small bowel of the rabbit by a modification of the method of Kasai and Burrows.[91] Serial 3-fold dilutions of serum were incubated with a constant amount of crude cholera toxin before injection into the loops. The endpoint was the highest serum dilution showing little or no accumulation of fluid in the loop after 16 h. The titer of antitoxin was determined by comparison of the endpoint with that of an antitoxin standard, arbitrarily valued at 100 units/ml, which was similarly titrated in the same rabbit. Titrations were considered valid only if a control loop injected with saline alone was negative and a control loop injected with cholera toxin alone was positive.

Craig et al.[92] developed a skin test with cholera toxin in man that could be safely used as an indicator of previous immunologic experience with cholera toxin. The correlation between this vascular skin permeability factor assay in rabbits and ELISA was found to be statistically significant ($P < 0.001$).[88] However, ELISA was more sensitive than the toxin neutralization assays in detecting both subclinical and overt cholera infections.[93] Serological tests for serum antibacterial and antitoxin antibodies have been extensively used for studies on the immunology and epidemiology of cholera. A large proportion of children living in endemic areas have detectable vibriocidal titers in their sera which persist throughout life, probably due to repeated exposure (either asymptomatic infection or with mild diarrhea) to V. cholerae.[81] Similarly, measurement of serum antitoxin response may be helpful in assessing the prevalence of infection in the community[87] in the developing countries. In fact, use of serologic tests could detect additional cases of cholera retrospectively[82] and identify asymptomatic ones.[80] However, there are serious limitations of the serological tests for the routine diagnosis of cholera, particularly in the endemic areas.

7. LABORATORY DIAGNOSIS OF CHOLERA CARRIERS

The only known natural reservoir for cholera is man. In an endemic area the cycle of transmission is maintained from person to person through the surrounding environment. Although an infected individual excretes vibrios for only a few days, the high rate of inapparent infection permits this cycle to be maintained.[12,13] During the course of a community study in Calcutta some of the carriers were found to excrete V. cholerae intermittently over long periods.[13] Out of the 127 carriers, 33(26.0%) were found to have excreted vibrios more than once, spread over a period of days, with 6–15 days being the most common. Studies on cholera carriers in Delhi also revealed that the carrier rate among families of hospitalized cholera patients was 4.5%, whereas the rate among persons living in a cholera-affected community was 1.5%. In comparison to observations made in highly endemic areas like Calcutta, no carrier was detected during the inter-epidemic period in Delhi.[94]

Carriers of V. cholerae, including convalescents and contacts in the families or households of such cases, generally excrete 10^2 to 10^5 organisms per gram of formed feces, which occasionally also contain large numbers of commensals.[2] This makes laboratory diagnosis of the carrier state much more difficult than that of the active case. In a community, sometimes the carriers can be traced by analyzing night soil,[95] community latrines,[12,94] or water sources, followed by examination of the users. The success of detection will depend on how quickly the carriers are identified after the initial detection of the index cases or environmental sources.

7.1. Collection of Samples

Freshly voided stool specimens are preferred for detection of carriers. During the cholera-carrier studies conducted in Calcutta, small earthenware containers were given to each household for collection of the feces from all the individual members. Each member of a household was told to keep the specimen away from sunlight, properly covered and labeled. In a cholera-carrier study conducted in Delhi, the family members were asked to defecate on a piece of paper and the formed stool samples were collected from the upper part of the feces with the help of a stick.[94]

The collection of freshly voided specimens often poses considerable difficulty, particularly when large numbers of persons have to be screened. The rectal swab is a very practical method for collecting specimens but it may not be the best method, since the vibrios probably multiply in the upper part of the small bowel and in the absence of diarrhea may be overgrown by normal intestinal flora of the large bowel. As rectal swabs generally contain a small amount of the material, it is desirable that they should be directly inoculated into alkaline peptone water or alkaline taurocholate tellurite trypticase broth in which the presence of even a few vibrios can be detected by careful enrichment and plating. Convalescent carriers have been diagnosed by routine stool or rectal swab examination, which showed that they were excreting vibrios intermittently.[96] For persons who had recovered from cholera and had stopped excreting V. cholerae in their stools, purging with 15 to 30 grams magnesium sulphate is helpful.[90,97,98] In cases of chronic or long-term carriers, duodenal intubation is very helpful in demonstrating the presence of V. cholerae in the bile,[90,96,98] the organism is probably harbored in the gall bladder of such carriers.

7.2. Isolation of V. cholerae 01

Enrichment plays a vital part in isolating V. cholerae 01 from the carriers. The specimen (either stool or rectal swab) may be inoculated in either alkaline peptone water or alkaline taurocholate trypticase tellurite broth for enrichment for a period of 6–8 h at 37°C, followed by plating on a selective medium such as TCBS agar. An amount of 0.1 to 0.2 ml of enrichment culture may be transferred to 10–15 ml fresh alkaline peptone water or alkaline taurocholate trypticase tellurite broth for secondary enrichment followed by plating. Second enrichment helps in detection of a larger number of carriers.[58,99]

Plates from both the primary and secondary enrichment cultures are screened for the characteristic colonies of V. cholerae and the organisms are identified and characterized in the same manner as described for cases. Takeya et al.[100] recommended a phage-enrichment method for the detection of carriers of El Tor vibrios and of cases receiving antimicrobials that has not been used very widely.

7.3. Serological Diagnosis

Contact carriers develop a high antibody titer[2] but the serological procedure involving paired sera taken initially and at a later stage of infection is not practicable for laboratory diagnosis of carriers.[43] A high antibody titer has been seen to persist in the long-term carrier reported by Azurin et al.[96] for more than 8 years in absence of vaccination. The Joint ICMR–GWB–WHO Cholera Study Group[13,73] investigating household contacts of cholera cases in a highly endemic focus in Calcutta demonstrated an almost similar serological pattern in carriers and bacteriologically negative contacts, indicating that in such endemic areas, where large numbers of individuals may have a relatively high antibody titer with or without bacteriologically detectable infection, serological investigation is not helpful for detection of carriers.

8. ISOLATION OF *V. CHOLERAE* 01 FROM ENVIRONMENTAL SAMPLES AND FOOD

Examination of food, water, and sewage, etc. for *V. cholerae* 01 is an essential component of cholera surveillance.[99,101-104]

8.1. Water

Samples of water from suspected sources should be collected in 1 or 2 liter sterile bottles with adequate precaution to prevent contamination from the fingers of the collector and then sent to the laboratory as soon as possible. If delay of more than 2 h is unavoidable, common salt should be added to final concentration of about 1%. The sample can be processed by passing it through millipore filter membrane of pore size of 0.45 μm. If the water is turbid, it should be filtered through several layers of ordinary gauze or filter paper and then the filtrate is filtered through sterile millipore filter membrane (Millipore Filter Corporation, USA) using a slow vacuum suction. The membrane should be transferred aseptically to a flask containing 20 ml of alkaline peptone water (APW) and incubated at 37°C for 8 h. A second enrichment by transferring of 0.2 to 0.5 ml enriched culture into a fresh APW is advisible before plating onto a selective medium. A quantitative examination is also possible using a grid-marked membrane for filtration and a solid medium for culture.

If millipore filter membrane is not available, concentrated alkaline peptone water can be used for collection of water. For this purpose 500-ml bottles containing 50 ml of concentrated APW containing peptone (5 g) and NaCl (5 g) may be used for collection of 450 ml of water samples. After 6 to 8 h incubation at 37°C, a second enrichment is to be done by transferring about 1 ml of enriched culture into 10 ml of a fresh APW and incubated for further 6–8 h before plating onto a selective medium. Isolation of *V. cholerae* 01 from polluted water sources can be very difficult. See also Chapter 2 for the laboratory procedures.

The millipore filter membrane technique has been found to be superior to the concentrated APW double enrichment method.[5,99,105]

8.2. Sewage

A sample of sewage is usually collected in a bottle and diluted with sterile normal saline so that it can be filtered through layers of sterile gauze to remove the suspended material. The filtrate is treated in the same manner as a water sample by double enrichment in alkaline peptone water. Sampling of sewage or running water can preferably be made with the help of Moore swabs.[106] The Moore swab can be made by cutting pieces of cotton gauze (15 cm wide and 60–120 cm long), folding them, lengthwise, several times to form light cylindrical rolls and tying the center with a strong wire. The swab can be wrapped in brown paper and autoclaved. The wires holding the swabs are tied to a nylon fishline, suspended by the line in the sewage or water to be tested and left in place for 1 or 2 days.

The swabs, after removal, should be dipped in 250 to 500 ml of alkaline peptone water in a jar and transported to the laboratory in ice chest. In the laboratory, the swabs in APW are to be incubated for 6–8 h after adjustment of pH. A second or even third enrichment in APW may be required for improved isolation of *V. cholerae* 01. (See also Chapter 2.) The technique has been successfully used by Isaacson[103] and Barret et al.[104] for cholera surveillance.

8.3. Food Stuffs

Samples of the suspected food should be collected in properly labeled sterile glass containers. The samples may have to be ground throughly before being mixed with alkaline peptone water in 1 in 10 proportion and incubated at 37°C for 6–8 h. A second enrichment may be rewarding. A loopful of the culture from the surface of the flask is then streaked on a selective medium for proper isolation and identification of *V. cholerae* 01.[99] Liquid food may have to be filtered and the filtrate examined for *V. cholerae* 01 as described for water.

8.4. Flies

A pooled collection of flies from an infected household or locality can be collected in a bottle and washed in alkaline peptone water, which can then be incubated for 6–8 h at 37°C and then subcultured on selective medium like TCBS. The collection of large numbers of flies within a short period can be achieved with the help of fly-baits ("Tugan," an organic phosphorus compound which attracts flies) spread on a piece of newspaper. About 100 to 200 flies can be collected in course of 10 to 15 min. This organic phosphorus compound does not have any antibacterial property.[5]

REFERENCES

1. Smith HL Jr, Freter R, Sweeney FJ Jr: Enumeration of cholera vibrios in faecal samples. *J Infect Dis* 109:31–34, 1961
2. Dizon JJ, Fukumi H, Barua D, et al: Studies on cholera carriers. *Bull WHO* 37:737–743, 1967
3. Gorbach SI, Banwell JG, Jacob B, et al: Intestinal microflora in Asiatic cholera. I. Rice-water stool. *J Infect Dis* 121:32–37, 1970
4. Venkatraman KV, Ramakrishnan CS: A preserving medium for the transmission of specimens for the isolation of *Vibrio cholerae*. *Indian J Med Res* 29:681–684, 1941
5. Pal SC, Murty DK, Murti GVS, et al: Bacteriological investigations of cholera epidemics in Gurgaon district and in Delhi during 1965–66. *Indian J Med Res* 55:810–814, 1967
6. Zafari Y, Zarifi A, Zomorodi F: A comparative study of sea water and Cary–Blair media for transportation of stool specimens. *J Trop Med Hyg* 71:178–179, 1968
7. Cary SG, Blair EB: New transport medium for shipment of clinical specimens. 1. Faecal specimens. *J Bacteriol* 88:96–98, 1964
8. Gaines S, Haque SU, Paniom W, et al: A field trial of a new transport medium for collection of faeces for bacteriological examination. *Amer J Trop Med* 14:136–140, 1965
9. DeWitt WE, Gangarosa EJ, Huq I, et al: Holding media for the transport of *Vibrio cholerae* from field to laboratory. *Amer J Trop Med Hyg* 20:685–688, 1971
10. Pal SC, Deb BC, Sen Gupta PG, et al: A controlled field trial of an aluminum phosphate-absorbed cholera vaccine in Calcutta. *Bull WHO* 58:741–745, 1980
11. Sen D, Saha MR, Nair GB, et al: Etiological spectrum of acute diarrhoea in hospitalized patients in Calcutta. *Indian J Med Res* 82:286–291, 1985
12. Sinha R, Deb BC, De SP, et al: Cholera carrier studies in Calcutta in 1966–67. *Bull WHO* 37:89–100, 1967
13. Joint ICMR–GWB–WHO Cholera Study Group: Cholera carrier studies in Calcutta, 1968. *Bull WHO* 43:379–387, 1970
14. Deb BC, Sen Gupta PG, De SP, et al: Effect of sulfadoxine on transmission of *Vibrio cholerae* infection among family contacts of cholera patients in Calcutta. *Bull WHO* 54:171–175, 1976
15. Sen Gupta PG, Sircar BK, Mondal S, et al: Effect of doxycycline on transmission of *Vibrio cholerae* infection among family contacts of cholera patients in Calcutta. *Bull WHO* 56:323–326, 1978
16. Monsur KA: Bacteriological diagnosis of cholera under field conditions. *Bull WHO* 28:387–389, 1963

17. Huq MI: A simple laboratory method for the diagnosis of V. cholerae. Trans R Soc Trop Med Hyg 73:553–556, 1979

18. Huq MI, Sanyal SC, Samadi AR, et al: Comparative behaviour of classical and El Tor biotypes of Vibrio cholerae 01 isolated in Bangladesh during 1982. J Diar Dis Res 1:5–9, 1983

19. Samadi AR, Huq MI, Shahid N, et al: Classical Vibrio cholerae biotype displaces El Tor in Bangladesh. Lancet i:805–807, 1983

20. Dold H, Ketterer M: Zeitsch Hygn Infectionskr 125:441, 1944

21. Bailey WR, Bynoe ET: "Filter paper" method for collecting and transporting stools to laboratory for enteric bacteriological examination. Can J Pub Hlth 44:468, 1953

22. Barua D, Gomez CZ: Blotting-paper strips for transportation of cholera stools. Bull WHO 37:798, 1967

23. Huq MI, Rahaman MM: Blotting paper strip for the transport of stool specimens. Indian J Med Res 78:765–768, 1983

24. Bandi I: Le epidemic coleriche delle Puglie e di Napoli. Riv Crit Clin Med 11:770, 785, 802, 1910

25. Cossery GN: The value of Bandi's test in the rapid diagnosis of cholera. Unpublished working document WHO/Cholera/14, p 3, (Quoted from Pollitzer, 1959).

26. Ghosal SC, Paul BM: The value of Bandi's test in the rapid diagnosis of cholera. Bull WHO 7:371–373, 1952

27. Lam SYS: A rapid test for the identification of Vibrio cholerae in stool. J Diar Dis Res 2:87–89, 1983

28. Benenson AS, Islam MR, Greenough III WB: Rapid identification of Vibrio cholerae by darkfield microscopy. Bull WHO 30:827–831, 1964

29. Greenough WB III, Benenson AS, Islam MR: Experience of darkfield examination of stools from diarrheal patients, in Proceedings of the Cholera Research Symposium (Jan 24–29, 1965, Honolulu). Public Health Service Publication No. 1338. US Government Printing Office, Washington DC, 1965, pp 56–58

30. Finkelstein RA, LaBrec EH: Rapid identification of cholera vibrios with fluorescent antibody. J Bacteriol 78:886–891, 1959

31. Finkelstein RA, Gomez CZ: Comparison of methods for the rapid recognition of cholera vibrios. Bull WHO 28:327–332, 1963

32. Sack RB, Barua D: The fluorescent antibody technique in the direct examination of cholera stool, in Proceedings of the Cholera Research Symposium (Jan 24–29, 1965 Honolulu). Public Health Service Publication No. 1328, U.S. Government Printing Office, Washington DC, 1965, pp 50–56

33. Zinnaka Y, Shimodori S, Takeya K: Application of fluorescent antibody technique to the detection of cholera vibrio. Jpn J Infect Dis 39:51–58, 1965

34. Lankford CE: The Henry oblique light technique as an aid in bacteriologic diagnosis of cholera. J Microbiol Soc Thailand 3:10–12, 1959

35. Barua D: Laboratory diagnosis of cholera cases and carriers, in Principles and Practices of Cholera Control, Public Health Paper No. 40. Geneva, World Health Organization, 1970, pp 47–52

36. Jasudason MV, Thangavelu CP, Lalitha MK: Rapid screening of fecal samples for Vibrio cholerae by coagglutination technique. J Clin Microbiol 19:712–713, 1984

37. Rahman M, Sack DA, Wadood A, et al: A low cost and rapid slide agglutination test for diagnosis of cholera using faecal samples. Abstract of the paper presented at the 23rd Joint Conference of Cholera. US–Japan Cooperative Medical Science Program, Virginia, Nov 10–12, 1987, p 88

38. Sack RB, Barua D: A comparative study of bile-salt agar and gelatin–taurocholate–tellurite agar in the bacteriologic diagnosis of cholera. Bull Calcutta Sch Trop Med 12:56–58, 1964

39. Gangarosa EJ, DeWitt WE, Huq I: Laboratory methods in cholera: isolation of V. cholerae (El Tor and classical) on TCBS medium in minimally equipped laboratories. Trans Roy Soc Trop Med Hyg 62:693–699, 1968

40. Pal SC, Murti GVS, Pandit CG, et al: A comparative study of enrichment media in the bacteriological diagnosis of cholera. Indian J Med Res 55:318–324, 1967

41. Pollitzer R: Cholera, Monograph Series No 43. Geneva, World Health Organization

42. Felsenfeld O: A review of recent trends in cholera research and control. Bull WHO 34:161–195, 1966

43. Barua D: Laboratory diagnosis of cholera, in Barua D, Burrows W, (eds): Cholera. Philadelphia, WB Sannders, 1974, pp 85–126

44. Lankford CE, Burrows W: Oblique light microscopy as an aid to rapid detection of enteric pathogens, in Proceedings of the Cholera Research Symposium (Jan 24–29, 1965, Honolulu). Public Health Service Publication No. 1328. U.S. Government Printing Office, Washington DC, 1965, pp 45–50

45. Kobayashi T, Enomoto S, Sakazaki R: A new selective isolation medium for the vibrio group on a modified Nakanishi's medium (TCBS agar medium). Jpn J Bacteriol 18:387–392, 1963

46. Tamura K, Shimoda S, Prescott LM: Vibrio agar: a new plating medium for isolation of V. cholerae. Jpn J Med Sci Biol 24:125–127, 1971

47. De SP, Sen D, De PC, et al: A simple selective medium for isolation of vibrios with particular reference to V. parahaemolyticus. Indian J Med Res 66:398–399, 1977

48. Finkelstein RA, Mukherjee S: Haemagglutination: A rapid method for differentiating V. cholerae and El Tor vibrios. Proc Soc Exp Biol Med 112:355–359, 1963

49. Barua D, Mukherjee AC: Direct bacterial haemagglutination test for differentiating El Tor vibrios from V. cholerae. Bull Calcutta Sch Trop Med 11:85–86, 1963

50. Zinnaka Y, Shimodori S, Takeya K: Haemagglutinating activity of Vibrio comma. Jpn J Microbiol 8:97–103, 1964

51. Barua D, Mukherjee AC: Haemagglutinating activity of El Tor vibrios and its nature. Indian J Med Res 53:399–404, 1965

52. De SN, Ghosh CR, Mukherjee B: Interesting variation observed in a strain of V. cholerae. J Ind Med Assn 44:520–524, 1965

53. Rizvi S, Huq MI, Benenson AS: Isolation of haemagglutinating non-El Tor cholera vibrio. J Bacteriol 89:910–912, 1965

54. Neogy KN, Sanyal SN, Mukherjee MK, et al: Haemagglutinating activity of classical V. cholerae. Bull Calcutta Sch Trop Med 14:1–3, 1966

55. Sehgal PN, Misra BS, Pal SC, et al: An epidemic of classical cholera in the south eastern districts of Madhya Pradesh in 1970. Indian J Med Res 60:7–14, 1972

56. Gan KH, Tjia SK: A new method for the differentiation of Vibrio comma and Vibrio El Tor. Amer J Hyg 77:184–186, 1963

57. Roy C, Mridha K, Mukherjee S: Action of polymyxin on cholera vibrios: techniques of determination of polymyxin-sensitivity. Proc Soc Exp Biol Med 119:893–896, 1965

58. Barua D, Gomez CZ: Observation on some tests commonly employed for the characterization of El Tor vibrios. Bull WHO 37:800–803, 1967

59. Pal SC, Gugnani HC, Misra BS, et al: Varients of Vibrio cholerae in Delhi. Indian J Med Res 61:649–652, 1973

60. Gugnani HC, Pal SC: Variation in polymyxin sensitivity among colonies in primary plate cultures of Vibrio El Tor. J Med Microbiol 7:535–536, 1974

61. Mukherjee S: The bacteriophage-susceptibility test in differentiating Vibrio cholerae and Vibrio El Tor. Bull WHO 28:333–336, 1963

62. Nobechi K: On the methods to differentiate classical cholera and El Tor vibrios and further the latter into their subgroups, in Proceedings of the Seventh International Congress on Tropical Medicine and Malaria, 1963 Vol III Rio de Jeneiro, Grafica Olimpica Editora, 1964, pp 27–29

63. Rizvi S, Benenson AS: Phage resistance in Vibrio cholerae. Bull WHO 35:675–680, 1966

64. Swanson RW, Gillmore JD: Biochemical characteristics of recent cholera isolates in the Far East. Bull WHO 31:422–425, 1964

65. Pollitzer R, Burrows W: Problems in immunology, in Pollitzer R (ed): Cholera, Monograph Series No 43. Geneva, World Health Organization, 1959, pp 202–372

66. Goodner K, Smith Jr HL, Stempen H: Serological diagnosis of cholera. J A Einstein Med Cent 8:143–147, 1960

67. Barua D, Sack RB: Serological studies on cholera. Indian J Med Res 52:855–864, 1964

68. Sakazaki R, Donovan TJ: Serology and epidemiology of Vibrio cholerae and Vibrio mimicus, in Bergan T (ed): Methods in Microbiology, Vol 16. London, Academic Press, 1984, pp 271–289

69. Bhattacharya FK: The agglutination reactions of cholera vibrios. Jpn J Med Sci Biol 30:259–268, 1977

70. De SN, Lahiri-Chaudhury PK, Ghosh ML, et al: A study of the technique for demonstration of 'O' and 'H' agglutinins in the serum of cholera patients. Indian J Med Res 46:351–358, 1958

71. Dey SK, Kusari J, Ghose AC: Detergent induced enhancement of antibody mediated flagellar agglutination of Vibrio cholerae. IRCS Med Sci 11:908, 1983

72. Benenson AS, Saad A, Paul M: Serological studies in cholera. 1. Vibrio agglutinin response of cholera patients determined by microtechnique. Bull WHO 38:267–276, 1968c

73. Joint ICMR–GWB–WHO Cholera study Group: Study on Vibrio cholerae infection in a small community in Calcutta. Bull WHO 43:401–406, 1970

74. Finkelstein RA: Vibriocidal antibody inhibition (VAI) analysis: A technique for the identification of the predominant vibriocidal antibodies in serum and for the detection and identification of V. cholerae antigens. J Immunol 89:264–271, 1962

75. Miles AA, Misra SS, Irwin JJ: The estimation of the bacteriocidal powers of the blood. *J Hyg (Camb)* 38:732–748, 1938

76. McIntyre OR, Feeley JC: Passive serum protection of the infant rabbit against experimental cholera. *J Infect Dis* 114:468–475, 1964

77. Sack RB, Barua D, Saxena R: Vibriocidal and agglutinating antibody patterns in cholera patients. *J Infect Dis* 116:630–640, 1966

78. Majumdar AS, Ghose AC: Evaluation of the biological properties of different classes of human antibodies in relation to cholera. *Infect Immun* 32:9–14, 1981

79. Benenson AS, Saad A, Mosley WH: Serological studies in cholera. 2. The vibriocidal antibody response of cholera patients determined by a microtechnique. *Bull WHO* 38:277–285, 1968

80. Clements ML, Levine MM, Young CR, et al: Magnitude, kinetics and duration of vibriocidal antibody responses in north Americans after ingestion of *Vibrio cholerae*. *J Infect Dis* 145:465–473, 1982

81. Glass RI: Epidemiologic studies of cholera in rural Bangladesh. Ph.D. thesis, University of Goteborg, Sweden, 1984

82. Snyder JD, Allegra DT, Levine MM, et al: Serologic studies of naturally acquired infection with *Vibrio cholerae* serogroup 01 in the United States. *J Infect Dis* 143:182–187, 1981

83. Feeley JC: Comparison of vibriocidal and agglutinating antibody responses in cholera patients, in *Proceedings of the Cholera Research Symposium (Jan 24–29, 1965, Honolulu)*, Public Health Service Publication No. 1328. Washington DC, U.S. Government Printing Office, 1965, pp 220–222

84. Engyall E, Perlmann P: Enzyme-linked immunosorbent assay ELISA. III. Quantitation of specific antibodies by enzyme-labelled anti-immunoglobulin in antigen-coated tubes. *J Immunol* 109:129–135, 1972

85. Holmgren J, Svennerholm AM: Enzyme-linked immunosorbent assays for cholera serology. *Infect Immun* 7:759–763, 1973

86. Sears SD, Richardson K, Young CR, et al: Evaluation of the human immune response to outer membrane proteins of *Vibrio cholerae*. *Infect Immun* 44:439–444, 1984

87. Levine MM, Young CR, Hughes TP, et al: Duration of serum antitoxin response following *Vibrio cholerae* infection in north Americans: relevance for seroepidemiology. *Am J Epidemiol* 114:348–354, 1981

88. Young CR, Levine MM, Craig JP, et al: Microtiter enzyme-linked immunosorbent assay for immunoglobulin G cholera antitoxin in humans: Method and correlation with rabbit skin vascular permeability factor technique. *Infect Immun* 27:492–496, 1980

89. Benenson AS, Saad A, Mosley WH, et al: Serological studies in cholera. 3. Serum toxin neutralization—rise in titer in response to infection with *Vibrio cholerae* and the level in the "normal" population of East Pakistan. *Bull WHO* 38:287–295, 1968

90. Pierce NF, Banwell JG, Gorbach SL, et al: Convalescent carriers of *V. cholerae*, detection and detailed investigation. *J Infect Dis* 72:359–364, 1970

91. Kesai GJ, Burrow W: The titration of cholera toxin and antitoxin in the rabbit ileal loop. *J Infect Dis* 116:606–614, 1966

92. Craig JP, Eichner ER, Hornick RB: Cutaneous responses to cholera skin toxin in man. I. Responses in immunized American males. *J Infect Dis* 125:203–215, 1972

93. Rabins-Browne R, Young CR, Levine MM, et al: Mictotiter enzyme-linked immunosorbent assay for immunoglobulin G cholera antitoxin in humans: sensitivity and specificity. *Infect Immun* 27:497–500, 1980

94. Pal SC, Misra BS, Arora DD, et al: Studies on cholera carriers in Delhi. *Indian J Med Res* 61:495–502, 1973

95. Vande Linde PAM, Forbes GI: Observations on the spread of cholera in Hong Kong 1961–63. *Bull WHO* 32:515–530, 1965

96. Azurin JC, Kobari K, Barua D, et al: A long term carrier of cholera: Cholera Dolores. *Bull WHO* 37:745–749, 1967

97. Gangarosa EJ, Saghari H, Emile J: Detection of *Vibrio cholerae* biotype El Tor by purging. *Bull WHO* 34:363–369, 1966

98. Wallace CK, Pierce NF, Anderson PN, et al: Probable gallbladder infection in convalescent cholera infection. *Lancet* i:865–868, 1967

99. Deb BC, Sircar BK, Sen Gupta PG, et al: Intra-familial transmission of *Vibrio cholerae* in Calcutta slums. *Indian J Med Res* 76:814–819, 1982

100. Takeya K, Shimodori S, Gomez CZ: Kappa-type phage detection as a method for the tracing of cholera El Tor carriers. *Bull WHO* 37:806–810, 1967

101. Goh KT, Lam S, Kumarapathy S, et al: A common source food borne outbreak of cholera in Singapore. *Int J Epidemiol* 13:210–215, 1983

102. Khan M: Presence of vibrios in surface water and their relation with cholera in a community. *Trop Geogr Med* 36:335–340, 1984

103. Isaacson M: Practical aspects of a cholera survaillance programme. *S Afr Med J* 49:1699–1702, 1975

104. Barret TJ, Blake PA, Morris GK, et al: Use of Moore swabs for isolating *Vibrio cholerae* from sewage. *J Clin Microbiol* 11:385–388, 1980

105. De SP, Banerjee M, Deb BC, et al: Distribution of vibrios in Calcutta environment with particular reference to *V. parahaemolyticus. Indian J Med Res* 65:21–28, 1977

106. Moore R: The detection of Paratyphoid carriers in towns by means of sewage examination. *Mon Bull Min Health Pub Health Lab Serv* 7:241, 1948

107. Shimada T, Sakazaki R, Fujimara S, et al: A new selective differential agar medium for isolation of *Vibrio cholerae* 01: PMT (Polymixin Mannose–Tellurite Agar). *Jap J Med Sci Biol* 43:37–41, 1990

108. Oku T, Uesaka Y, Hirayama T, et al: Development of a highly sensitive Bead ELISA to detect bacterial protein toxins. *Microbiol Immunol* 32(8):807–816, 1988

109. Ramamurthy T, Pal Amit, Nair GB, et al: Experience with a toxin bead–ELISA in cholera outbreak. *Lancet* ii(336):375–376, 1990

110. Almeida RJ, Hickmann Branner FW, Sowers EG, et al: Comparison of latex agglutination assay and an enzyme linked immunosorbent assay for detecting cholera toxin. *J Clin Microbiol* 28(1):128–131, 1990

13

Clinical Management of Cholera

Dilip Mahalanabis, A. M. Molla, and David A. Sack

1. INTRODUCTION

Cholera patients who receive adequate treatment will almost always recover fully and rapidly. For a disease capable of spreading in epidemic fashion and causing case–fatality rates of 50% or more, the development of successful, simple, and inexpensive therapy constitutes one of the most dramatic success stories of modern medical research and its application to a major public-health scourge. Using rapid rehydration, a seriously ill patient in profound shock with no detectable pulse or blood pressure is able to sit, talk, and eat within a few hours and can return to work within two to three days. Furthermore, this life-saving and dramatic treatment can be rendered at a very low cost. A sequence of dehydration-rehydration can be seen in Figure 1.

This chapter describes the development of the strategies for clinical management, the basis of optimum therapy, and a treatment plan for cholera patients. Since cholera affects largely underprivileged populations in developing countries, the recommended management plan attempts to be simple yet scientifically appropriate. Because treatment of cholera patients in remote areas presents special challenges, a description of the treatment of patients in the home or in "makeshift" rehydration centers is also included.

Manifestations of severe cholera are due almost entirely to the loss of salts and water in the stool and in the vomit, although other complications of cholera may occur if effective rehydration is not accomplished. Objectives of treatment are: (1) rapid replacement of water and salts already lost; (2) maintenance of normal hydration until diarrhea ceases by replacing further fluid losses as they occur; (3) reduction of the magnitude and duration of diarrhea with suitable antibiotics; and (4) prompt introduction of a normal diet to minimize the adverse nutritional effects from the illness.

Cholera, edited by Dhiman Barua and William B. Greenough III. Plenum Medical Book Company, New York, 1992.

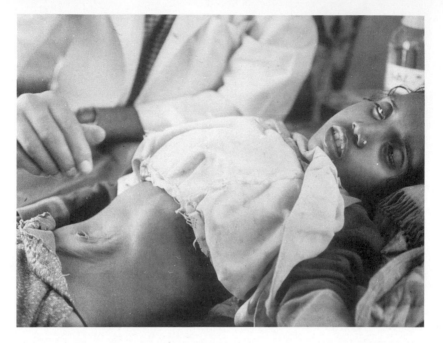

FIGURE 1A. Rehydration of a patient with cholera. The girl shown in this series of photographs has many of the features of cholera. Note the sunken eyes and poor skin turgor in photograph A. The hand shown above the abdomen had just released a fold of skin and the skin remains tented. The same patient is seen a few hours later in photograph B. C and D show the same girl on the second and third day following rehydration therapy.

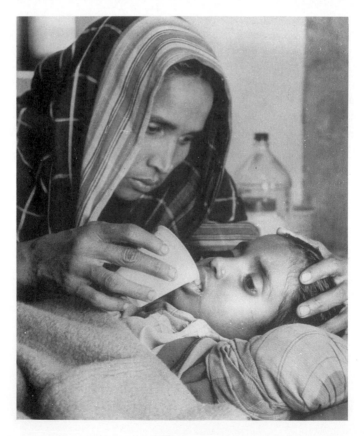

FIGURE 1B.

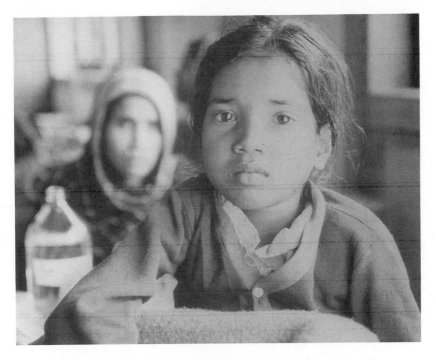

FIGURE 1C.

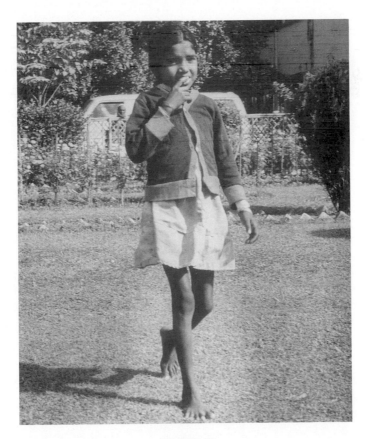

FIGURE 1D.

TABLE 1
Landmarks in the Treatment of Cholera

1. Hermann (1830) observed hemoconcentration in cholera patients and proposed the idea of injecting fluid into their veins.
2. O'Saughnessy (1831–1832) accurately described "deficient saline matters" after carefully examining blood from cholera patients.
3. Latta (1832) treated 15 moribund cholera patients and 5 survived; *Lancet* considered the treatment to be life saving.
4. Rogers (1908–1909) treated cholera patients with sufficient volumes of intravenous hypertonic saline using aseptic precautions; mortality dropped from 70% to 30%.
5. Sellards (1910) described acidosis in cholera and used alkali; Rogers added alkali to regimen and mortality dropped to 20%.
6. Phillips, Watten, Carpenter, Gordon (1958–1964) measured exact loss of water and electrolytes in cholera; developed details of I.V. clinical management using isotonic saline and alkali plus oral water; mortality dropped to less than 1%.
7. Phillips, Pierce, Hirschhorn (1964–1968) established that cholera patients can absorb electrolytes and water if glucose is included in the oral solution, thus establishing the scientific basis for oral rehydration therapy.

2. DEVELOPMENT OF CHOLERA TREATMENT

The history of cholera and its treatment has been described in Chapter 1. Some of the landmarks in the development of appropriate fluid replacement of cholera are given in Table 1. Historically, mortality from cholera among inpatients declined steadily as the therapy employed the type of fluid replacement that more closely met the actual needs with respect to volume, rate of delivery, and electrolyte content. The most recent landmark in cholera therapy was the development of oral rehydration therapy (ORT) using solution containing glucose and appropriate salts. According to a *Lancet* editorial, the discovery that glucose facilitated the intestinal transport of sodium and water may have been the most important medical discovery of the century.[1] This discovery and its application to public health has led to the development of a practical, simple, safe, available, inexpensive, and effective means of treating dehydration from cholera and other dehydrating diarrheal diseases. Being a powerful tool, ORT (along with appropriate feeding) has emerged as one of the foundations for diarrheal diseases control programs worldwide.

Through the ages, many can claim to have used oral rehydration therapy, beginning at least as far back as Hippocrates. Certainly many cultures of the world have given various types of fluids to their children during bouts of diarrhea. These fluids have ranged from apple juice to yogurt (we could not identify a fluid beginning with "z"). While these traditional fluids were undoubtedly helpful in many cases, the basic understanding of the mechanisms of absorption, the need for rehydration, and the appropriate types of fluids to be used were lacking. Consequently they could not be used effectively in cholera patients nor in those with other forms of severe diarrhea in whom rehydration was critical. After the fluid and electrolyte requirements were known for cholera and a highly effective treatment regime based on intravenous therapy was developed, attention could be turned towards more cost-effective ways of delivering these rehydration fluids.

2.1. Glucose-Facilitated Absorption of Salts and Water

Physiologists have long studied the relationship between glucose and sodium absorption from the small intestine. Some examples of these research efforts relevant to the development of ORT include the following: (1) In 1902, Waymouth Reid, a Scottish physiologist, demonstrated enhanced sodium absorption in the presence of glucose by the mammalian small intestine using dog intestinal loops[2]; (2) Barany and Sperber, in 1939, and Fisher and Parsons, in 1953, confirmed these findings using rabbit small intestine[3,4]; (3) Riklis and Quastel showed in 1958 that sodium ion was linked to glucose absorption,[5] and Schultz and Zalusky[6] described the mechanism of this linkage (4) Schedl and Clifton, in 1963, using intestinal intubation techniques in human volunteers, demonstrated a dramatic improvement in sodium chloride and water absorption from Ringer's solution in both the jejunum and ileum with the addition of 1 g% glucose[7]; (5) Subsequently, *in vivo* studies in normal human small intestine defined the quantitative relationships of glucose with enhanced sodium and water absorption.[8-10]

More recently, it was hypothesized that this intestinal glucose-facilitated absorption of sodium and water from the small intestinal lumen remained largely intact during cholera. Phillips first validated this approach in a few profusely purging adult cholera patients.[11,12] In contrast to earlier studies[13] in which an oral electrolyte solution, but without glucose, did not lead to absorption of the fluid, the glucose-containing electrolyte solution was absorbed from the small intestine and led to a positive fluid and sodium balance. Deaths occurred during these early trials of oral therapy, however, and Phillips did not believe that a practical form of therapy had been discovered. Nevertheless, this demonstration may be regarded as the beginning of the scientific development of oral rehydration therapy.

Subsequently, Pierce[14,15] in Calcutta and Hirschhorn[16] in Dhaka evaluated isotonic oral rehydration salt solutions containing glucose and sodium in approximately equal concentrations and dramatically demonstrated the substantial decrease in the requirement for intravenous fluids, indicating that absorption was taking place across the small intestine. Studies in animal models[17] showing that glucose-mediated absorption took place in the intestines of dogs challenged with cholera toxin helped to confirm these findings.

To be useful as a public health tool, this physiologic observation had to be extended to larger numbers of patients with both cholera and noncholera diarrhea. This was carried out in Dhaka by Cash and Nalin[18] and later in refugee camps in India.[19] During the war of independence of Bangladesh, refugees fled across the border into India. In these conditions of poor sanitation and scarce medical resources, oral rehydration therapy was used as a matter of necessity and it performed extremely well. Case–fatality rates of about 3% were not as low as they would have been with adequate intravenous supplies; still, ORT saved most of the patients and proved that oral rehydration was a powerful tool for controlling epidemics. This helped to convince the health planners and public health workers of its obviously important role as a public health weapon.

Soon to follow were independent studies from Calcutta and Dhaka that provided additional evidence for the usefulness of ORT in cholera patients.[20-23] Demonstration of the success of ORT in adult cholera patients was then followed by a series of clinical trials in children with cholera,[24] in infants and small children with diarrhea due to rotavirus,[25] enterotoxigenic *E.coli,* and other etiologic agents.[26]

Another demonstration of the power and versatility of oral rehydration in a practical setting was the decrease in diarrhea mortality following the introduction of an ORT program in a village in southern Bangladesh.[27] Here, ORT was provided by a packet distribution program in which depot holder families maintained a supply of ORS packets and were trained how to make the solution for their neighbors. Furthermore, the village members knew where to obtain the fluids in their own village and were taught the value of rehydration. Thus, rehydration could begin at an early stage in the illness.

With such clinical and public health demonstrations as those cited above, ORT emerged as a major therapeutic tool with the ability to correct dehydration and maintain hydration in acute diarrhea in all but the most severe cases and in all ages regardless of etiologic agents.

2.2. Composition of Oral Rehydration Solutions

Early trials of ORS in cholera used solutions containing sodium, 90–120 mmol; potassium, 10–25 mmol; sodium bicarbonate, 30–48 mmol; and glucose, 110–120 mmol per liter of solution.[26] In 1971, the World Health Organization (WHO) began recommending an ORS containing 90 mmol of sodium, 20 mmol of potassium, 80 mmol of chloride, 30 mmol of bicarbonate, and 111 mmol of glucose per liter of water. This ORS (now modified with citrate, see below) has been successfully adapted and extensively tested both under controlled hospital conditions as well as in the field. It meets the varying needs of rehydration therapy in all ages suffering from acute diarrheas due to many etiologic agents including cholera.

Several factors were considered in devising the appropriate formulation. It was known that the cholera patient loses bicarbonate and potassium in addition to sodium and water in the isosmotic stool. Thus, the replacement solution should replace these losses with a solution of similar concentration of electrolytes to correct the acidosis and potassium deficiency. Furthermore, sodium and glucose absorption are coupled and are thus absorbed on an equimolar basis. Therefore, it was appropriate to have similar concentrations of glucose and sodium. Finally, the solution should not be excessively hypertonic since an excessive osmotic load is associated with a lessened absorption and increased diarrhea. Two grams of glucose appeared to be optimal for absorption[16]; higher concentrations increase the osmolality excessively and are counterproductive.

2.2.1. ORS Formulations Containing Trisodium Citrate

A base is needed in the ORS to replace the bicarbonate lost in the cholera stool and correct the resulting metabolic acidosis. Sodium bicarbonate was originally selected for ORS[26]; however, ORS packets with sodium bicarbonate have a short shelf life (a few months), especially in hot and humid tropical climates. It, therefore, seemed appropriate to select a different base for ORS. Laboratory studies demonstrated that ORS containing 2.9 g of trisodium citrate dihydrate in place of 2.5 g of sodium bicarbonate was the most stable of the candidate formulations evaluated, and it seemed likely that citrate would perform as well as bicarbonate in the solution.[28] Subsequently, clinical trials were undertaken to compare the efficacy of an ORS containing citrate with ORS containing bicarbonate.[29–32] Among those studies undertaken in adults and older children with cholera with dehydration and acidosis, the acidosis of those receiving the citrate ORS was corrected at a rate equal to that of those patients receiving bicarbonate ORS. In one of the studies in adults with cholera, diarrhea stool output was significantly decreased in the group receiving citrate ORS and in two other studies there was a similar trend. Among studies undertaken in infants and children below two years of age with moderate to severe dehydration from noncholera diarrhea, citrate ORS was found to be uniformly as effective as bicarbonate ORS in correcting acidosis and dehydration. No reduction in diarrhea stool output, however, was observed in these children. In conclusion, ORS with citrate was found to be at least as effective as ORS with bicarbonate but to have a significant advantage in its improved shelf life. However, one should not hesitate to use ORS with bicarbonate when the situation requires it since this is also highly

TABLE 2
ORS Solution[a]

A. Composition by weight of oral rehydration salts (ORS) (quantities shown for preparation of *one liter* of ORS Solution)

Ingredient	Weight (g)
1. Sodium chloride	3.5
2. Trisodium citrate, dihydrate	2.9
or	
Sodium hydrogen carbonate (sodium bicarbonate)	2.5
3. Potassium chloride	1.5
4. Glucose, anhydrous[b,c]	20.0

B. Molar concentration of components of ORS Solution

Component	Citrate-containing solution (mmol/liter of water)	Bicarbonate-containing solution (mmol/liter of water)
Sodium	90	90
Potassium	20	20
Chloride	80	80
Citrate	10	—
Bicarbonate	—	30
Glucose	111	111

[a]The formula for Oral Rehydration Salts (ORS) recommended by WHO, and first used in 1971, is shown in Part A. The quantities shown under A are for the preparation of one liter of ORS Solution and the concentrations of the components of this solution are shown under B.
[b]Or glucose, monohydrate, 22.0 g; or sucrose, 40.0 g.
[c]50 g rice powder can replace 20 g glucose. To prepare a rice powder solution: put 50 g rice powder (i.e., rice flour) in 1100 ml of water and bring it to boil. Continue boiling for approximately 7 min when the mixture becomes opalescent. Allow it to cool, add and mix the three salts. Serve the solution warm. After 8 h discard and prepare a fresh batch.

effective in the treatment of dehydration. Presently, all centrally produced and distributed ORS packets by UNICEF, WHO, and other agencies are citrate based.

The currently recommended composition of ORS with citrate is shown in Table 2.

2.2.2. Sucrose as a Substitute for Glucose in ORS Formulation

Since glucose is not locally manufactured in many countries and is not available in many households, studies were conducted to evaluate sucrose (table sugar) as a possible alternative to glucose. Sucrose is broken down by the intestinal brush-border enzymes into glucose and fructose, and it was expected that glucose should be available to participate in the absorptive process. It was possible, however, that sucrase activity would be insufficient during diarrhea, and that this would result in a sucrose malabsorption and a worsening of the diarrhea. Also, it was known that fructose, which is much less efficient than glucose in its absorption, might create an osmotic load leading to increased diarrhea. Hence, the studies showing the effectiveness of sucrose as an alternative were reassuring.[25,33,34]

Although the studies comparing sucrose with glucose show them to be nearly equivalent, all studies have suggested a slight trend in favor of glucose. Also, occasional patients have been documented to have a sucrose malabsorption and these patients will need a glucose solution for severe diarrhea. In spite of these relative deficiencies, the availability of sucrose in most homes, its local production and economy, and its efficacy for the vast majority of patients make it an acceptable alternative to glucose for ORS. However, when preparing packets for mass distribution, the slight advantage of glucose suggests that glucose is preferred since, in this situation, glucose can generally be obtained at a price similar to that for sucrose. If sucrose is used, one should use 40 g/liter in order to obtain a yield of 20 g of glucose.

2.2.3. Starches and Cereals in ORS

As an extension of the desire to make ORT available and acceptable to the people who use it, the use of cereals, especially rice, has been evaluated as the substrate in place of glucose. Rice has many attributes which make it attractive for ORT in addition to its cultural familiarity. Starches and proteins in cereals, when broken down by the digestive processes in the intestinal tract, release glucose, amino acids, and short-chain peptides, all of which are organic solutes that may enhance the absorption of sodium and water. In addition, cereals may also be used in larger quantities, thus providing some additional calories with little or no osmotic penalty.

Molla, using retrospective controls, demonstrated that rice-powder ORS (30 g per liter) was as effective as sucrose-based ORS (40 g sucrose per liter) in adults and older children with cholera.[35] Subsequently, Patra demonstrated in a controlled clinical trial in children with cholera and noncholera diarrhea that rice-powder-containing ORS (50 g precooked rice powder per liter) could reduce the volume and the duration of diarrhea.[36] A follow up clinical trial by Molla in adults and older children, predominantly with cholera, confirmed that a rice-powder (80 g rice powder per liter) ORS (in comparison to standard ORS) could reduce diarrhea stool volumes and ORS requirement.[37] In a more recent clinical trial in children with cholera and noncholera diarrhea, Patra used a combination of cooked rice power (50 g per liter packet) and glycine (111 mmols per liter) in ORS and showed that adding glycine to rice did not further improve its efficiency.[38]

In studies conducted so far, rice-based ORS has proved to be at least as efficacious as glucose in rehydrating patients with cholera and other diarrheal diseases. In addition, the use of rice rather than a sugar as the carbohydrate source may be associated with a reduction in the total diarrheal stool output.[35,36,39]

Starches other than rice may also be used, as demonstrated by Alam and colleagues, who found that a well-hydrolyzed wheat-based oral rehydration solution also significantly reduced the diarrhea stool output in children with cholera.[40] The wheat product used, which contained 11.5 g % protein and 87 g % carbohydrate (60% maltose, 15% maltotriose, and 10% maltodextrins), was completely soluble in water and did not require cooking. Finally, preliminary analysis of trials with ORS based on other cereals such as wheat and maize have shown that these may also be used as substrates to promote absorption (unpublished data from studies at ICDDR,B).

Practical constraints of the currently used rice-based ORS formulations include the need for cooking prior to use and a short shelf life of the prepared solutions particularly in hot and humid conditions (6 to 12 h). Although the need for cooking makes rice and other cereal-based ORS less suitable as a prepackaged product (unless a precooked stable cereal-based ORS can be produced), the results of studies with cereal-based solutions should also be very

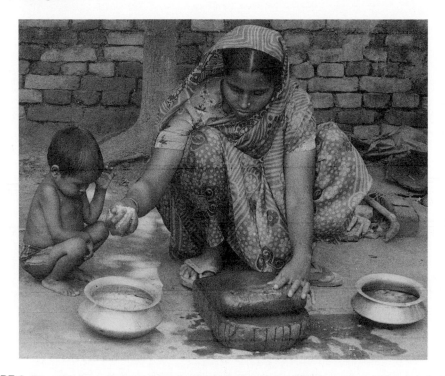

FIGURE 2. Five steps for making cereal-based oral rehydration therapy (ORT) in a village in Bangladesh. Photos by Asem Ansari, ICDDRB, courtesy of Dr. A. Majid Molla. Step 1: Take one fistful of dry rice grain (20-25g) Wash and soak the rice in some water until soft.

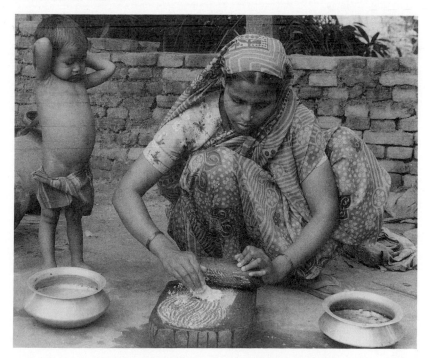

FIGURE 2. (cont.) Step 2: Grind the soaked rice with a pestle and mortar (or any grinder) until it becomes a paste.

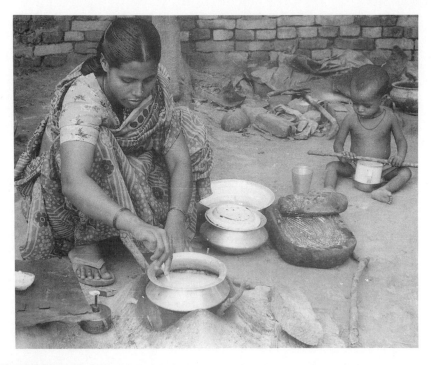

FIGURE 2. (cont.) Step 3: Put two and a quarter glasses of water (about 600 ml) in a cooking utensil and mix with the paste.

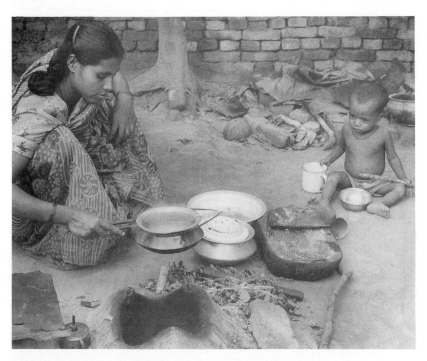

FIGURE 2. (cont.) Step 4: Stir well and bring the mixture to a boil until the first bubble appears. Take the pan off the fire and allow to cool.

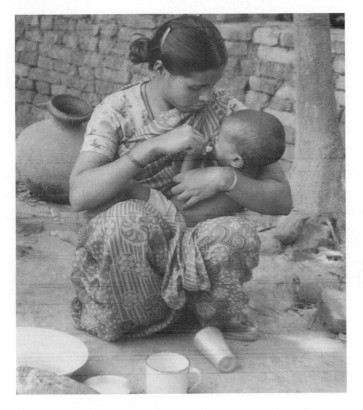

FIGURE 2. (cont.) Step 5: Add one "three-finger" (up to the first crease of the finger) pinch of salt to the mixture and stir well. The rice-based oral rehydration solution is now ready for feeding to the diarrheal patient. Do *not* overcook. This solution should be stored in a cool and clean place. Once prepared, the solution should be used within 6–8 h, after which it should be discarded.

useful proxy indicators for the efficacy of cereal-based home fluids for early home therapy (Fig. 2).

In summary, cereal-based ORS formulations tested so far are highly encouraging. Based on these results and the acceptability of a rice-based formula in Bangladesh, the ICDDR,B currently uses a rice-based ORS (50 g per liter of rice powder) as its routine rehydration solution at its treatment centers. Rice-based ORT is not seen as competing with the glucose formulation; rather, both are acceptable and either can be used depending on local circumstances. If a packet formulation can be prepared with an economical and stable rice powder which does not require cooking, the rice-based formula will likely become much more popular.

2.2.4. Improved ORS Formulations (Super ORS)

Oral rehydration therapy with the present ORS formulation is intended to rehydrate the patient but, with the possible exception of cereal-based ORS, does not reduce the volume, frequency, or duration of diarrhea. This raises the practical problem of its acceptance by patients and by parents of ill children who would like to see a dramatic reduction in the severity of the diarrheal symptoms. This desire leads to a continuing demand for antidiarrheal medication.

It has been postulated that a super ORS formulation could be developed that could utilize a combination of pathways of absorption, which in turn would lead to a net decrease in diarrhea volume.[39,41] Such a super ORS could theoretically induce reabsorption of the endogenous secretion, in addition to facilitating the absorption of the fluids administered, and thus it would become an antidiarrheal medication as well as a form of rehydration.

The mechanisms that could be utilized in a super ORS include the following: (a) organic nutrient–linked absorption; (b) the use of glucose polymers rather than glucose; (c) weak organic acid–linked absorption; and (d) colonic salvage of salts and water by short-chain fatty acids.

Glucose is one organic nutrient that is linked to absorption; however, other D-hexoses and certain amino acids, e.g., glycine and L-alanine, also can be utilized. Early studies in adults and older children with cholera and noncholera diarrhea indicated that an ORS prepared with a combination of glucose and glycine (110 mmols per liter) could substantially reduce the stool volume and duration of diarrhea.[42] Subsequently, a double-blind, controlled clinical trial of glucose-and glycine (111 mmols of each per liter)-based ORS in children with cholera and noncholera diarrhea showed that the stool volume, duration of diarrhea, and volume of ORS requirement were reduced compared with controls receiving the standard glucose ORS formula.[43] A recent double-blind, clinical trial in Indonesia confirmed that a glucose- and glycine-containing ORS formulation reduced diarrhea stool output in actively purging adult cholera patients (Moechtar et al., unpublished data). Finally, results from a similar clinical trial of ORS with L-alanine in older children and adults with cholera showed a marked reduction in stool output and duration of diarrhea among patients receiving the L-alanine ORS compared to the standard ORS controls.[44] When glucose is administered in a free form, the upper limit of its effective concentration is about 2 g per 100 ml; higher concentrations are associated with an increase in the diarrhea. One way to effectively increase the concentration of glucose while minimizing the risk for the osmotic penalty is to use a suitable polymer(s) of glucose which releases glucose on digestion at a rate favorable for its absorption. These glucose polymers include the maltodextrins of various grades as well as natural foods containing starch and protein.

The suggestion that weak acids might increase fluid absorption was alluded to when discussing citrate ORS above. Weak organic acids, e.g., acetate, n-butyrate, and propionate, are rapidly absorbed from both the small and large intestine. These weak acids are exchanged for bicarbonate; and sodium and potassium are absorbed in the process. Sodium citrate has also been shown in a rabbit model to stimulate absorption of sodium and potassium.[45]

Whether these physiologic improvements in ORT will result in a substantially better oral rehydration formulation is not yet known. If additional substrates are to be added to the standard ORS packet, its formulation will depend on a clinically significant improvement in efficacy while not adding appreciably to the cost of the solution. At present, the cereal-based formulae come the closest to meeting these requirements.

2.2.5. Incomplete Oral Rehydration Solutions

The practical considerations that led to the development of sucrose ORS have also been extended further to consider simple "sugar–salt" rehydration solutions that contain neither potassium nor added base and, thus, can be prepared from ingredients normally found in the home. Since these solutions do not have a base or potassium, patients who receive only this solution have an increased risk for both continued acidosis and hypokalemia.[46] For the more common noncholera diarrheal illnesses which tend to be less severe and are generally the focus of community health problems, the incomplete simple solutions can be used effectively.[47] However, they should be used with a diet supplemented with potassium-rich foods during and after diarrheal episodes to compensate for the potassium loss.

For heavily purging cholera patients, however, the incomplete formula is not sufficient and should be used only as a temporary measure until an appropriate complete solution can be obtained. Diarrhea treatment centers, clinics, and hospitals should always prepare a complete solution including a base and potassium since patients receiving assistance from these sources tend to be more ill and require the complete solution.

3. USE OF INTRAVENOUS FLUIDS

The alternative appropriate intravenous rehydration solutions are described briefly in Table 3 and their compositions are shown in Table 4. The issues that had to be addressed in the development of the I.V. solutions were similar to those described for ORT, namely, replacement fluids were needed which replaced diarrheal losses of water and electrolytes during cholera. Although many of the basic concepts were learned in the early 1800s, they were not widely held until this century and were not utilized until mid century.

In spite of the importance and success of ORT, intravenous rehydration still plays a critical role in the treatment of cholera. For cholera patients who present with severe dehydration and shock, rapid infusion of appropriate I.V. fluid is life saving. For diarrheal diseases other than cholera, patients with such profound and rapid dehydration are unusual, but for cholera, especially during epidemics, it occurs frequently. Since cholera usually occurs in geographic areas with few medical resources, ORT conserves the limited I.V. supplies that are available.

The composition of a standard I.V. solution for cholera patients is based on the concept that the fluid given should replace the losses of the cholera stool which, in a severely purging cholera patient, contains sodium (100–140 mmol per liter), bicarbonate (30–50 mmol per liter), and potassium (15–30 mmol per liter) with an osmolality close to that of plasma. A suitable polyelectrolyte solution for intravenous use should, therefore, contain (per liter)

TABLE 3
Solutions for Intravenous Infusion

Ringers lactate: This is the best commercially available solution. Lactate yields bicarbonate for correction of the acidosis. Although its potassium concentration is low, prompt introduction of ORT during maintenance provides adequate amount of potassium.

Special solutions (e.g., Dhaka Solution or DTS): Dhaka solution is produced in Bangladesh and is in routine use for all patients with diarrhea and dehydration. Acetate is the preferred base because it is more stable during storage than lactate. This and similar other special diarrhea treatment solutions are not available commercially. Some national diarrheal diseases control programs are producing similar special solutions suitable to treat diarrheal dehydration in all age groups. [48,49]

Normal saline: Also called physiological isotonic saline, this solution is often readily available. It will not correct acidosis and will not replace potassium. This is a poor choice but may be used if it is the only solution available. Normal saline in 5% dextrose is also often available. The same comments apply for this as for normal saline.

5% Dextrose in water: Do not use for the treatment of dehydrating diarrheal diseases.

TABLE 4
Comparison of Cholera Stools in Adults and Children, and of Intravenous
and Oral Fluids Used in Cholera Treatment

	mmol/liter				
Cholera stools	Na$^+$	K$^+$	Cl$^-$	HCO$_3^-$	Glucose
Adults	130	15	100	45	—
Children	105	25	90	30	—
Intravenous fluids					
Ringer's lactate					
(Hartmann's fluid)	131	4	111	29	—
Diarrhea treatment					
solution (DTS)[49]	118	13	83	48	50
Dhaka solution[48]	113	13	98	48	—
2 Saline : 1 lactate[50]	158	—	103	56	—
Normal saline	154	—	154	—	—
Half-Darrow's solution					
with 2.5% Glucose[a]	61	17.5	52	26	150
Oral rehydration solution as					
recommended by WHO	90	20	80	30	111
					(10 as citrate)

[a]Full-strength Darrow's solution contains too much potassium, while half-strength has too little sodium for correcting dehydration in cholera.

sodium (110 to 140 mmol), potassium (10–15 mmol), a base (30–50 mmol), and chloride (70–100 mmol). Lactated Ringer's (Hartmann's fluid) is one of the recommended fluids because it is the one commercially available I.V. solution with a suitable composition. In cholera-endemic areas special polyelectrolyte fluids may be prepared especially for diarrhea treatment, e.g., the "Dhaka Solution,"[48] or "DTS"[49] (diarrhea treatment solution), or others.[50] Fluids such as normal saline or normal saline containing glucose should only be used if a more suitable polyelectrolyte solution is not available and if the I.V. fluids are critical to treat a patient in shock. If this less-desirable solution is used, complete ORS should be instituted as early as possible to replace the base and potassium not included in saline. 5% dextrose in water (D5W) is not suitable for a patient with cholera.

Treatment with intravenous fluids is recommended only for patients with severe dehydration and signs of hypovolemia. For these patients intravenous fluids are given to completely rehydrate the patient, and this can generally be accomplished within 2 to 4 h. After this complete initial rehydration most patients can be maintained with oral rehydration therapy, although about 10–15% of hospitalized patients may need an additional short course(s) of intravenous therapy due to high purging rate and recurrence of signs of dehydration. Generally, these patients who again become dehydrated while on oral rehydration therapy will be those whose purging rate is in excess of 10 ml/Kg/hour.[34]

Extensive experience indicates that a single intravenous solution may be used for all age groups with cholera, as well as with noncholera diarrhea, who require such I.V. rehydration. Except for the rare case of a complicated patient in which electrolyte balance has been compromised by inappropriate fluids already given, it is not necessary to tailor-make a solution for the individual patient. This saves a great deal of effort in not having to prepare separate solutions for individual patients and it allows paramedics and nurses (rather than physicians) to largely manage patients.

4. ANTIBIOTICS

4.1. Antibiotic Therapy of Patients

The purpose of giving antibiotics to cholera patients is to decrease the volume and duration of purging.[51,52] Antibiotics are not "life-saving" for cholera patients as they are for many other severe infections. In cholera the use of tetracycline will: (a) reduce the duration of diarrhea by about 50% to an average of about 2 days; (b) reduce the volume of diarrhea after initiation of treatment by about 60%; and (c) reduce the duration of vibrio excretion to an average of one day and a maximum of 48 h. Thus, the use of appropriate antibiotics lessens the expense and duration of treatment, which in turn allows for the treatment of more patients when supplies and personnel are limited. It also increases the success rate with oral rehydration therapy since such therapy need not be so prolonged.

Antibiotics are given orally and are usually started after completing initial rehydration, i.e., about 4 to 6 h after starting therapy in a dehydrated patient. It is neither urgent nor of additional benefit to use injectable antibiotics.

Tetracycline is the antibiotic of choice. The dose for adults is 500 mg every 6 h for 48 to 72 h (some use 250 mg every 6 h for 3 days) while the dose for children is 50 mg/kg/day in four divided doses for 48 to 72 h. Doxycycline, a long-acting tetracycline, can also be used in a single dose of 300 mg for adults and 4 to 6 mg per kg of body weight for children below 15 years of age.[53-55] Doxycycline may cause nausea but this is lessened considerably if patients eat some food before taking the drug.

If tetracycline cannot be used, one may use furazolidone, 100 mg every 6 h (for children, 5 mg/kg/day in four divided doses) for 72 h; erythromycin, 250 mg every 6 h (for children, 30 mg/kg/day in three divided doses) for 72 h; or trimethoprim-sulfamethoxazole (8 mg of trimethoprim and 40 mg of sulfamethoxazole per kg per day, in two divided doses for 72 h). For young children tetracycline syrup may not be available in some countries, in which case liquid preparations of furazolidone, erythromycin, or trimethoprim-sulfamethoxazole can be used. Sulfadoxine (fanasil) has been used in one dose for the treatment of cholera. However, resistance to it has been found in a few countries in Africa and potentially serious adverse reactions (e.g., Stevens–Johnson syndrome) can occur following a single dose. Chloramphenicol is also effective and can be given in the same dosage as tetracycline but it has no advantage over tetracycline and may have serious side-effects.

Though not an antibiotic, the use of cholera phage as a treatment for cholera should be mentioned.[56] Orally administered cholera phage have been tested as a way to eliminate the *V. cholerae* from the intestine of patients. Although the phage were safe and had an anti-vibrio biological effect, tetracycline was much more effective clinically, as well as being more practical.

4.2. Prophylactic Antibiotics

When cholera epidemics occur there is sometimes pressure to provide prophylactic antibiotics to family contacts of cholera patients and even to whole communities. Tetracycline or doxycycline, when given to family contacts, can prevent secondary cases from occurring.[57] The difficulty in giving prophylactic antibiotics, however, is in developing and implementing a policy of providing antibiotics to high-risk individuals selectively without giving massive amounts of antibiotics to whole communities. Prophylactic antibiotics for cholera can create enormous antibiotic pressure in the community leading to the emergence of antibiotic-resistant strains. While family contacts are at higher risk for developing cholera during an epidemic, treatment of family members would represent only a small fraction of those who will become infected. Also, the risk of cholera for those living in cholera-endemic areas extends over a prolonged time period and this also makes prophylactic antibiotics impractical. Considering the cost of such a program, it becomes even more impractical. Hence, the use of prophylactic antibiotics is not recommended.

4.3. *V. cholerae* Resistant to Multiple Antibiotics

Resistance of *V. cholerae* to tetracycline and other antibiotics has been reported from East Africa[58] and Bangladesh.[59] In these two geographic areas resistance was mediated by conjugative plasmids bearing resistance to multiple antibiotics; however, the resistance patterns of the strains from the two areas were different from each other. With time the epidemic strains seemed to disappear, to be replaced once again by sensitive ones. In Africa there had been excessive use of prophylactic tetracycline for cholera and it was postulated that this encouraged the emergence of the resistant strain.

Clinically, the presence of resistant strains may be suspected by an inadequate clinical response after administration of the antibiotic. Thus, it may be important to determine the antibiotic susceptibility of representative strains periodically and to be aware of the resistance pattern of the organism in adjacent geographical areas. Since *V. cholerae* which are resistant to one antibiotic are frequently multiply resistant, it is necessary to define the sensitivity pattern of the local strains to determine which of the effective antibiotics should be used.

5. ANTIDIARRHEAL AND ANTISECRETORY AGENTS

Kaolin, pectin, activated charcoal, and bismuth sub-salicylate have not been shown to be of value in the treatment of cholera. In one study charcoal interfered with the beneficial effect of tetracycline.[60] In another, a charcoal-gm1 ganglioside preparation which was documented to have bound lumenal cholera toxin was used in an attempt to block absorption of the toxin to the mucosa. This therapy led to a moderate reduction in the rate of purging in cholera patients, but only for a short period early in the illness.[61] Opiates and opiatelike compounds and other inhibitors of intestinal motility are useless and may be harmful in cholera.

There has been considerable enthusiasm for the development of antisecretory drugs which would, through an understanding of the cellular mechanisms of the secretory processes, turn off intestinal secretion in cholera patients. Such an effective antisecretory agent might simplify the treatment of the cholera patients since it would further shorten the duration of the illness and decrease the course of rehydration needed.

Several drugs have been shown to have an antisecretory effect in experimental animal studies, and some of these have been tested in patients. Chlorpromazine, a phenothiazine with antisecretory properties in animal models, also proved to significantly reduce the stool volume of cholera patients if they were rehydrated with and maintained on intravenous fluids and were not given antibiotics.[62,63] A follow-up study was carried out to determine if this physiologic observation could be confirmed using a study design in which chlorpromazine was added to a routine treatment regimen, including antibiotics and ORT. In this follow-up study there was no overall difference between treatment groups; though, there was a suggestion that chlorpromazine did have some antisecretory effect in severely purging children.[64] Unfortunately, children taking chlorpromazine also developed somnolence which interfered with the administration of oral rehydration fluid; hence, chlorpromazine is not recommended. If another phenothiazine could be identified which retains the antisecretory activity of chlorpromazine without producing somnolence, it might still be useful.

Berberine, an alkaloid used extensively as a traditional remedy in Asia for diarrhea, has also been shown to have an antisecretory effect in animal studies.[65] However, controlled clinical trials testing the effectiveness of the drug in patients with cholera have not been definitive. In two studies among adults with cholera or choleralike diarrhea it had either no effect upon the rate of stool output or reduced the rate minimally.[66,67] In another trial involving patients with enterotoxigenic *E. coli* diarrhea, it had a more markedly beneficial effect.[68] So far, it has had no side-effects which would limit its usefulness. Additional studies, perhaps using other dose schedules, are needed to determine if it has a clinical use in secretory diarrhea.

Other drugs that have been tested in patients include nicotinic acid,[69] aspirin,[70] indomethacin,[71] chloroquine,[71] and somatostatin.[72] Nicotinic acid showed a possible but marginal effect, but the others showed no benefit.

In summary, although antisecretory drugs could potentially assist in the treatment of cholera patients, none so far have proved to be of use in routine clinical management.

6. FEEDING DURING CHOLERA

Over the last 20 years a large number of studies have introduced early feeding as part of the standard treatment. Subsequently, a series of studies vindicated this clinical wisdom. This conclusion is based on the observation that food does not interfere with recovery from cholera, that it can be absorbed even during an episode of cholera, and that food may provide substrate for ORT.

Molla showed that children with cholera are able to eat and that the mean caloric intake during the acute phase was 75 calories per kg per 24 h. This increased to 111 calories per kg per 24 h two weeks later.[73] Further, he showed that macronutrients can be absorbed by children during cholera. 70% of the fat intake, 47% of the protein intake, 88% of the carbohydrate intake, and 81% of the calories (mean values) were absorbed during the acute phase of the illness. This increased two weeks later to 90%, 74%, 93%, and 91%, respectively.[74] Additionally, trypsin and amylase activities in adult cholera patients during a basal period and after a stimulation by Lund's test meal is well preserved during the acute phase of the disease.[75]

In a group of young children (1–2 years) with cholera, a nitrogen-balance study during the acute phase showed that a positive nitrogen balance could be promptly achieved with liberal milk feeding even before diarrhea was controlled, even in clinically severe cases. [76] Finally, in a controlled clinical trial, Dr. Khin Muang U, in Burma, compared a group of severely dehydrated children with cholera served with rice meals along with appropriate fluid therapy (initial I.V. followed by ORT) to a control group, who received no food for 24 h.[77] The group receiving rice meals showed a significant increase in the diarrhea stool output but demonstrated a better weight gain compared to the controls. Recovery was uneventful.

In conclusion, early liberal feeding of cholera patients assists nutritional recovery and is compatible with a rapid and uneventful recovery. The concept of early feeding appropriate for age is complimentary with that of the improved ORS. In both situations, additional substrates are provided early in the illness. In one case, they are provided for their nutritive value; in the other, they are provided to increase absorption of electrolytes and water. It may be that the introduction of appropriate food with the variety of nutrients thereby provided, may, in fact, convert the standard ORS into an improved ORS.

7. CLINICAL MANAGEMENT

7.1. Diagnosis and Assessment of Patients at a Treatment Center

The diagnosis of patients with severe cholera (*cholera gravis*) is usually not difficult because of the sudden and dramatic signs and symptoms. Patients usually come for treatment after only a few hours with diarrhea, vomiting, thirst and giddiness, and weakness. The onset is sudden and the diarrhea is generally described as painless, in contrast to shigellosis, in which defecation is associated with many cramps. The diarrhea stool is at first loose, then it becomes more watery and takes on the appearance of "rice water." Likewise the vomit has the same appearance. As the disease worsens and the dehydration becomes more severe, the patient's voice becomes weak, his level of consciousness fades, and he is too weak to hold himself upright. The breathing is noticeably labored. The patient may complain of a dry mouth, and urine flow stops.

On examination the cholera patient appears extremely weak, hoarse, and thirsty, often experiencing severe muscle cramps. There is evidence of dehydration, e.g., decreased skin turgor, sunken eyes, dry mucous membranes, and a weak or undetectable radial pulse. Kussmaul respirations may be evident. The dramatic aspect of the disease is the rapidity with which a healthy person can become so sick. The appearance is sometimes described as cadaveric.

The case described above is typical of cholera, but much less severe episodes of cholera are more common and the mild cases cannot be distinguished clinically from other acute watery diarrheal diseases. Also, a few other etiologic agents can also cause a *cholera gravis* syndrome, most notably the enterotoxigenic *E. coli*. For management of the individual patient, however, it is not necessary to know with certainty whether the acute diarrheal syndrome was due to a *Vibrio cholerae* or another agent. The rehydration therapy is the same.

The assessment of the patient with the acute dehydrating diarrhea syndrome consists of evaluating him for signs of dehydration, estimating the severity of the dehydration, and then estimating the fluid requirements. This must be accomplished rapidly since the severely dehydrated patient may literally be within minutes of death unless hydration is instituted immediately. One estimates the degree of dehydration through a clinical assessment of the signs of dehydration. Laboratory tests (hematocrit, plasma specific gravity, or serum proteins) are useful in research studies for comparing groups of patients, but the clinician must formulate a treatment plan for the individual patient based on the clinical examination.

As a guide, the severity of dehydration is categorized into four categories: none, mild, moderate, and severe. Patients with no objective signs of dehydration are categorized as "none" while realizing that at least 5% of the body weight must be lost before signs of dehydration develop. Patients with some evidence of dehydration, mildly decreased skin turgor, for example, will be categorized as having mild dehydration and their fluid deficit will be estimated at 5%. Moderately dehydrated patients, whose deficit is estimated at 7.5%,

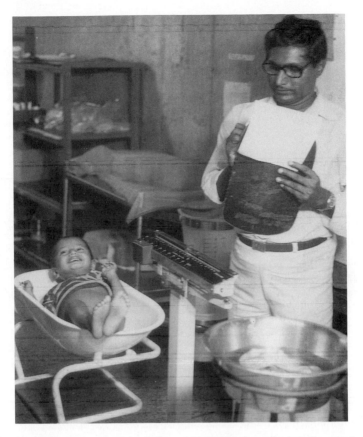

FIGURE 3. The photograph shows a simple scale for weighing babies immediately before rehydration begins. The weight gain during therapy is an excellent way to assess rehydration status.

have obvious signs of dehydration with dry mucous membranes, somewhat sunken eyes, and poor skin turgor. The radial pulse of these patients will be diminished and rapid, but will be palpable. Severely dehydrated patients, whose deficit is estimated at 10%, are extremely weak with poor level of consciousness, very poor skin turgor, very sunken eyes, and a barely perceptible or absent pulse. Although no one sign should be used to the exclusion of others, among the various signs of dehydration, many experienced clinicians find palpation of the radial pulse to be the most helpful in differentiating between moderate and severe dehydration. Skin turgor must be interpreted with caution in elderly patients or malnourished children since the skin may have lost its elasticity from the underlying condition.

To guide rehydration therapy and assist in the clinical follow up, each patient should be weighed on admission. This need take only a minute and is extremely helpful in calculating the patient's net fluid balance (Fig. 3).

7.2. Rehydration

Rehydration is the first form of treatment for a patient with cholera or with acute diarrheal dehydration of any etiology. For mild to moderate degrees of dehydration, this can generally be accomplished with oral rehydration, but patients with severe dehydration (i.e., with evidence of shock) need intravenous rehydration therapy. As a first step to therapy, one calculates the estimated volume needed to rehydrate the patient. A practical method to determine this volume is to first determine the patient's weight in kilograms and then estimate the percent dehydration. By multiplying the percent dehydrated by the body weight, one arrives at the volume of fluid required for rehydration. For example, a severely dehydrated adult weighing 40 kg will require four liters of rehydration fluid to correct dehydration (10% of 40 kg = 4 kg = 4 liters). Similarly a mildly dehydrated child weighing 10 kg will require 500 ml of rehydration fluid for initial rehydration.

When intravenous fluids are needed, they should be given rapidly to cholera patients in order to quickly restore circulating volume. As an approximate guide half the estimated volume of fluid requirement in a severely dehydrated patient should be given over the first hour, initially as fast as possible until radial pulse is palpable; such a patient should be fully hydrated in 2–4 h, at which time the I.V. line can be removed. Sometimes, it may be necessary to start an I.V. line at several sites simultaneously to restore circulation quickly. The composition of the appropriate I.V. fluids is displayed in Tables 3 and 4. As soon as the patient can tolerate oral fluids, administration of ORT can begin since usually the cholera patient will continue to pass watery stool and this loss must be replaced as soon as possible with oral solution. ORS is then used to continue to replace the ongoing stool losses as they occur until the diarrhea is over.

Oral rehydration, rather than intravenous, can be given both for initial rehydration as well as for replacement of ongoing fecal losses for most patients with mild or moderate dehydration. The composition of the oral rehydration salt solution is shown in Table 2.

Early in the treatment patients may continue to vomit and this may be a constraint to ORS administration. However, with persistence and with small, frequent feedings, most patients will retain enough fluid to become rehydrated. Small children may prefer teaspoon amounts at a time, while older patients can drink from cups. Usually family members (especially mothers) are the best providers of oral therapy solution, and nurses should primarily provide supervision, encouragement, and guidance to the family in the treatment of a patient rather than giving it themselves.

The adequacy of fluid replacement should be assessed by the following simple bedside methods: (1) return of pulse to normal strength and rate, the pulse rate will be below 90 per min in adults; (2) return of normal skin turgor, if skin turgor has returned to normal but pulse remains rapid, other causes of shock such as sepsis and cardiac infarction should be sought; (3) the return of a feeling of comfort to the patient with the disappearance of cyanosis, muscular cramps, nausea, and vomiting, children who are drowsy or in stupor may not become fully alert for 12–18 h despite adequate rehydration; (4) return of normal fullness to the neck veins; (5) weight gain, a severely dehydrated patient should gain 8–10% in body weight after rehydration, this is an especially useful guide in small children; (6) return of urine output, this usually occurs within 12–20 h of initial rehydration.

7.3. Maintenance Therapy

After the initial fluid and electrolyte deficit have been corrected (i.e., the signs of dehydration have disappeared), it is important to replace ongoing abnormal losses of fluids and electrolytes that are associated with continuing diarrhea—this is maintenance therapy. For severely dehydrated patients who receive I.V. fluids for rehydration, ORT should begin as soon as the patient can begin taking fluids. The principle is to provide ORS in a volume to match the volume of fluid lost by diarrheal stools and vomiting, and in addition, to provide hypotonic fluids for the body's normal daily fluid requirements. For older children and adults fluids normally consumed (e.g., water) can be given as desired in addition to ORS solution. For infants and young children breast feeding should be continued, and in non–breast fed babies other fluids should be offered at regular intervals.

Patients are most easily treated while lying on a cholera cot (see Fig. 4) since this allows collection and measurement of stool most efficiently. A calibrated bucket beneath the central hole in the cot, into which the stool collects, allows sufficiently accurate measurement of stool output to guide the subsequent administration of maintenance hydration. One simply measures the volume of the stool output periodically (e.g., every 4 h) and assures that an equivalent amount of oral rehydration solution is taken by the patient and that the rate of intake approximately matches the output. The patients should be given bedside urinals and instructed to pass urine separately from the stool. Children's beds can be similar to the adult cholera cots although separation of urine from stool in children is more difficult but will need to be estimated. A simple input–output chart at bedside (as shown in Fig. 5) should be maintained showing amounts of intravenous and oral solutions and the volume of stool output. In a few of the hospitalized cholera patients, signs of dehydration may recur while on oral maintenance therapy. If dehydration occurs, additional intravenous fluids are needed, following which oral maintenance should be resumed.

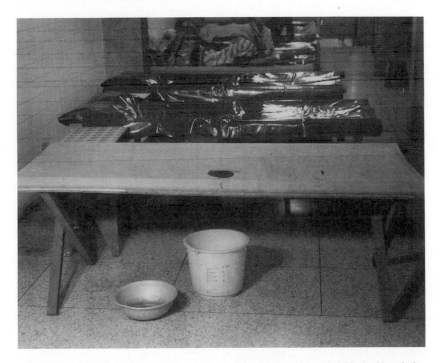

FIGURE 4. Maintenance of intake and output records as well as nursing care are simplified with a cholera cot. The cot in the foreground has the plastic sheet removed to show the simple construction. In the background are cots with the plastic sheets. A sleeve in the plastic sheet guides the diarrhea stool into a plastic bucket underneath the cot so that its volume can be measured periodically. Patients can be covered with a cotton sheet to maintain modesty. A vomit basin should also be available.

BEDSIDE INTAKE–OUTPUT CHART

Patient's name: _____ Number: _____

Date of admission: _____ Time of admission: _____

Age: _____ Sex: _____ Body Weight: _____ Kg

Initial Fluid Deficit _____ % Rehydration volume _____ ml

		Intake			Output			
Date	Time	I.V.	ORS	Other	Stool	Vomit	Urine passed (Y/N)	Net balance

FIGURE 5.

Antibiotics should be started within 3–6 h of starting fluid therapy as indicated earlier. Use of antibiotics conserves intravenous fluids and maximizes the use of the available ·hospital beds and substantially reduces demand on trained staff.

7.4. Diet

Cholera patients should be offered food appropriate for age during maintenance therapy with the choice of food guided by the patient's appetite (Fig. 6). Food should not be withheld from cholera patients; there is no benefit in "resting the bowel."

A summary of treatment for cholera patients is shown in Table 5.

8. COMPLICATIONS OF CHOLERA

Complications of cholera are rare if correct treatment is rapidly provided, since most complications result from delay in therapy or provision of inappropriate fluids. Case–fatality rates for cholera patients at the ICDDR,B is less than 0.5% and these low rates are re-

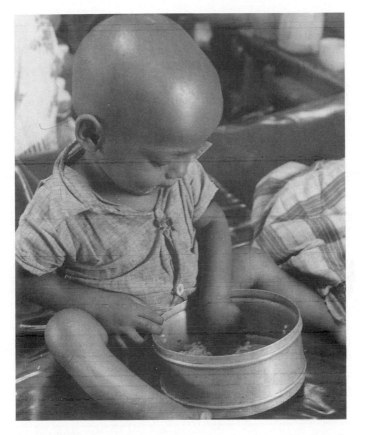

FIGURE 6. Feeding is an important part of the treatment of diarrhea patients. Usually patients can begin eating within a few hours of beginning treatment.

produced in other simple treatment centers. The few cholera patients who die are those who arrive at the treatment center after death has already occurred or are those whose death was due to another underlying condition or disease, e.g., malnutrition or pneumonia.

Complications that may be seen include the following:

1. Persistence or recurrence of signs of dehydration and hypovolemic shock. This may occur due to inadequate volume replacement. In a cholera patient the cause is almost always inadequate fluid replacement although other causes of shock should be kept in mind. Occa-

TABLE 5
Summary of Clinical Management of Cholera Patients

1. *Rehydrate:* Estimate degree of hydration and rapidly replace water and electrolytes already lost with appropriate oral or I.V. solution, depending on severity.
2. *Maintain hydration:* Replace ongoing abnormal stool losses with ORT and provide water for normal evaporative and urinary losses.
3. *Antibiotics:* Give to shorten the severity and duration of diarrhea.
4. *Nutrition:* Do provide food appropriate for age as soon as a patient is able to take it. Do not wait for the diarrhea to stop.

sional cholera patients will pass only small volumes of stool while accumulating intestinal secretions in their gut lumen. These patients with so called "cholera sicca" may develop signs of shock sometimes with a swollen abdomen suggestive of an acute peritonitis. These patients require rehydration with I.V. fluids to restore the circulating volume while waiting for stool to pass. A rectal tube may be helpful.

2. Persistence of vomiting. Vomiting is part of the cholera syndrome and can interfere with ORT. If it continues more than a few hours, it is likely due to the persistence of acidosis and/or hypovolemia. Usually, ORS can be given in small amounts frequently to maintain a positive balance, but if this is not possible, I.V. fluids should be used.

3. Acute renal failure.[78] Mildly elevated blood urea is seen commonly in cholera patients due to the dehydration (pre-renal azotemia), but acute renal failure is much less common than it was formerly because the usual treatment practice now includes rapid rehydration. When acute renal failure occurs it is usually seen in those who have had repeated or prolonged episodes of hypotension as a result of inadequate fluid replacement. This may happen for example, when there is a shortage of I.V. fluids or when the trip to the treatment center takes several hours and the patient receives just enough fluids on the way to keep him alive but not enough to restore circulating volume. When acute renal failure develops the patient should be treated for acute tubular necrosis by managing fluids and electrolytes. Dialysis may be required in a few patients. When the diuretic phase of the renal failure occurs, care must be given to insure adequate fluid intake to match urinary output. Unless the urine flow rate becomes excessively large, the hydration of these patients can be maintained with oral rehydration solution, though the electrolyte content of this solution will have to be adjusted to balance the urinary losses. Two percent glucose in the solution should still be used to facilitate absorption.

4. Hypokalemia. Hypokalemia may occur if the potassium losses of a heavily purging patient are not replaced by potassium in the rehydration fluids. Although rarely symptomatic in adults, it can cause severe symptoms in children, e.g., abdominal distension, paralytic ileus, urinary retention, muscular weakness, cardiac arrhythmias, and even death.

5. Overhydration. This results from excessive intravenous (or less commonly oral) fluid replacement and is manifested by swelling of the eye lids, full neck veins, slow full pulse. Excessive I.V. fluids can even lead to frank cardiac failure, but this has not occurred with ORT.

6. Acute pulmonary edema. Pulmonary edema can occur due to overreplacement of intravenous electrolyte solutions as mentioned above, but has been reported especially when the metabolic acidosis was left uncorrected (e.g., overuse of normal saline I.V. rather than an I.V. fluid with a base).[79]

7. Hypoglycemia. Normally, patients with cholera have a fall in their blood sugar during treatment for cholera. This is likely a nonspecific response to the correction of the stress. Severe hypoglycemia on the other hand occurs rarely, nearly always in children, and is usually manifested as the sudden onset of seizures. The mechanism of this complication is not understood, but it does not seem related necessarily to malnutrition. If seizures should occur, a blood sample should be obtained for glucose determination and an intravenous bolus of glucose should be given immediately (without waiting for the glucose results). If hypoglycemia is confirmed, the patient should continue on intravenous fluids with glucose, and follow-up blood samples should be obtained to document that blood-glucose levels are in a normal range.

8. Abortion and stillbirth. Women in the third trimester of pregnancy may abort if they become severely dehydrated. The treatment principles of pregnant women are the same as for other patients.

9. Fever. Rigor and fever occurring early in therapy may be due the administration of incorrectly prepared fluids or the repeated use of I.V. administration sets. This can be avoided by using pyrogen-free fluids and disposable administration sets.

During cholera epidemics other serious illnesses associated with diarrhea may be diagnosed clinically as cholera. Such illnesses may include meningitis, septic shock, myocardial infarction, and typhoid fever.

9. CHOLERA IN REMOTE AREAS

9.1. Rural or Community Diarrhea Treatment Centers

Treatment of severe diarrheal disease and cholera can be provided at relatively modest treatment centers. Examples of such treatment centers exist in several countries and may be, but do not have to be, associated with other hospitals. Oral therapy can be provided in the home for patients with no or mild dehydration (Fig. 7); however, there is no question that moderately dehydrated patients will receive more effective care in a treatment center where treatment can be supervised. In one example of a treatment center assisted by the ICDDR,B, a community provides a small house and trained volunteers (paid a subsistence salary) and these volunteers care for the patients. The ICDDR,B provides training to the volunteers (Fig. 8) and some logistic support, but the treatment center itself is nearly self-supporting from a small fee It receives from its patients. Another example of a treatment center is one operated as a unit of a hospital. Here under physician's overall supervision, paramedics treat the patients who visit. In both situations case–fatality rates for cholera have been the same as it is

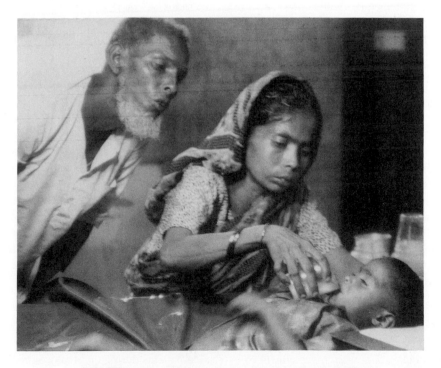

FIGURE 7. Oral rehydration therapy should involve the family.

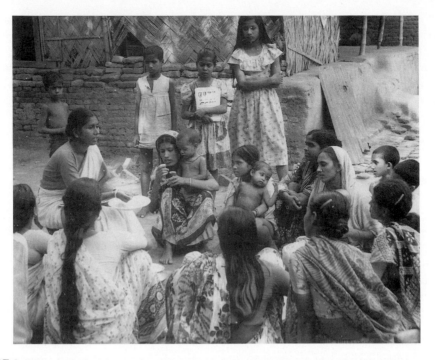

FIGURE 8. Oral rehydration therapy is a component of primary health care and should be taught to mothers everywhere. Shown here is a community health worker teaching a group of mothers in Bangladesh how to make ORS.

when physicians provide the care. The success of these treatment centers has depended on the training received by the paramedics and on continued logistic support (provision of rehydration supplies, antibiotics, and periodic in-service training) from physicians and other institutes, but the treatment provided can be extremely cost-effective.

9.2. Recognition of an Epidemic

Since cholera occurs most often in remote areas, and since surveillance systems for diarrheal disease are usually nonexistent in these areas, many outbreaks of cholera go undetected. Where surveillance systems have been established through clinic or hospital records for diarrhea, seasonal changes are noted frequently. Where such records are not kept, an outbreak is often detected when a cluster (2 or 3) of adults die of acute watery diarrhea. (In developing countries diarrhea-associated deaths in young children are all too common; hence, childhood diarrhea deaths often do not lead to outbreak investigations.) Other simple but more sensitive mechanisms are needed to identify cholera in remote areas and to transmit this information to central health authorities. Once identified, management of outbreaks can be relatively inexpensive and can prevent many unnecessary deaths.

9.3. Management of a Cholera Outbreak

Principles of clinical management of individual patients during outbreaks of cholera are the same as already described. If treatment centers are already established, efforts may have to be made to increase the inventory of rehydration supplies and to reorganize the medical staff to handle an increased load. If a treatment center is not available within a reasonable distance, an assessment will need to be made as to the advisability of establishing a temporary treatment center. For this, readers are referred to *"Guidelines for cholera control,* WHO/CDD/SER/80.4 REV.1(1986)" available from WHO.

If an outbreak is detected, a team should be formed to organize the available resources and provide treatment to the people. A plan for this organization may already be a part of a national diarrhea control program or it may have to be formulated by the health or community authorities. The team will have several functions: (1) to quickly assess the nature and severity of the problem; (2) to obtain the needed resources for establishing a treatment center if this is appropriate; (3) to work with the community leaders to assist with the cholera control plans; (4) to provide training to persons (usually local physicians and/or village volunteers) who will be providing care (Fig. 9); (5) to ensure that the surrounding people know of the availability of treatment; (6) to continue to assist the community by "trouble shooting." Records should be kept on these outbreaks to help in the monitoring of cholera and in assisting future teams with managing such situations.

Often the arrival of a team experienced in the treatment of cholera will help to allay the panic that understandably accompanies a cholera epidemic. The team will need to bring hydration supplies (I.V. and ORS packets) and antibiotics, and these can often be obtained through the Health Ministry. Most of the other resources are likely to be available in the community and one of the challenges for outbreak teams is to help the community to mobilize their own resources. Establishment of a treatment center can occur in nearly any facility. School buildings, community centers, huts, or houses can be used, and in some

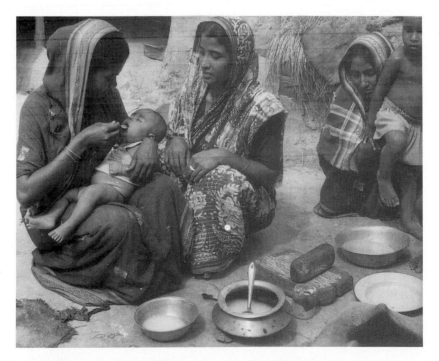

FIGURE 9. The best time to teach oral rehydration therapy is when it is needed. Here, a community health worker assists a mother in preparing and administering a rice-based, homemade solution and gives it to her child with diarrhea.

TABLE 6
Equipment and Supplies for a Makeshift Diarrhea Treatment Center[a]

Rehydration supplies
  240 liters I.V. polyelectrolyte solution, e.g., lactated Ringer's solution (480 bags
    of 0.5 liters each) with giving sets
  10 disposable syringes (5 or 10 ml)
  10 needles (18 g) for adults
  20 needles (21–23 g) for children
  10 scalp vein sets
  10 naso-gastric tubes (adult size 16 fr. 20 inch long, child size 8 fr. 15 inches
    long)
  1300 packets ORS (for one liter each)

Antibiotics
  For adults and older children: 3200 capsules tetracycline, 250 mgm (16 caps per
    case) or 600 caps doxycycline, 100 mg (3 caps per case) and furazolidone
    tablets (for pregnant women)
  For younger children: doxycycline syrup or furazolidone syrup

Other supplies
  Two large water dispensers with tap (marked at 5-, 8-, 10-liter intervals) for
    making ORS solution in bulk
  20 bottles (1 liter) for ORS solution (e.g., I.V. bottles)
  20 bottles (0.5 liter)
  40 tumblers, 200 ml
  3 kidney dishes
  5 spirit lamps
  Flashlights (2) (or hurricane lantern)
  Cotton (5 kg)
  Alcohol (250 ml)
  Adhesive tape (3 reels)
  Soap
  Disinfectant
  Bleaching powder

If possible
  Cholera cots (adults)
  Cholera cots (infant)
  Plastic drain sheets
  Plastic buckets
  Patient scales

---

[a]These suggestions are based on approximately 200 cases (typical for an outbreak in a total
population of 100,000) assuming that 40 cases will require initial intravenous fluid followed by
ORT and that the remaining 160 cases can be managed exclusively with ORT.

climates, no buildings are needed at all. A list of supplies for establishing a treatment center
is shown in Table 6.

Prophylactic antibiotics are not indicated during such outbreaks although persons should
be taught to drink safe water if possible. Boiled water is the safest water for drinking, though
this may not always be practical. Immunization with the current injectable cholera vaccine is
not a cost-effective way to control a cholera outbreak and such a program may divert effort
from more effective actions.

ACKNOWLEDGMENT. The photographs were taken by Mr. Asem Ansari of the International
Centre for Diarrhoeal Disease Research, Bangladesh.

REFERENCES

1. Editorial: Water with sugar and salt. *Lancet* ii:300–301, 1978
2. Reid EW: Intestinal absorption of solutions. *J Physiol (London)* 18:241–250, 1902
3. Barany EH, Sperber E: Absorption of glucose against a concentration by the small intestine of the rabbit. *Scand Arch Physiol* 81:290–297, 1939
4. Fisher RB, Parsons DS: Glucose movements across the wall of the rat small intestine. *J Physiol* 119:210–223, 1953
5. Riklis E, Quastel JH: Effects of cations on sugar absorption by isolated surviving guinea pig intestine. *Can J Biochem Physiol* 35:347–362, 1958
6. Schultz SG, Zalusky R: Ion transport in isolated rabbit ileum, II. the interaction between active sodium and active sugar transport. *J Gen Physiol* 47:1043–1059, 1964
7. Schedl HP, Clifton JA: Solute and water absorption by the human small intestine. *Nature (London)* 199:1264–1267, 1963
8. Malawar SJ, Enton M. Fordtran JS, et al: Interrelation between jejunal absorption of sodium glucose and water in man. *J Clin Invest* 44:1072, 1965
9. Levison RA, Schedl HP: Absorption of sodium, chloride, water and simple sugars in rat small intestine. *Am J Physiol* 211:939–942, 1966
10. Fordtran JS, Rector FC, Carter NW: The mechanism of sodium absorption in the human small intestine. *J Clin Invest* 47:1264–1267, 1968
11. Phillips RA: Water and electrolyte losses in cholera. *Fed Proc* 23:705–712, 1964
12. Phillips RA, Wallace CK, Blackwell RQ: Water and electrolyte absorption by the intestine in cholera, in: *Proceedings of the Cholera Research Symposium, Honolulu, Hawaii, Jan. 24–29.* U.S. Government Printing Office, Washington, D.C., 1965, pp 299–311
13. Phillips RA, Wallace CK, Blackwell: *Failure of an oral solution comparable to stool in volume and electrolyte composition to replace stool losses in cholera.* Research Report MR005.09-1040.1.14. US Naval Medical Research Unit No 2. September 24, 1963
14. Pierce NF, Banwell JG, Mitra RC, et al: Oral maintenance of water–electrolyte and acid–base balance in cholera: a preliminary report. *Indian J Med Res* 56:640–645 1968
15. Pierce NF, Banwell JG, Mitra RC, et al: Effect of intragastric glucose–electrolyte infusion upon water and electrolyte balance in Asiatic cholera. *Gastroenterol* 55:333–343, 1968
16. Hirschhorn N: Decrease in net stool output in cholera during intestinal perfusion with glucose containing solution. *N Engl J Med* 279:176–88, 1968
17. Carpenter CCJ, Sack RB, Feeley JC et al: Site and characteristics of electrolyte loss and effects of intraluminal glucose in experimental canine cholera. *J Clin Invest* 47:1210–1220, 1968
18. Cash RA, Nalin DR, Rochar T, et al: A clinical trial of oral therapy in a rural Cholera-Treatment Center. *Am J Trop Med Hyg* 19(4):653–656, 1970
19. Mahalanabis D, Choudhuri AB, Bagchi NG, et al: Oral fluid therapy among Bangladesh refugees. *Johns Hopkins Med J* 132:197–205, 1973
20. Pierce NF, Banwell JG, Mitra RC, et al: Oral replacement of water and electrolyte losses in cholera. *Indian J Med Res* 57:848–855, 1969
21. Nalin DR, Cash RA, Islam R, et al: Oral maintenance therapy for cholera in adults. *Lancet* ii:370–373, 1968
22. Nalin DR, Cash RA: Oral or nasogastric maintenance therapy for diarrhoea of unknown aetiology resembling cholera. *Trans Roy Soc Trop Med Hyd* 64:769–771, 1970
23. Pierce NF, Sack RB, Mitra RC, et al: Replacement of water and electrolyte losses in cholera by an oral glucose electrolyte solution. *Ann Intern Med* 70:1173–1181, 1969
24. Mahalanabis D, Sack RB, Jacobs B, et al: Use of an oral glucose electrolyte solution in the treatment of pediatric cholera—a controlled study. *J Trop Pediatr* 20:82–87, 1974
25. Sack DA, Chowdhury AKMA, Eusof A, et al: Oral hydration in rotavirus diarrhoea: A double-blind comparison with sucrose with glucose electrolyte solution. *Lancet* ii:280–283, 1978
26. *Oral Rehydration Therapy: An Annotated Bibliography.* 2nd Edition. Geneva World Health Organization/Pan American Health Organization (WHO/PAHO), 1983, pp 9–54
27. Rahaman MM, Aziz KMS, Patwari Y, et al: Diarrhoeal mortality in two Bangladeshi villages with and without community-based oral rehydration therapy. *Lancet* ii:809–812, 1979
28. Siewart M, Gnekow H: Uberdie stabilitat von glucose–elektrolyte–Mischungen (oral rehydration salts:ORS) zur therapie von Durchfallerrkrankungen. *Pharmazeutische Zeitung* 128:1169–1174, 1983
29. World Health Organization Diarrhoeal Diseases Control Programme (WHO/CDD): *Oral Rehydration Salts (ORS) Formulation Containing Trisodium Citrate.* WHO/CDD/Ser/84.7 Rev.1, 1985

30. Islam MR, Samadi AR, Ahmed SM, et al: Oral rehydration therapy: efficacy of sodium citrate equals to sodium bicarbonate for correction of acidosis in diarrhoea. *Gut* 25:900–904, 1984

31. Hoffman SL, Moechtar MA, Simanjuntak CH, et al: Rehydration and maintenance therapy of cholera patients in Jakarta: Citrate-based versus bicarbonate-based oral rehydration solution. *J Infect Dis* 152:1159–1165, 1985

32. Salazar-Lindo E, Sack RB, Chea-Woo E, et al: Bicarbonate versus citrate in oral rehydration therapy in infants with watery diarrhea: a controlled clinical trial. *J Pediatr* 108:55–60, 1986

33. Palmer DL, Koster FT, Rafiqul Islam AFM, et al: Comparison of sucrose and glucose in the oral electrolyte therapy of cholera and other severe diarrheas. *N Engl J Med* 297:21107–1110, 1977

34. Sack DA, Islam S, Brown KH, et al: Oral therapy in children with cholera: A comparison of sucrose and glucose electrolyte solutions. *J Pediatr* 96:20–25, 1980

35. Molla AM, Sarkar SA, Hossain M. et al: Rice-powder electrolyte solution as oral therapy in diarrhoea to *Vibrio cholerae* and *Escherichia coli. Lancet* i:1317–1319, 1982

36. Patra FC, Mahalanabis D, Jalan KN, et al: Is oral rice electrolyte solution to glucose electrolyte solution in infantile diarrhea? *Arch Dis Child* 57:910–912, 1982

37. Molla AM, Ahmed SM, Greenough WB III: Rice-based oral rehydration solution decreases the stool volume in acute diarrhoea. *Bull WHO* 63:751–756, 1985

38. Patra FC, Mahalanabis D, Jalan KN, et al: A controlled clinical trial of rice and glycine containing oral rehydration solution in acute infantile diarrhoea. *J Diar Dis Res* 4:16–9, 1986

39. Mahalanabis D, Merson M: Development of an improved formulation of oral rehydration salts (ORS) with antidiarrhoeal and nutritional properties: A "super ORS," in Holmgren J, Kindberg A, Mollby R (eds): *Development of Vaccines and Drugs against Diarrhoea.* Sweden, Studentlitteratur, 1986, pp 240–256

40. Alam AN, Sarker SA, Molla AM, et al: Hydrolysed wheat based oral rehydration solution for acute diarrhea. *Arch Dis Child* 62:440–444, 1987

41. Khin-Maung-U: *In vitro* determination of intestinal amino acid (^{14}C-L-glycine) absorption during cholera. *Am J Gastroenterol* 81:536–539, 1986

42. Nalin DR, Cash RA, Rahman M, et al: Effect of glycine and glucose on sodium and water absorption in patients with cholera. *Gut* 11:768–772, 1970

43. Patra FC, Mahalanabis D, Jalan KN: In search of a super solution: Controlled clinical trial of glycine–glucose oral rehydration solution in infantile diarrhoea. *Acta Paediatr Scand* 73:18–21, 1984

44. Patra FC, Sack DA, Islam A, Alam AN, Mazumder RN: Oral rehydration formula containing alanine and glucose for treatment of diarrhoea: a controlled trial. *Brit Med J* 298:1353–1356, 1989

45. Newsome PM, Burgess MN, Holman GD: Stimulation of ileal absorption by sodium citrate. *Scand J Gastroenterol* 18:119–121, 1983

46. Islam MR, Greenough WB, III, Rahman MN, et al: Labon-gur (common salt and brown sugar) oral rehydration solution in the treatment of diarrhoea in adults. *J Trop Med Hyg* 83:41–45, 1980

47. Ellerbrock TV: Oral replacement therapy in rural Bangladesh with some home ingredients. *Trop Doct* 11:179–183, 1981

48. Cash RA, Toha KMM, Nalin DR, et al: Acetate in the correction of acidosis secondary to diarrhoea. *Lancet* ii:302, 1969

49. Rahman MM, Majid MA, Monsur: Evaluation of two intravenous rehydration solutions in cholera and non-cholera diarrhoea. *Bull WHO* 57:977–981, 1979

50. Carpenter CCJ, Mondal A, Sack RB, et al: Clinical studies in Asiatic Cholera. H. Development of 2 : 1 saline lactate regimen: Comparison of this regimen with traditional methods of treatment. *Bull Johns Hopkins Hosp* 118:174–196, 1966

51. Greenough WB III, Rosenberg IS, Gordon RS, et al: Tetracycline in the treatment of cholera. *Lancet* i:355–357, 1964

52. Carpenter CCJ, Barua D, Sack RB, et al: Clinical Studies in Asiatic Cholera. IV. Antibiotic therapy in cholera. *Bull Johns Hopkins Hosp* 118:230–242, 1966

53. Rahman, MM, Majid MA, Alam AKMJ, et al: Effects of doxycycline in actively purging cholera patients: a double blind trial. *Antimicrob Agents Chemother* 10:610–612, 1976

54. Sack DA, Islam S, Rabbani H, et al: Single dose doxycycline for cholera. *Antim Chemother* 14:462–464, 1978

55. Alam AN, Alam NH, Ahmed T, Sack DA: Randomised double blind trial of single dose doxycycline for treating cholera in adults. *Brit Med J* 300:1619–1621, 1990

56. Monsur KA, Rahman MA, Huq F, et al: Effect of massize doses of bacteriophage on excretion of Vibrios, duration of diarrhoea and output of stools in acute cases of cholera. *Bull WHO* 42:723–732, 1970

57. Gupta PGS, Sircar BK, Mondal S, et al: Effect of doxycycline on transmission of *Vibrio cholerae* infection among family contacts of cholera patients in Calcutta. *Bull WHO* 56:323–326, 1978

58. Mhalu FS, Muari PW, Ijumba J: Rapid emergence of El Tor *Vibrio cholerae* resistant to antimicrobial agents during first six months of fourth cholera epidemic in Tanzania. *Lancet* i:345–347, 1979

59. Glass RI, Huq I, Alim ARMA, et al: Emergence of multiply antibiotic resistant *Vibrio cholerae* in Bangladesh. *J Inf Dis* 142:939–942,1980

60. Sack RB, Cassells J, Mitra R, et al: The use of oral replacement solutions in the treatment of cholera and other severe diarrhoeal disorders. *Bull WHO* 43:351–360, 1970

61. Stoll B, Holmgren J, Bardhan PK, et al: Binding of intraluminal toxin in cholera: trial of GM 1 ganglioside charcoal. *Lancet* ii:888–891, 1980

62. Rabbani GH, Greenough WB III, Holmgren J, et al: Chlorpromazine reduces fluid loss in cholera. *Lancet* i:410–412, 1979

63. Rabbani GH, Greenough WB III, Holmgren J, et al: Controlled trial of chlorpromazine as antisecretory agent in patients with cholera hydrated intravenously. *Brit Med J* 284:1361–1364, 1982

64. Islam MR, Sack DA, Holmgren J, et al: Use of chlorpromazine in the treatment of cholera and other severe acute watery diarrheal diseases. *Gastroenterol* 82:1335–40, 1982

65. Sack RB, Froehlich JL: Berberine inhibits intestinal secretory response of *Vibro cholerae* and *Escherichia coli* enterotoxin. *Infect Immun* 35:471–475, 1982

66. Butler T, Rabbani O, Knight J, et al: Antisecretory activity of berberine sulfate in acute cholera. *Clin Res* 32:511A, 1984

67. Khin-Maung-U, Myo-Khin, Nyunt-Nyunt Wai, et al: Clinical trial of berberine in acute watery diarrhoea. *Brit Med J* 290:1601–1605, 1985

68. Rabbani GH, Butler T, Knight J, et al: Randomized controlled trial of berberine sulfate therapy for diarrhea due to enterotoxigenic *Escherichia coli* and *Vibrio cholerae*. *J Infect Dis* 155:979–984, 1987

69. Rabbani GH, Butler T, Bardhan PK, et al: Reduction of fluid loss in cholera by nicotinic acid: a randomized controlled clinical trial. *Lancet* ii:1439–1442, 1939

70. Islam A, Bardhan PK, Islam MR, et al: A randomized double blind trial of aspirin versus placebo in cholera and non-cholera diarrhoea. *Trop Geogr Med* 38:221–225, 1986

71. Rabbani GH, Butler T: Indomethacin and chloroquin fail to inhibit fluid loss in cholera. *Gastroenterol* 89:1035–1037, 1985

72. Molla AM, Gyr K, Bardhan PK, et al: Effect of intravenous somatostatin on stool output in diarrhea due to *Vibrio cholerae*. *Gastroenterol* 87:845–847, 1984

73. Molla M, Molla AM, Sarkar SA, et al: Whole-gut transit time and its relationship to absorption of macronutrients during diarrhoeas and after recovery. *Scand J Gastroenterol* 8:537–543, 1983

74. Molla A, Molla AM, Rahim A, et al: Intake and absorption of nutrients in children with cholera and rotavirus infection during acute diarrhea and after recovery. *Nutr Res* 2:233–242, 1982

75. Molla A, Gyr K, Majid AM, et al: Preserved exocrine function in patients with acute cholera and acute non-cholera diarrheas. *Intern J Pancret* 1:259–264

76. Mahalanabis D: Nitrogen balance during recovery from secretory diarrhea of cholera in children. *Am J Clin Nutr* 34:1548–1551, 1981

77. Khin Muang U, Nyunt Nyunt Wai, Myo Khin, et al: Effect of boiled rice feeding in childhood cholera on clinical outcome. *Hum Nut Clin Nut* 40C:249–254, 1986

78. Benyajati C, Keoplug M, Beisel WR, et al: Acute renal failure in Asiatic cholera: clinicopathologic correlations with acute tubular necrosis and hypokalemic nephropathy. *Ann Int Med* 52:960–975, 1960

79. Greenough WB III, Hirschhorn N, Gordon RS Jr, et al: Pulmonary oedema associated with acidosis in patients with cholera. *Trop Geogr Med* 28:86–90, 1976

14

Immunity and Vaccine Development

Myron M. Levine and Nathaniel F. Pierce

1. INTRODUCTION

Public health authorities would like to have at their disposal a safe, practical, inexpensive, and highly effective vaccine to provide long-term protection against cholera. The Diarrheal Diseases Control Programme of the World Health Organization has targeted the development of an improved vaccine against cholera as a high priority.[1] Such a vaccine to combat cholera is not yet in the public health armamentarium but, as shown in this chapter, several promising candidates are on the horizon.

There are many reasons why high priority is being given to the development of an improved vaccine against cholera. Like most bacterial diarrheal diseases, the transmission of cholera occurs most readily in less-developed areas of the world where sanitation and hygiene are primitive or compromised. However, cholera is special in that it is one of the few diarrheal diseases that is capable of causing rapidly fatal dehydration in adults, as well as children. Furthermore, cholera typically occurs in explosive outbreaks and periodically in world-wide pandemics. While the case fatality-rate for cholera can be kept below 1%, even under field conditions, by the judicious use of oral and intravenous rehydration, stricken patients must first reach health-care facilities where there must be available sufficient quantities of rehydration supplies to cope with the demand and health workers trained to use these materials effectively. Unfortunately, these conditions are often not achieved in the least-developed areas of the world. For example, from sub-Saharan Africa there continue to appear reports of case fatality rates of 10–20% during cholera outbreaks.[2,3] For these reasons, public health authorities seek a highly effective, safe, practical, and inexpensive cholera vaccine that would provide long-lasting protection, especially against the severe forms of the

Cholera, edited by Dhiman Barua and William B. Greenough III. Plenum Medical Book Company, New York, 1992.

disease. Such a vaccine might be administered to infants in endemic areas through the auspices of national Expanded Programs on Immunization, but would also be used in older children and adults. Whether a vaccine would be useful in controlling epidemics, which are often explosive in onset but relatively brief, would need to be determined.

In this chapter the history of cholera vaccination will be reviewed and progress toward the development of several new cholera vaccines, some of which make use of the most modern techniques of biotechnology, will be described.

2. HISTORICAL ASPECTS

The first recorded attempt at vaccination against cholera was that of Ferran[4,5] in 1884, barely one year after the initial isolation of *Vibrio cholerae* by Koch.[6] Ferran's vaccine, which consisted of broth cultures containing "attenuated" vibrios, was inoculated parenterally into about 30,000 individuals who eagerly sought protection during the 1884 epidemic of cholera in Spain.[5,7] This experience generated much interest internationally, and commissions from several countries came to inspect and evaluate Ferran's work. Perhaps the most influential committee, that sponsored by the Pasteur Institute, Paris, criticized Ferran's vaccine and argued that no convincing proof was provided to support his claims for a prophylactic effect.[7] Furthermore, it was reported that Ferran's live vaccine was heavily contaminated with other microorganisms and that only a small proportion of the bacteria were *V. cholerae*[8,9]; this contamination may have accounted for the severe adverse reactions associated with this vaccine and its apparent lack of efficacy.[5,7]

Haffkine, who joined the Pasteur Institute in Paris in 1890 as an assistant to Roux, was asked by Pasteur in 1891 to carry out research to develop an immunizing agent against cholera.[7] Following Pasteur's general dictum that live vaccines elicit better protection than do killed-microorganism vaccines, Haffkine prepared two modified *V. cholerae* strains for use as live vaccines. The first strain was attenuated by growth at 39°C with continuous aeration; in contrast, the second strain underwent multiple intraperitoneal passages in guinea pigs in an attempt to increase its pathogenicity. Following Pasteur's example, Haffkine utilized these strains sequentially as parenteral immunizing agents; the attenuated strain was inoculated first, followed six days later by the strain of enhanced virulence. Typical side reactions following vaccination included fever, malaise, headache, and pain and swelling at the injection site. Uncontrolled trials with this vaccination regimen were carried out by Haffkine in different sites in India in 1893 and 1894, involving 42,197 individuals and from 1895 to 1896 involving an additional 30,000 persons.[10-12] However, the most important applications of his vaccine involved relatively small groups of individuals residing in prisons and on tea plantations[10-12]; some authorities believe that these were the first attempts to determine vaccine efficacy by controlled field trials.[12] As reviewed by Cvjetanovic,[12] Haffkine concluded that to properly assess the efficacy of his cholera vaccine, equally sized groups of individuals, who are randomly allocated to receive vaccine or to serve as unimmunized controls, and who are at essentially identical risk of exposure to natural infection, should be compared. In his later vaccinations, Haffkine abandoned the initial inoculation with the "attenuated" vibrio and administered to humans only the pathogenic strain, without an increase in adverse reactions. Although statistical analysis suggested that the vaccines were efficacious, notable drawbacks to Haffkine's vaccine included difficulty in standardizing it and in producing it in large quantities.[8,13]

In 1896, Kolle[8,13] recommended the use of agar-grown, heat-inactivated whole *V.*

cholerae organisms for parenteral immunization. This nonliving vaccine was notably easier to prepare and to standardize and so it eventually replaced Haffkine's live parenteral vaccine; by 1911 Haffkine was also utilizing inactivated vibrios as a vaccine with 0.5% phenol as a preservative. Kolle-type vaccines were first used on a large scale during the 1902 cholera epidemic in Japan.[14]

The use of nonliving whole cell *V. cholerae* as oral vaccines in humans also had an early start, with the first report published in 1893[15] describing the oral immunization of two investigators and a student with multiple doses containing billions of inactivated vibrios. In the 1920s and 1930s, field trials of a killed oral *V. cholerae* vaccine combined with bile (the so-called bilivaccine) were carried out in India[16-18] and in Indochina[19] with significant protection apparently having been achieved. In the Indian trials the oral vaccine was also compared with a parenteral, killed whole-cell vaccine. However, it is not certain that the vaccine and control (nonvaccinated) groups were properly randomized to achieve equal risk of infection. Nevertheless, the oral bilivaccine provided 82% protection and the parenteral vaccine 80% protection during the period of surveillance.[16-18] The bilivaccine was administered in a total of three doses on consecutive days; the vaccinee first ingested a bile tablet followed in 15 min by a bilivaccine tablet containing 70 billion dried vibrios. Because of the bile component, the bilivaccine commonly caused adverse reactions, including nausea, vomiting, and acute diarrhea; presumably as a consequence of these reactions, further work with the bilivaccine was abandoned.

The next few decades represented a relatively quiet period in cholera vaccine research, as the inactivated whole-cell parenteral vaccines were widely used during the 1940s and 1950s in military and civilian populations. In the 1960s there occurred a resurgence in cholera vaccine research culminating in a series of carefully executed, controlled field trials in Bangladesh and the Philippines that assessed the efficacy of the parenteral killed whole-cell and other vaccines.

3. DEMONSTRATION OF INFECTION-DERIVED IMMUNITY

Among bacterial diseases cholera is now recognized as one of the most striking examples wherein an initial clinical infection gives rise to a high level of enduring protection. However, this was not well appreciated until challenge studies were carried out in volunteers. Cash *et al.*[20] first demonstrated that an initial infection with classical *V. cholerae* 01, Inaba serotype, provides solid protection for at least one year against rechallenge with the homologous organism. Levine *et al.*[21-25] expanded these observations to show that an initial clinical infection with classical biotype *V. cholerae* 01 provides 100% protection against illness following rechallenge with classical biotype organisms of either serotype and that this protection persists for at least three years,[24] the longest duration tested; these investigators also showed that an initial clinical infection with El Tor biotype *V. cholerae* 01 provided 90% protection against rechallenge with El Tor organisms of either Inaba or Ogawa serotype.[23,24] One difference between the classical and El Tor *V. cholerae* 01 revealed by these studies is that in homologous rechallenge experiments involving the former, it was not possible to recover vibrios in direct cocultures of rechallenged volunteers.[21] In contrast, it was possible to cultivate *V. cholerae* 01 from cocultures of approximately one third of the volunteers who were challenged and subsequently rechallenged with El Tor vibrios[23,25] (Table 1). It is not clear whether these results reflect a lesser immune stimulation by El Tor vibrios or whether this biotype is better able to survive in small numbers in the intestinal tract

TABLE 1
Protective Efficacy Conferred by Prior Clinical Infection with Pathogenic *Vibrio cholerae* 01
of Classical or El Tor Biotype

Immunizing *V. cholerae* biotype	Attack rate for diarrhea[a]		Protective efficacy	Isolation of *V. cholerae* from direct coprocultures	
	Controls	"Vaccinees"[b]		Controls	"Vaccinees"
Classical	24/27 (89%)	0/16 (0%)	100%	26/27 (96%)	0/16 (0%)
					p = 0.012
El Tor	32/37 (86%)	2/22 (9%)	90%	34/37 (92%)	8/22 (36%)

[a]Challenge with 10^6 pathogenic *V. cholerae* 01 given with $NaHCO_3$.
[b]Includes both serotype-homologous and serotype-heterologous challenges. Volunteers who developed diarrhea following ingestion of *V. cholerae* 01 on initial challenge were rechallenged 4–6 weeks later with *V. cholerae* 01 of either the same or the heterologous serotype within the identical biotype.

in the presence of antagonistic normal colonic flora,[26] thus allowing the challenge organism to be recovered in coprocultures.

From Bangladesh, Woodward[27] reported the occurrence of 14 bacteriologically proven cases of cholera reinfection, seven of which were subclinical. Woodward interpreted these data as suggesting that in rural Bangladesh cholera is not a highly immunizing disease; however, it was not clear from this report what rate of infection was expected and whether the rate of reinfection was similar or less. Subsequently, Glass *et al.*[28] examined data from the same area of Bangladesh, Matlab Bazaar, using a life-table analysis technique and concluded that an initial episode of clinical cholera is indeed a very potent immunizing event that diminishes by approximately 90% the risk of a second clinically apparent infection.

Taken together, these demonstrations of the magnitude and duration of infection-derived immunity, observed in an endemic area and in volunteers, indicate what should be expected of an ideal cholera vaccine with respect to both the level and duration of achievable protection.[25] It is against this yardstick that the efficacy of past, present, and future cholera vaccines will be measured in this chapter.

4. ANTITOXIC VERSUS ANTIBACTERIAL IMMUNITY

Recognizing the strong, long-lived immunity that occurs following cholera, even in immunologically naive persons from nonendemic areas,[20–25] it is appropriate to ask against what antigens of *V. cholerae* 01 the immune response is directed. The clinical syndrome of cholera gravis has been evoked in volunteers by the oral administration of highly purified cholera enterotoxin in single doses as low as 5.0 μg.[25] That observation suggests that the *V. cholerae* 01 organism serves as a sophisticated delivery system for cholera toxin and that neutralizing antitoxin present at the mucosal surface might, therefore, be able to prevent the clinical manifestations of cholera gravis. On the other hand, the observation that *V. cholerae* 01 is only rarely recovered from coprocultures of rechallenged volunteers[21,25] suggests the presence of competent protective mechanisms that interfere with bacterial survival or growth. This may be due largely to interference with the process of mucosal colonization in the small intestine. If *V. cholerae* 01 are prevented from colonizing the small intestine they cannot proliferate and elaborate toxin; if they are then removed by peristalsis to the large intestine, the vibrios may be unable to survive in the unfavorable environment created there by the indigenous bowel microflora.

Considerable direct and indirect evidence from epidemiologic studies,[29-48] research using animal models,[49-74] and studies of experimental cholera in volunteers[20-25,75] points to the existence of both antibacterial and antitoxic immunity and further suggests that the most complete immunity achievable probably involves a synergistic interplay between antitoxic and antibacterial immune mechanisms.[48,70-73]

4.1. Protective Mechanisms against Cholera: Inferences from Volunteer Studies and Field Trials

4.1.1. Antibacterial Immunity

Both volunteer studies and field trials provide incontestable evidence that antibacterial immune mechanisms by themselves can provide significant protection against cholera. In volunteers, killed whole-cell vaccines administered either parenterally[20] or orally[20,76] have, in comparison with unimmunized controls, significantly reduced attack rates, and the severity of clinical illness was also reduced after oral vaccination. Perhaps the most compelling evidence comes from volunteer studies[75] involving the oral administration of a genetically engineered vaccine strain, JBK 70, from which the genes encoding both the A and B subunits of cholera toxin were deleted by recombinant DNA techniques.[77] A single dose of this live oral vaccine (*vide infra*) colonized the intestine, elicited very high levels of vibriocidal antibody in serum (but no antitoxin response), and provided significant protection against subsequent challenge with a wild toxigenic strain of *V. cholerae* 01.[75]

Similarly, in controlled field trials, killed whole-cell vaccines administered parenterally [31-47] or orally,[48] which evoke no antitoxin response, have provided significant protection against cholera. These observations all support a fundamental role for antibacterial immune mechanisms in protection against cholera.

4.1.2. Antitoxic Immunity

The induction of antitoxin by immunization with purified cholera toxin, or toxoids derived from the toxin, may be similarly regarded as a direct way of answering the question of the protective role of pure antitoxic immunity. Although cholera occurs naturally only in humans and all the available animal models are subject to some criticisms, studies in animal models have provided insights that have sometimes proven helpful in guiding the development of cholera vaccines. For example, studies in animals have shown that high levels of serum antitoxin, induced by parenteral immunization with toxin, toxoids, or B subunit, were protective but the protection was short-lived as the serum antitoxin declined rapidly.[59-62,68] Further studies showed that intestinal secretory antitoxin was also protective against experimental cholera and that such a response could be induced safely in animals using the purified B subunit of cholera toxin given orally or enterally.[59-61,63-69]

In man, two separate field trials of parenteral toxoid vaccines in Bangladesh[78] and the Philippines[79] provided little, if any, evidence of protection. Similarly, a glutaraldehyde cholera toxoid administered by oral or enteral routes to North American volunteers was not protective under experimental challenge conditions.[21,22,25] In contrast, oral B subunit, given in conjunction with oral, killed whole-vibrio vaccine, evoked significant serum and intestinal antitoxin responses and significantly enhanced the protective effect of an oral, killed whole-cell vaccine during the first six months of observation in a large-scale field trial in Bangladesh[48] (Table 2). However, this enhancing effect was not detectable beyond the first six months of surveillance[80,81] (Table 2). To further support the argument for the existence of antitoxic immunity in man, in the same field trial in Bangladesh, it was found that the B subunit/whole-vibrio combination vaccine also provided significant protection against diarrhea due to *Escherichia coli* that elaborate heat-labile enterotoxin (LT), a toxin closely related antigenically to cholera toxin.[82]

4.1.3. Synergy of Antibacterial and Antitoxic Immunity

Considerable evidence has been generated from several groups of investigators working with different animal models that shows that when bacterial and toxin-derived antigens are combined for immunization, the level of protection observed is greater than what can be achieved by each antigen alone; moreover, the protection induced by the antigen combination is not just additive but is synergistic.[67,70–73]

Synergistic protection is believed to be operative in man, although there is little direct evidence to support this contention. The strongest evidence comes from the recent, controlled field trial in Bangladesh[48] where, during the first six months of surveillance, persons immunized with the combination vaccine consisting of inactivated vibrios plus purified B subunit had a significantly lower attack rate from cholera than participants who received only the inactivated vibrios. However, it cannot be definitively ascertained whether the short-term superiority of the combination vaccine was due to an additive or a synergistic effect over antibacterial immunity, since a group immunized only with oral B subunit was not included in the trial. In volunteer studies with these two vaccines a significant advantage was not detected for the combination vaccine.[76]

4.2. The Protective Antigens of *V. cholerae*

4.2.1. Inferences from Seroepidemiology

4.2.1.1. Vibriocidal Antibody and Protection

V. cholerae 01 is a noninvasive enteropathogen that colonizes the mucosal surface without invading enterocytes or destroying brush borders. It is reasonable to conclude, therefore, that protection against cholera is mediated almost entirely by antibodies that reach the mucosal surface, most of which would be locally produced secretory antibodies of the IgA type. Therefore, it is curious that the level of serum vibriocidal antibody correlates so strongly with protection. Studies in rural Bangladesh have shown that the prevalence and the geometric mean titer of naturally acquired vibriocidal antibody increases with age, as the incidence of cholera falls.[36,37] For every two-fold increase in geometric mean vibriocidal titer, the incidence of cholera falls by approximately one-half.[36,37] Vibriocidal antibody in unvaccinated rural Bangladeshis is presumed to be derived from subclinical and mild infections. The relationship between vibriocidal titer and protection against cholera also holds for parenteral whole-cell cholera vaccines tested in endemic areas.[37,39]

Glass *et al.*[30] carried out prospective family-based studies in rural Bangladesh to assess the rates of *V. cholerae* 01 colonization and of clinical cholera in family contacts of index

TABLE 2

Occurrence of Cholera after 6, 12, and 36 Months of Surveillance of Recipients of Oral B Subunit/Whole-Cell Combination Vaccine (BS/WCV), Oral Whole-Cell Vaccine (WCV) Alone, or Placebo, in a Large-Scale Randomized, Controlled Field Trial in Bangladesh

Group	Subjects	1st 6 mos.			1st 12 mos.			1st 36 mos.		
		No. cases	Incidence per 10^4	Vaccine efficacy	No. cases	Indicence per 10^4	Vaccine efficacy	No. cases	Incidence per 10^4	Vaccine efficacy
BS/WCV	21,141	4[a]	1.89	85%	41[b]	19.4	63% (62–94)[c]	131	619.6	50.8% (39–60)
WCV	21,137	11[d]	5.20	58% (14–79)	52[e]	24.6	53% (34–66)	127	600.8	52.3% (41–61)
Placebo	21,120	26[f]	12.25		110[g]	52.1		266	1259.5	

[a] BS/WCV vs. placebo at 6 mos., p <0.0001; BS/WCV vs. WCV at 6 mos., p <0.04.
[b] BS/WCV vs. placebo at 12 mos., p <0.0001; BS/WCV vs. WCV at 12 mos., NS.
[c] 95% confidence intervals of vaccine efficacy.
[d] WCV vs. placebo at 6 mos., p <0.01.
[e] WCV vs. placebo at 12 mos., p <0.0001.

cases, in relation to preexisting levels of vibriocidal antibody. Both colonization and clinical cholera were significantly more common in persons with low circulating titers of vibriocidal antibody (reciprocal titer <20) than in family members with higher titers, and the relationship was independent of age.

Most authorities believe that vibriocidal antibody in serum is not by itself protective against cholera but is rather a marker for the existence of intestinal antibodies which may be directed against the same antigenic specificities as the serum vibriocidal antibodies. Therefore, an analysis of vibriocidal antibodies may offer some insight into identification of the critical antigens involved in protection against cholera.

Most of the vibriocidal antibodies are directed against lipopolysaccharide antigens of *V. cholerae* 01.[25,50,70,71,83] Nevertheless, there also exist, albeit in lesser amount, vibriocidal antibodies directed against protein antigens of the bacterial surface.[25,50,83,85] Unfortunately, the precise nature of these protein antigens is still not clear, despite considerable research on the subject.[25,83,84,85] In endemic areas vibriocidal antibodies are present in both mercaptoethanol-sensitive (IgM) as well as in mercaptoethanol-insensitive (IgG/IgA) fractions.[86–88] In contrast, that small percentage of persons from nonendemic areas, such as Czechoslovakia and the U.S., who have naturally occurring low titers of vibriocidal antibody,[79,89] generally have it solely within the IgM class.[79]

The environment of the gut is not usually considered to be compatible with the action of vibriocidal antibodies, at least as mediated by the usual complement-dependent mechanisms.[90] Furthermore, SIgA is not usually thought to be involved in bactericidal actions. Nevertheless, there are reports of the occurrence of vibriocidal antibodies within intestinal fluids and bile.[91–94]

4.2.1.2. Anti-LPS and Protection

Some experiments in animal models show that anti-LPS antibodies play a role in preventing adhesion of *V. cholerae* 01 to the gut mucosa[95,96] suggesting that this might be a mechanism of action of such antibodies in the human intestine. Based on work in animal models, Holmgren and Svennerholm[68] concluded that virtually the entire antibacterial component of immune sera was directed against LPS and could be removed by absorption with purified LPS.

However, the family-based studies of Glass *et al.*[30] showed no correlation between the level of serum IgM anti-LPS antibody and protection against colonization or against clinical cholera in family contacts of index cholera cases. Rather, when exploring the components in breast milk that were protective against cholera in breast-fed children in Bangladesh, Glass *et al.*[31] found an inverse correlation between the titer of SIgA anti-LPS antibodies in breast milk and the development of cholera. Interestingly, the presence of high titers of SIgA anti-LPS antibody in breast milk did not appear to prevent intestinal colonization with *V. cholerae 01*.

Further evidence for a protective role for LPS antibodies comes from a field trial in which individuals immunized with a parenteral vaccine consisting of purified LPS were significantly protected against clinical cholera, in comparison with unimmunized controls[39] (Table 3).

4.2.1.3. Antitoxin and Protection

Following clinical cholera, including experimental cholera in North American volunteers, a substantial serum IgG antitoxin response occurs and persists for several years.[97–100] Considerable data from a series of studies in animal models suggest that antitoxin can neutralize the biological effects of cholera toxin *in vivo.*[59–69] Curiously, however, seroepidemiological studies do not show a correlation of serum antitoxin with protection. Studies by Benenson *et al.*[97] in East Pakistan (now Bangladesh) first noted that, in contrast with vibriocidal antibody, the prevalence and titer of serum antitoxin do not progressively increase with age in inverse correlation with the incidence of cholera. Other seroepidemiological studies have since confirmed those early results. Most recently, family-based studies have failed to show protection against development of cholera in contacts who have high levels of serum antitoxin.[29]

In contrast, it has been found that protection of breast-fed children against cholera is highly correlated with the presence of SIgA antitoxin in breast milk.[30] This suggests that local SIgA antitoxin, rather than serum antitoxin, may be the mediator of antitoxic protection and that serum antitoxin levels may not necessarily predict the capacity for mucosal antitoxin production.

4.2.2. Newly Identified, Possible Protective Antigens of *V. cholerae* 01

In animal models several vibrio surface antigens have been shown to be protective including LPS, flagellar protein, flagellar sheath protein, and a cell-associated hemag-glutinin.[55–58,74] As reviewed by Levine *et al.*,[25] many antigens have been proposed to function as the colonization factor of *V. cholerae* 01, usually without strong supportive data. In 1987, however, Taylor *et al.*[101] convincingly described a fimbrial antigen of *V. cholerae* 01 that is almost certainly the long-sought colonization factor. This pilus (fimbrial) antigen is composed of subunits, is 6–7 nm in diameter, and is not associated with hemagglutination (Fig. 1). Notably, along with the structural genes encoding the A and B subunits of cholera toxin (*ctxAB*), the expression of these pili is controlled by the same regulator gene, *toxR,* that controls expression of cholera toxin[102]; this accounts for the name given to the fimbriae: TCP, for toxin coregulated pilus. Culture conditions that increase production of cholera toxin also increase expression of TCP.[103] Volunteer studies by Herrington *et al.*[104] have confirmed the role of these pili as a colonization factor in man. Volunteers were fed genetically engineered mutants in which either the *toxR* gene (strain JJM443[101]) or the *tcpA* structural gene (strain TCP2[105]) was inactivated, resulting, respectively, in vibrios that had a greatly diminished or a total lack of expression of TCP. These mutants were unable to colonize the human intestine; in contrast, the parent strain from which they were derived, 0395-N1, a genetically engineered A⁻B⁺ mutant of classical Ogawa 395, readily colonized volunteers.[104]

5. THE INTESTINAL SECRETORY IMMUNE SYSTEM AND IMMUNIZATION AGAINST CHOLERA

It is not appropriate in this chapter to provide an extensive general review of the secretory immune system of the intestine; such reviews exist elsewhere.[90,106] However, recent advances in vaccination against cholera have paralleled and benefited from increasing knowledge of the intestinal secretory immune system. Therefore, a brief summary is provided of relevant aspects of the intestinal secretory immune system as it relates to immunization against cholera. This includes consideration of how to prime and boost intestinal immunity, mucosal immunologic memory, the cell types involved in a SIgA response, and the mechanisms by which SIgA antibodies mediate protection.

TABLE 3
Summary of Controlled Field Trials of Efficacy of Parenteral Inactivated Whole-Cell and Bacterial Vaccines[a]

| Site & dates | Vaccine (no. of doses) | Age group (years) | No. inoculated | | Period of surveillance (months) | Incidence of cholera/10³ | | Percent vaccine efficacy |
			Cholera vaccine	Control vaccine		Vaccinees	Controls	
Bangladesh 1963–1966[33,34]	Classical Inaba + Ogawa whole cell (one dose)	0–9	2,777	2,834	0–6	2.2	9.1	77
					17–18	6.1	13.3	55
					19–30	1.8	2.5	29
		≥ 10	4,179	4,264	0–6	0.5	1.7	71
					7–18	0.5	2.8	82
					19–30	0.2	0.7	71
Bangladesh 1964–1966[34]	Classical Inaba + Ogawa whole cell (one dose)	0–9	3,304	3,381	0–8	3.0	10.9	72
					9–20	1.5	2.4	60
		≥ 10	5,153	5,072	0–8	0.6	2.0	70
					9–20	0.4	0.4	0
Bangladesh 1964–1966[34]	Purified Ogawa LPS (one dose)	0–9	3,304	5,702	0–8	7.6	10.9	30
					9–20	3.6	2.4	33
		≥ 10	5,153	5,072	0–8	0.4	2.0	80
					9–20	0.4	0.6	33
Bangladesh 1966–1967[38,40]	Classical Inaba + Ogawa whole cell (one dose)	0–4	3,818	3,793	0–3	2.9	4.2	31
					4–7	1.3	1.3	0
		5–14	6,202	6,130	0–3	0.3	1.6	81
					4–7	0.3	0.7	51
	(two doses)	0–4	7,636	3,793	0–3	0.4	4.2	91
					4–7	1.4	1.3	8

Location / years	Vaccine	Age (yr)	No. vaccinated	No. controls	Period			% protection
Bangladesh 1968–1969[39,41]		5–14	12,283	6,130	0–3	0.4	1.6	75
					4–7	0.5	0.7	25
	Monovalent classical Ogawa whole cell (one dose)	0–4	4,145	4,145	0–7	4.8[b]	4.3[b]	0
		5–14	7,346	7,285	0–7	1.6	2.6	38
	Monovalent classical Inaba whole cell (one dose)	0–4	4,180	4,145	0–7	0.5	4.3	89
		5–14	7,255	7,285	0–7	0.0	2.6	100
	Purified Inaba LPS/protein antigen (one dose)	0–4	4,143	4,145	0–7	1.2	4.3	72
		5–14	7,272	7,285	0–7	0.3	2.6	88
Philippines 1964–1965[42,43]	Classical Inaba + Ogawa whole cell (one dose)	0–70[c]	145,500	146,800	0–18	0.9[d]	1.2[d]	23
	El Tor Inaba + Ogawa whole cell (one dose)	0–70	148,100	146,800	0–18	0.8	1.2	35
	Classical vibrios + oil adjuvant (one dose)	0–70	143,600	146,800	0–18	0.6	1.3	50
Indonesia 1973–1975[47]	Classical Inaba + Ogawa whole cells (one dose)	1–70[e]	156,300	158,500	0–6	0.12	0.23	51
					7–12	0.12	0.19	35
					13–18	0.11	0.22	49
	Inaba/Ogawa whole cells absorbed to aluminum hydroxide adjuvant (one dose)	1–70[e]	155,600	158,500	0–6	0.06	0.23	73
					7–12	0.13	0.19	32
					13–18	0.09	0.22	49
India 1975–1977[46]	Classical Inaba/Ogawa whole cells adsorbed to aluminum phosphate	1–4	7,159	7,132	0–12	0.14	1.26	89
					13–18	0.0	0.42	100
					19–24	0.28	0.28	0
		>5	93,937	93,898	0–12	0.18	0.42	56
					13–24	0.16	0.23	30

[a] This is not a comprehensive list of all field trials but is a selected summary to illustrate major points in the text.
[b] Classical Inaba cases only.
[c] 72% < 25 years of age.
[d] El Tor cases only.
[e] 60% < 25 years of age.

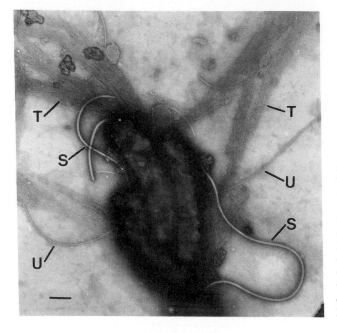

FIGURE 1. This electron photomicrograph of *Vibrio cholerae* 01 classical Ogawa strain 395 shows TCP fimbriae (T) (pili) bundles emanating from the surface of the vibrios. The individual fimbrial filaments are 6-7nm in diameter and can reach 10-15 micrometers in length. Also demonstrated are sheathed (S) and unsheathed (U) flagellae (Bar=200nm). Photomicrograph courtesy of Dr. Robert Hall, Center for Vaccine Development, University of Maryland School of Medicine.

The intestine is a major immunologic organ, having within its lamina propria as many lymphoid cells as the spleen. Among these are B lymphocytes, T lymphocytes (involved in modulating the immune response), and plasma cells (most of which produce dimeric secretory IgA, SIgA). Peyer's patches are follicular aggregations of lymphoid cells present in the submucosa. The epithelium overlying the Peyer's patches contains M cells, which are specialized for sampling antigen from the gut lumen and presenting it to underlying lymphocytes and macrophages in the patches.

In individuals immunologically naive to a specific antigen, ingestion of that antigen results in its uptake by the Peyer's patches and interaction with B lymphocytes capable of responding to the antigen. These lymphocytes proliferate, some transforming to plasmablasts that enter the efferent lymphatic vessels. Others become memory cells that remain in the Peyer's patches or circulate through organized gut lymphoid tissue and the lamina propria. When a second exposure to the antigen occurs, as in the second dose of an inactivated oral vaccine, these sensitized cells rapidly undergo blast transformation, cellular proliferation, and migration as IgA plasmablasts.[106,107] The cells first migrate to the mesenteric lymph nodes and then reach the systemic circulation via the thoracic duct. During this migration, some of these gut-derived plasmablasts reach the lamina propria of other mucosa, such as the respiratory and urinary tracts, as well as the ductal epithelium of the mammary and salivary glands.[106,108,109] However, most "home in" on the lamina propria of the intestine where they take on the typical morphology of plasma cells and produce IgA antibody until they die and are replaced. The distribution of gut-derived plasma cells to the mammary gland and other mucosal sites explains why certain body fluids, such as saliva or breast milk, can sometimes be used as a proxy for intestinal fluid to monitor SIgA antibody responses following oral immunization or following natural infection.[110–112] When the intestinal secretory immune system undergoes prolonged exposure, as might occur during a natural infection with *V. cholerae* 01 or following ingestion of a colonizing live oral vaccine, the features of the primary and secondary immune responses merge to appear as a single, progressive immune process. In the lamina propria, the plasma cells secrete a 9S dimeric IgA that enters enterocytes in the intestinal crypts. Combination of the IgA dimers with secretory pieces elaborated by the crypt cells results in the 11S secretory IgA antibodies that are secreted to the mucosal surface. Dimeric IgA that escapes this secretory process enters the circulation but is rapidly extracted in the liver and is secreted as SIgA in the bile; this represents a second pathway by which IgA antibodies reach the bowel lumen. SIgA antibodies against *V. cholerae* 01 antigens are readily detectable in intestinal fluid and breast milk after clinical cholera.[111,112] These antibodies can neutralize cholera toxin and, by binding to critical surface antigens, can agglutinate and immobilize vibrios and prevent them from adhering to the gut mucosa, thereby interfering with mucosal colonization.

An important feature of the mucosal secretory immune system, recognized during the past decade, is its long-lasting memory. Once stimulated, memory persists even after specific SIgA antibodies can no longer be detected in intestinal secretions.[24,66,67,113−115] Immunologic memory is apparently responsible for rapid anamnestic responses, which are characterized by accelerated antibody production and are probably responsible for the enduring immunity that follows an episode of cholera. Immunologic memory to some antigens following cholera or immunization with cholera vaccines has been shown to endure for at least several years in animal models and in man.[115,116]

Perhaps the most important observation to come from studies of the secretory immune system is that, to maximize the secretory intestinal immune response, antigen must be delivered directly to the mucosal surface; in practical terms, this means that vaccines against enteric infections must be given orally. In immunologically primed individuals, parenteral administration of an antigen can result in a significant increase in gut SIgA antibodies but this is short-lived[117,118]; a similar phenomenon does not usually occur in unprimed persons.[119] Moreover, this phenomenon may not be repeatable and additional parenteral inoculations can actually suppress the secretory antibody response.[119,120] In contrast, oral immunization primes the intestinal immune system so that subsequent oral administrations of antigen act as boosters, eliciting rapid and enhanced secondary SIgA responses.

6. VACCINES DEVELOPED OR TESTED SINCE 1960

Since 1960, many candidate cholera vaccines have been tested in various animal models and protective effects have been demonstrated.[25] Some of these vaccines were aimed at stimulating primarily antibacterial and others at evaluating purely antitoxic immunity. Other studies in animal models clearly demonstrate a synergistic effect resulting from the interplay of antibacterial and antitoxic immune responses.[25,70−73]

However, as cholera occurs naturally only in humans and an increasing number of vaccine-related studies have been carried out in man, this review will focus on immunizing agents that have been, are being, or will shortly be evaluated in clinical trials in humans.

6.1. Parenteral Vaccines

From the turn of the century when the first cholera vaccines were developed until the toxoid vaccines produced in the early 1970s, most cholera vaccines were given parenterally. However, by the mid-1970s, with the recognition that *V. cholerae* 01 is a noninvasive pathogen, with increasing examples of the efficiency of the intestinal immune system and with awareness that antigens must be administered orally to maximally stimulate the intestinal immune response, studies on oral vaccines were given priority over parenteral ones. Nevertheless, in view of the important historical role that parenteral vaccines have played in immunoprophylaxis against cholera, they will be reviewed first.

6.1.1. Killed Whole-Cell Vaccines

Since the late 19th century, heat-killed and chemically inactivated whole *V. cholerae* 01 organisms have been utilized as parenteral vaccines. It is only since the early 1960s, however, that well-designed, randomized, controlled trials of their efficacy have been carried out. The studies up to 1980 have been reviewed by Benenson,[31] Feeley and Gangarosa,[32] and Joo.[33] The results of these field trials, summarized in Table 3, show quite clearly that killed whole-cell vaccines can provide at least moderate (and occasionally much higher) levels of protection, although usually for only a few months. In several controlled field trials, the level of vaccine-induced protection was age-related, being lowest in young children (the population at greatest risk of cholera) and highest in adults; this suggested that the vaccines worked best in immunologically primed populations by boosting underlying immunity.

Immunization with killed whole-cell vaccines prepared from classical biotype *V. cholerae* 01 protected against El Tor vibrios of the same serotype.[121] While Inaba vaccine protected against both Inaba and Ogawa cholera,[41,121] monovalent Ogawa vaccine did not protect against Inaba disease.[41]

In a few trials killed whole-cell vaccines were administered with adjuvants that prolonged the duration of protection for up to 12–18 months.[42,43,46,47] Unfortunately, some of these adjuvants led to serious local reactions, including sterile abscesses, and were therefore not suitable for widespread public health use.[42,43]

6.1.2. Toxoid Vaccines

The toxoid vaccines were intended to protect by stimulating antitoxic immunity. Those tested in man included formaldehyde-treated cholera toxin (i.e., formaldehyde cholera toxoid), glutaraldehyde-treated cholera toxin (i.e., glutaraldehyde cholera toxoid), procholeragenoid (i.e., heat-aggregated cholera toxin), and B subunit.

6.1.2.1. Formaldehyde Cholera Toxoid

Formaldehyde treatment of purified cholera toxin was found to eliminate its toxicity in animals without eradicating its ability to stimulate neutralizing antibodies. When the prototype formaldehyde cholera toxoid was given to monkeys and humans as a parenteral vaccine in phase 1 clinical studies, however, the toxoid reverted to partial toxicity, leading to unacceptable adverse reactions at the site of inoculation.[122] Further studies with this first cholera toxoid were abandoned.

A nonreverting formaldehyde cholera toxoid was prepared by investigators at the Wellcome Research Laboratories in the United Kingdom. This toxoid was administered with alum adjuvant to Bangladeshi volunteers, including lactating mothers.[123,124] In contrast with the earlier product, this formaldehyde toxoid did not elicit severe local reactions and stimulated significant increases in serum IgG and breast milk SIgA antitoxin.[123,124] However, an intended field trial to test the efficacy of this parenteral toxoid was never initiated.

Ohtomo *et al.*[125] prepared a toxoid (termed "lot 11") using formalin and glycine. This toxoid was immunogenic in humans and did not cause unacceptable reactions at the site of inoculation. A large-scale field trial of this parenteral toxoid vaccine was carried out in the Philippines to assess its efficacy but no beneficial effect was detected[79]; consequently, no further field trials were pursued.

6.1.2.2. Glutaraldehyde Cholera Toxoid

A method for the large-scale preparation of glutaraldehyde cholera toxoid that yielded a product free of contaminating somatic antigen was described by Rapoport et al.[126] It was anticipated that this antigen could be used to assess the protective role of purely antitoxic immunity. In 1974, a large-scale field trial of this parenteral toxoid, which was absorbed to aluminum phosphate, was carried out in Bangladesh.[78] The toxoid elicited high titers of serum antitoxin. Two waves of epidemic cholera, first El Tor Inaba, then El Tor Ogawa, struck the field area, permitting a fair evaluation of the efficacy of the vaccine. Protection could be demonstrated in only one age group and was restricted to the period of the Inaba epidemic (Table 4). Thus, the glutaraldehyde cholera toxoid alone provided little protection as a parenteral vaccine and was notably inferior to a series of parenteral killed whole-cell and subunit vaccines tested in similar field trials in the same population. Accordingly, no further field studies were carried out with this parenteral toxoid.

6.1.2.3. Procholeragenoid

Procholeragenoid is a high molecular weight (circa 10^3 kDa) toxoid that results when cholera toxin is heated to 65°C for at least 5 min.[127-129] Procholeragenoid is highly immunogenic, while retaining less than 1% of the biological activity of the parent toxin. This minimal residual toxin activity could be completely abolished by treatment of procholeragenoid with formaldehyde. The formaldehyde-treated procholeragenoid was found to be as potent as the parent toxin in stimulating serum antitoxin following parenteral immunization of rabbits. Swiss volunteers exhibited marked serum antitoxin responses following parenteral immunization with 10, 30, or 100 mcg of the formaldehyde-treated procholeragenoid[129]; no notable adverse reactions were reported. Further studies of procholeragenoid as a parenteral vaccine have not been performed.

6.1.2.4. B Subunit

The B subunits of cholera toxin bind the enzymatically active A subunit to GM1 ganglioside receptors as a preliminary step in entrance of the A subunit into enterocytes. The B subunit is markedly more immunogenic than the A subunit and most of the neutralizing activity of cholera antitoxin is directed against the B subunit. Since B subunit in purified form is not toxic, does not activate adenylate cyclase, and does not lead to intestinal secretion, it represents an attractive immunogen to stimulate antitoxic immunity in humans.[130,131]

Purified B subunit has been administered to healthy Bangladeshis and Swedes, including lactating women, as an intramuscular toxoid in doses of up to 200 mcg.[116,132] This parenteral toxoid vaccine did not cause either local or systemic reactions and it elicited high levels of circulating antitoxin. Immunologically primed Bangladeshi women frequently showed rises in SIgA antitoxin in breast milk after parenteral inoculation with B subunit; however, such secretory antibody responses were rare in Swedish women who were immunologically naive with regard to this antigen.[116,132] A field trial of efficacy of the parenteral B subunit toxoid vaccine was not carried out.

TABLE 4
Results of a Controlled Field Trial in Bangladesh of the Efficacy of a Parenteral Glutaraldehyde Cholera Toxoid Vaccine:
Age-Specific and Serotype-Specific Protection

Days after first dose	Serotype	1–4 years			5–14 years			> 15 years			All ages		
		CT[a] (9671)	TT[b] (9517)	Vac. eff.[c]	CT (19,765)	TT (20,136)	Vac. eff.	CT (17,007)	TT (16,742)	Vac. eff.	CT (46,443)	TT (46,395)	Vac. eff.
14–97	Both	36	42	14%	30	61	51%[d]	30	31	3%	96	134 p<0.02	28%
	Inaba	18	26	31%	16	40	60%[d]	19	22	14%	53	88	40%
	Ogawa	18	16	0%	14	21	33%	11	9	0%	43	46	7%
98–365	Both	42	36	0%	49	44	0%	22	18	0%	113	98	0%
	Inaba	15	13	0%	17	17	0%	7	6	0%	39	36	0%
	Ogawa	27	23	0%	32	27	0%	15	12	0%	38	28	0%

[a]Cholera toxoid group (no. vaccinated); includes recipients of both one and two doses.
[b]Tetanus toxoid control group (no. vaccinated); includes recipients of both one and two doses.
[c]Percent vaccine efficacy. Statistical test was Chi square with Yates correction.
[d]$p < 0.002$.

6.1.3. Bacterial Subunit Vaccines

Subunit somatic antigen vaccines consisting of purified Ogawa LPS and Inaba LPS-protein extract were evaluated for safety, immunogenicity, and efficacy in controlled trials in Bangladesh in the 1960s.[35,39,41] These subunit somatic antigens were surprisingly well tolerated as parenteral vaccines and stimulated vibriocidal responses with geometric mean titers approximately one-third as high as those elicited by killed whole-cell vaccines of the same serotype. In controlled field trials of efficacy, the subunit vaccines conferred significant, albeit short-lived, protection in at least some age groups.[35,39,41] The level of protection conferred by the Ogawa LPS vaccine (43% vaccine efficacy) was somewhat lower than that conferred by the bivalent whole-cell vaccine (72% vaccine efficacy) in the same trial in East Pakistan, and protection was limited to individuals above 10 years of age. Curiously, the protection provided by the purified Ogawa LPS vaccine in individuals over 10 years of age during the first season of surveillance was against cholera caused by serotype Inaba. This was in contrast to results obtained with a monovalent killed whole-cell Ogawa cholera vaccine in another field trial in Bangladesh[37]; in that trial significant protection was encountered only against Ogawa cholera. Mosley et al.[39] hypothesized that the purified Ogawa LPS vaccine was effective in older residents of the field trial area because it boosted preexistent Inaba immunity by means of the portion of the LPS antigen that is common to both serotypes of V. cholerae 01.

In a controlled field trial, the Inaba LPS-protein subunit vaccine provided a level of protection as high as that conferred by the monovalent Inaba whole-cell vaccine[39,41] (Table 3).

6.1.4. Combination Killed Whole-Cell/Toxoid Vaccines

In the late 1970s in Bangladesh, evaluations of the safety and immunogenicity of three alum-adjuvanted parenteral vaccines prepared by the Wellcome Research Laboratories were carried out. These included a formaldehyde cholera toxoid, a killed whole-cell vaccine, and a combination killed whole-cell/toxoid vaccine[123]; tetanus toxoid served as the control in these clinical trials. All three cholera vaccines were judged to be satisfactorily safe. The combination vaccine stimulated excellent serum vibriocidal and antitoxin responses. These vaccines were not evaluated for efficacy in controlled field trials.

6.2. Oral Vaccines

In the first 90 years of immunization against cholera, vaccines were administered by the parenteral route. Nevertheless, as mentioned above in the historical review of early cholera vaccines, some oral vaccine candidates were developed and evaluated in field trials in the first quarter of this century.[16-19] However, these early attempts at oral immunization were empirical rather than being based on immunological principles. In contrast, a wealth of scientific evidence on the role of the intestinal immune system in protection against cholera and on the need to immunize orally in order to optimize the intestinal immune response, forms the basis of the modern approach involving oral cholera vaccines. This section reviews the immunizing agents that have been administered orally.

6.2.1. Killed Whole-Cell Vaccines

A series of clinical studies have demonstrated the safety, immunogenicity, and efficacy of inactivated *V. cholerae* 01 given in multiple, spaced doses as an oral vaccine. Modern studies using this approach to vaccination against cholera were begun by Freter and Gangarosa.[133,134] These investigators showed the innocuity of very large doses of inactivated vibrios administered per os. More importantly, for the first time, they demonstrated that the vast majority of recipients of an oral cholera vaccine manifested significant rises in coproantibodies against *V. cholerae* 01 antigens when appropriate assays were utilized. In his 1962 report on oral vaccination of North American volunteers with killed *V. cholerae* 01, Freter[133] wrote

> A measurable coproantibody response to oral vaccine in at least 77% of all subjects, as in the present study, appears sufficient for routine use. This removes one of the major obstacles to the acceptance of oral vaccine as a possible means of inducing prophylactic immunity. The evidence now available is strong enough to suggest that the next major step in the study of prophylactic immunity to enteric infections might profitably be a field trial of oral vaccine.

In their studies, Freter and Gangarosa gave 28 daily oral doses of killed vibrios; every seven days of vaccination were followed by five days without vaccine, until a total of 28 doses was administered.

Cash *et al.*[20] also immunized North American volunteers with inactivated vibrios; 1.6 × 10^{10} killed Ogawa and Inaba *V. cholerae* 01 were given daily with 2 g of NaHCO$_3$ for 10 days. When volunteers were challenged with 10^6 pathogenic *V. cholerae* 01 (strain 569B), the vaccine provided significant protection; diarrhea occurred in 5 of 16 vaccinees but in 47 of 58 controls ($p=0.0003$, 61% vaccine efficacy) (Table 5). Additional reports of the safety and immunogenicity of oral killed vibrios were published.[135–137]

A Swedish killed whole-cell oral vaccine consisting of a mixture of heat- and formalin-killed *V. cholerae* 01 of both serotypes and biotypes was extensively evaluated first in North American and Swedish adult volunteers and then in Bangladeshi adults and children.[48,76,100,138] The Swedish vaccine did not cause any notable adverse reactions.[76,138] Given in three doses spaced 14 days apart with each dose containing 2 × 10^{11} organisms, the vaccine stimulated modest but significant rises in serum vibriocidal titers in approximately 80% of vaccinees.[76] In an experimental challenge study in North American volunteers to assess the efficacy of the killed whole-cell oral vaccine, the attack rate in vaccinees was diminished (albeit not significantly) and the severity of the disease was significantly ameliorated[72] (Table 5).

Clemens *et al.*[138] found that administration of NaHCO$_3$ with the oral killed-vibrio vaccine did not improve the serum antibody response. In a large-scale controlled field trial still on-going in Bangladesh, the oral, killed whole-cell vaccine provided significant protection (52% vaccine efficacy) for at least 36 months. During the first 12 months of surveillance the vaccine conferred 53% protection overall against cases of cholera presenting at the treatment center in the field area (Table 2).[48,80] However, the protective effect during this first year of surveillance was markedly greater in individuals over five years of age (66% vaccine efficacy) than in children 2–5 years of age (31% protection). The vaccine was also shown to reduce the need to visit the treatment center for watery diarrhea of any cause. Thus, in vaccinees given the oral whole-cell vaccine, the number of cases of nonsevere diarrhea and of severe diarrhea seen in the treatment center were reduced by 35% and 32%, respectively, in comparison with the placebo group. Finally, during cholera epidemics in the field area the oral whole-cell vaccine was seen to have reduced by 33% the overall mortality in women 15

TABLE 5
A Summary of Volunteer Studies Evaluating the Efficacy of Inactivated *Vibrio cholerae* Whole-Cell Oral Vaccines in Experimental Challenges

Vaccine	Diarrhea	Vaccine efficacy	Mean diarrheal stool volume	Coprocultures
Monovalent Inaba[a]				
Vaccinees	5/16 (31%)	62%	NA[b]	9/16 (56%)
	$p < 0.001$			$p < 0.0013$
Controls	47/58 (81%)		NA	54/58 (93%)
Multivalent[c]				
Vaccinees	3/9 (33%)	56%	0.9 liters	7/9
	$p = 0.10$		$p < 0.05$	NS[d]
Controls	6/8 (75%)		2.1	8/8[e]

[a]Merck, Sharpe & Dohme lot # 4445G containing 8×10^9 vibrios per ml. Vaccinees received 2 ml daily for 10 days with $NaHCO_3$; some received five daily booster doses one month later. Volunteers were challenged with 10^6 enterotoxinogenic classical Inaba 569B.
[b]NA, data not available.
[c]Multivalent vaccine prepared by the Swedish Bacteriological Laboratories; each 8 ml dose had 5×10^{10} organisms each of classical Inaba and Ogawa and 1×10^{11} El Tor Inaba. A dose of vaccine was given on days 0, 14, and 28. Challenge was with 10^6 enterotoxinogenic El Tor Inaba 16961.
[d]NS, not significant.
[e]The mean excretion of organisms by the vaccines 9.9×10^5 vibrios per gram of stool was significantly less than the controls, 5.1×10^7 ($p < 0.05$). Statistical analyses were by Fisher's exact test or Student's t test.

years of age and older. Taken together, these observations from a large-scale field trial show that the multivalent oral killed vaccine exhibited impressive protective effects against cholera that translated into a considerable public health impact, including diminished morbidity, decreased mortality, and lessened pressure on treatment centers during cholera epidemics.

6.2.2. Bacterial Fraction Vaccine

A bacterial fraction vaccine, referred to as CH1 + 2, was prepared at the Pasteur Institute.[139,141] This antigenic complex, extracted from the outer membrane of *V. cholerae* 01 by treatment with trichloroacetic acid, followed by chromatography and ultracentrifugation, has not been extensively characterized; the extract contains specific polysaccharides, as well as proteins.[139,141] Administered as an oral antigen in two spaced doses, this vaccine was tolerated well and elicited serum vibriocidal antibodies and antibodies to *V. cholerae* 01 polysaccharide.[140–142]

Two doses of this vaccine were given to five children, 1–4 years of age, with extrahepatic bile duct obstruction several weeks prior to their undergoing surgical repair[92]; bile was collected during surgery, 1–12 days after the second dose of vaccine. Vibriocidal activity was demonstrable in bile, as well as in the serum of these children; in bile, specific anti-*V. cholerae* 01 polysaccharide antibodies were found exclusively in the IgA class.[92]

A field trial of a modified version of the CH1 + 2 oral vaccine was carried out in Zaire in an area where cholera was epidemic.[143] A total of 18,623 individuals were vaccinated in the trial. One group, comprising 6248 subjects, ingested two capsules (each containing 100 mcg) of vaccine antigen and, in addition, each subject was given a parenteral dose of tetanus toxoid; 8 days later, this group ingested two more capsules of vaccine and received another parenteral dose of tetanus toxoid. A second group of 6249 subjects received two doses of parenteral, killed whole-cell cholera vaccine, 8 days apart; at the time of each parenteral immunization these subjects also ingested two capsules containing placebo. A third group of 5766 individuals received oral vaccine 8 days apart without parenteral inoculations. It was not stated whether the subjects were randomly assigned to these three groups. There remained an additional 18,377 individuals in the area who received no vaccine of any kind. The age composition of the different groups and other relevant demographic data were not reported. Approximately 7 months after vaccination of these groups, an outbreak of cholera occurred in the field area. No mention was made in the report of whether suspect cholera cases were bacteriologically confirmed. The incidence of clinical cholera was 57 cases in the parenteral cholera vaccine group (9.1 cases/10^3 population), six cases in the combined group of 12,014 persons who received oral vaccine with or without tetanus toxoid ($0.5/10^3$), and 216 cases in the nonvaccinated group ($11.7/10^3$). Despite the substantial limitations in the design of this study as reported, when the incidence of clinical cholera cases in recipients of the oral vaccine is compared to the incidence in the recipients of parenteral cholera vaccine, the difference is highly significant ($p < 0.0001$). The nonvaccinated persons in the field area do not constitute a fair comparison group because they were not randomized (so it is not known if they were at equal, less, or greater risk than the vaccinated groups) and surveillance was not carried out in a blind manner to preclude the inadvertent introduction of biases. No other objective information is available on this oral vaccine candidate, which has not been evaluated for efficacy in volunteer studies or in additional field trials utilizing a stricter study design and bacteriological confirmation of cases.

6.2.3. Toxoids

Oral toxoid vaccines that have been administered alone in clinical studies include glutaraldehyde cholera toxoid[21,22] and B subunit.[116,132]

6.2.3.1. Glutaraldehyde Cholera Toxoid

The only oral toxoid that was given alone and evaluated for efficacy was the glutaraldehyde cholera toxoid.[21,22] North American volunteers were given three 2-mg doses enterally 1 month apart or three 8.0-mg oral doses with $NaHCO_3$ at 1-month intervals.[21,22] No adverse reactions were observed[21,22] and the immune response to the toxoid was enhanced when it was administered with $NaHCO_3$.[144] In experimental challenge studies to assess the protective efficacy of these regimens, no significant protection was observed.

6.2.3.2. B Subunit

Considerable data have been accumulated on the safety and immunogenicity of oral B subunit which has been evaluated extensively in Swedish and Bangladeshi volunteers.[116,132] Oral purified B subunit caused no adverse reactions and stimulated high titers of antitoxin in serum and in intestinal washings, breast milk, and saliva.

Administration with $NaHCO_3$ or other buffer to neutralize gastric acidity enhanced the immune response. The efficacy of purified B subunit given alone as a protective antigen has not been evaluated in man. As reviewed below, however, it has been given orally in combination with killed whole vibrios.[48,80]

6.2.4. Combination Oral Vaccines

6.2.4.1. Toxoid/Killed Whole-Cell Vaccines

Three different toxoid/killed whole-cell combinations have been evaluated as oral vaccines in clinical studies to assess their safety, immunogenicity, and efficacy.[25,76,100,110,111] These include glutaraldehyde cholera toxoid combined with alcohol-killed vibrios, procholeragenoid combined with heat- and formalin-inactivated vibrios, and B subunit combined with heat- and formalin killed vibrios.[25,76] All three combinations were well tolerated. The B subunit/whole-cell combination gave the best immune response. Significant rises in serum vibriocidal antibody were recorded in 89% of the B subunit/whole-cell vaccinees and antitoxin rises were seen in 100%[76]; three-fourths showed fourfold or greater rises in SIgA antitoxin in jejunal fluid.[76]

As summarized in Table 6, all three combination vaccines evoked significant protection, manifested in vaccinees as a reduced diarrhea attack rate, diminished stool volumes, or curtailed excretion of V. cholerae 01. For comparison, Table 5 shows the results of challenge of volunteers immunized with only the whole-cell component of the B subunit/whole-cell vaccine.

TABLE 6
A Comparison of the Efficacy of Three Inactivated Whole-Vibrio/Toxoid Combination
Oral Vaccines in Protection against Experimental Cholera in Volunteers

Whole-cell vaccine	Toxoid	Diarrhea	Vaccine efficacy	Mean diarrheal stool volume	Positive direct coprocultures
Alcohol-killed El Tor Inaba (5 × 10^{10}/dose)^a	Glutaraldehyde-toxoid (2 mg/dose)^a				
Vaccinees		2/9^b $p = 0.11$	67%	0.7 liter $p < 0.05$	2/9 $p < 0.01$
Controls		4/6		1.4	6/6
Multivalent vaccine (see Table 5)^c	Purified B subunit (5 mg/dose)^c				
Vaccinees		4/11 $p < 0.01$	64	0.70 $p < 0.05$	9/11 NS
Controls		7/7		3.5	7/7
Heat- and formalinized classical & El Tor vibrios (10^{11}/dose)^d	Procholeragenoid (50 mcg for 2 doses, 200 mcg for 3rd dose)^d				
Vaccinees		11/15 NS	27	1.6 $p < 0.05$	14/15 NS
Controls		6/6		9.4	6/6

^{a}Vaccinees received two doses of whole cell vaccine and one dose of toxoid weekly for four weeks and were challenged one month later with 10^6 enterotoxinogenic El Tor Inaba P27459.[25]
^{b}No positive/no. challenged.
^{c}Vaccinees received one dose of whole cell vaccine (2 × 10^{11} organisms) and one dose of B subunit on days 0, 14, and 28. One month later they were challenged with 10^6 enterotoxinogenic El Tor Inaba N16961.[70]
^{d}Vaccinees received one dose of whole cell vaccine and one of toxoid on days 0, 14, and 28 and were challenged one month later with 10^6 enterotoxinogenic El Tor Inaba N16961.[25] All doses of vaccine were administered with NaHCO$_3$ to neutralize gastric acid; recipients of B subunit and procholeragenoid also received cimetidine to suppress gastric acid production.

As previously mentioned, the B subunit/killed whole-cell combination vaccine and the oral whole-cell vaccine alone were tested for efficacy, in comparison with a placebo control consisting of killed *E. coli* K-12 organisms.[48,80,81] Results of this randomized, double-blind placebo-controlled trial involving 63,498 individuals in Bangladesh are summarized in Table 2. Vaccine or placebo was administered in a "cocktail" with a $NaHCO_3$/citric acid buffer to neutralize gastric acid. Several hallmark observations were made in the course of this well-designed and executed large-scale field trial. First of all, it was found that oral vaccines that elicited no adverse reactions could induce a moderate degree of protection (51% efficacy for the combination and 52% efficacy for the whole-cell vaccine) that endures for at least three years; this represents a significant new achievement in vaccination against cholera.

In addition, the combination vaccine demonstrated certain advantages over the killed whole-cell vaccine given alone. During the first six months of surveillance the level of protection provided by the combination vaccine was significantly greater (85% vaccine efficacy) than that conferred by the whole-cell component given alone (56% vaccine efficacy) (Table 2); by the eighth month of surveillance, however, the difference in efficacy between the groups was no longer significant and after 12 months of surveillance the combination vaccine showed 62% protection, with the whole-cell vaccine alone showing 53%.

Of further interest, during the first six months, the combination vaccine protected as well in young children as in older children and adults. This result differed from results of earlier trials in this area with parenteral inactivated whole-cell and bacterial fraction (lipopolysaccharide or lipopolysaccharide–protein complex) vaccines in which the level of protection was usually inferior in children less than five years of age. Unfortunately, after six months, the level of protection dropped appreciably in children less than six years of age. During the first year of surveillance, the combination vaccine was also shown to confer 37% protection against diarrheal disease due to LT-producing *E. coli;* however, in the first two months after vaccination there was an impressive 75% protection against LT-*E. coli* diarrhea.[82] Although the excellent protection of young children against cholera and the protective effect against *E. coli* LT diarrhea with this particular vaccine were quite short lived, the combination vaccine nevertheless clearly showed that the modern approach to cholera immunoprophylaxis, involving oral immunization with vaccines that elicit both antitoxic and antibacterial immunity, is a correct approach that can hopefully be further improved upon.

The B subunit/killed whole-vibrio oral vaccine represents the best cholera vaccine developed so far that has been evaluated in a well-designed, large-scale field trial. It is safe, provides a high level of protection (85%) for six months, even in young children, and confers moderate protection (51%) for at least 36 months. Other important observations made in this field trial provide important insights on the public health impact that an effective cholera vaccine might have in endemic areas of less-developed countries. The combination vaccine was more protective against disease caused by classical than El Tor biotype *V. cholerae* 01; the vaccine significantly and equally protected against both severe and milder forms of clinical cholera. The effect of the vaccine was also appreciated as a reduction in cases seeking treatment for watery diarrhea of any cause at the treatment center in the field area. In this analysis, the combination vaccine provided 28% and 51% protection, respectively, against diarrhea cases that were not severe or were severe. Lastly, mortality surveillance among trial participants showed that crude mortality from all causes in women 15 years of age or older was reduced by 45% in those who received the combination vaccine (and by 33% in recipients of the whole-cell vaccine alone). This protective effect against mortality was demonstrable only during the periods of cholera epidemics in the field trial area, when death rates approximately trebled overall. These data suggest that the oral combination vaccine, as well as the whole-cell component alone, averted deaths due to diarrheal dehydration during cholera epidemics, even though effective rehydration therapy was available to trial participants at local treatment centers in the field area.

Despite the significant advantages of the B subunit/whole-vibrio combination oral vaccine over previous cholera vaccines, it nonetheless has drawbacks that may ultimately limit its usefulness as a practical vaccine, particularly in less-developed countries. One of these is the observation that protection in young children was transient, only lasting for approximately six months; a similar pattern of protection would be expected in adults from nonendemic areas, such as travelers from industrialized countries who venture into cholera-endemic areas. Another possible drawback to the combination vaccine is that it may prove to be relatively expensive, due both to the large number of inactivated bacteria required and to the cost of preparing the B subunit. Thirdly, the requirement for multiple (at least two and possibly three) spaced doses to prime and boost the gut immune system would make achievement of immunity within a community appreciably more difficult than with an ideal, single-dose oral vaccine.

6.2.5. Live Oral Vaccines

Some investigators have for many years favored the concept of an attenuated strain of *V. cholerae* 01 as a live oral vaccine against cholera.[24,25] Until the advent of recombinant DNA technology, attenuated vaccine candidates consisted of naturally occurring environmental strains or chemically mutagenized strains, each suffering certain drawbacks. Beginning in the 1980s, it has been possible to attenuate pathogenic *V. cholerae* 01 by creating precise deletion mutants lacking genes that encode factors required for bacterial virulence but not necessary to induce immunity. These, and other approaches to developing a live oral cholera vaccine, are reviewed below.

6.2.5.1. Environmental Strains

Nonenterotoxinogenic *V. cholerae* 01 strains isolated from environmental sources in India and Brazil were evaluated in volunteers in India[145] and the U.S.[146,147] to assess their potential as live oral cholera vaccines; the results were disappointing. Although the strains tested were well tolerated, they colonized the intestine very poorly and elicited only feeble serologic responses.[146,147] Most importantly, in controlled experimental challenge studies in volunteers, the environmental strains conferred no protection.[146,147]

6.2.5.2. Chemically Mutagenized Attenuated Strains

In the early 1970s, a hypotoxinogenic strain, M13, was prepared from pathogenic classical Inaba 569B by mutagenesis with nitrosoguanidine.[148,149] In volunteers, the strain did not cause diarrhea but colonized poorly.[150] A moderate but significant level of protection against challenge with pathogenic enterotoxinogenic *V. cholerae* 01 was observed in volunteers who had been immunized with eight doses of vaccine. The hypotoxigenicity of mutant M13 has since been shown to be the consequence of a genetic lesion in the *toxR* gene which regulates the *ctxAB* structural gene.[102]

Texas Star-SR is an A−BR+ mutant of El Tor Ogawa strain 3083 that was also induced by treatment with nitrosoguanidine. In selecting this strain, Honda and Finkelstein[151] tested thousands of colonies to identify one that had a stable loss of holotoxin activity but continued to produce B subunit. Texas Star was extensively evaluated in clinical studies in volunteers.[152]

When Texas Star was given to volunteers in doses of 10^5 to 5×10^{10} viable organisms, mild diarrhea occurred in 24% of the 68 vaccinees; however, the total diarrheal stool volume exceeded 1.0 liter in only one individual. This attenuated strain colonized the intestine moderately well; hundreds of isolates recovered from stool cultures of volunteers were tested by sensitive assays for cholera toxin biological activity and all were negative. The vaccine provided moderate but significant protection against challenge with either serotype of El Tor vibrios.

While the clinical, immunological, and bacteriological studies with Texas Star provided invaluable data to support the concept of utilizing attenuated strains to stimulate anticolonizing and antitoxic immunity to cholera, this attenuated strain suffered from certain inherent drawbacks. First, mutagenesis with nitrosoguanidine is known to induce multiple mutations, not all of which are readily detectable but which may enfeeble the strain as a vaccine candidate. Second, the precise genetic lesion presumed responsible for the attenuation was not known. Therefore, there always remained the theoretical possibility that it could revert to virulence.

6.2.5.3. Vibriophage-Induced Mutants

Prior to the development of attenuated strains by recombinant DNA techniques, one method used to create nontoxigenic strains by gene deletions involved the use of mutagenic bacteriophages, as described by Mekelanos et al.[153] These investigators used vibriophages to prepare V. cholerae 01 mutants with deletions in DNA-encoding cholera toxin sequences. No mutants prepared by this method were evaluated in clinical studies because shortly after their description genetically engineered vaccine strains became available in which the gene deletions were prepared by more precise, recombinant DNA techniques.

6.2.5.4. Attenuated Mutants Prepared by Recombinant DNA Techniques

Three major approaches are being followed by various investigators to develop live oral vaccines to prevent cholera. The first involves the use of recombinant DNA techniques to delete from pathogenic V. cholerae 01 the genes encoding critical virulence properties that may not be necessary for protection. In the second approach, auxotrophic strains of V. cholerae 01 are prepared that are crippled in their ability to proliferate in the human intestine. The third involves the cloning of genes which encode putative protective antigens of V. cholerae 01[154] and their insertion and expression in attenuated Salmonella typhi strains, such as Ty21a or 541Ty, whose safety has been established in humans.[155–157]

6.2.5.4a. Attenuation of V. cholerae by Gene Deletions

Starting with strains of V. cholerae 01 whose pathogenicity and ability to confer immunity were well-established in volunteers, Kaper et al.[77,158] and Mekalanos et al.[159] prepared oral vaccine candidates by deleting the genes that encode only the A subunit or both the A and B subunits of cholera toxin. Several of these strains have been tested in volunteers.[75,160–163]

JBK 70. The A−B− strain JBK 70[77] was fed to volunteers in doses of 10^6, 10^8, or 10^{10}, organisms[75] (Table 7). Compared to the clinical response of 38 volunteers following ingestion of the toxigenic A+B+ parent strain, N16961, 35 of whom developed diarrhea with a mean diarrheal stool volume of 4.2 liters and of whom 10 (29%) each purged at least 5.0 liters, JBK 70 was greatly attenuated. Nevertheless, although severe diarrhea did not

TABLE 7

Clinical and Bacteriological Response of Volunteers Following Ingestion of A−B− EL Tor
Inaba Vaccine Strain JBK 70 Prepared by Recombinant DNA Techniques or Its Virulent Parent,
V. cholerae El Tor Inaba N16961

Dose ingested	No. of volunteers	No. (%) with diarrhea	Mean diarrheal stool volume per ill volunteer (ml)	No. (%) with stool volume ≥ 5.0 liter	Mean no. of loose stools per ill volunteer	Coprocultures	
						No. (%) positive	Geometric mean excretion[a]
JBK 70							
10^6	4	1 (25)	543	0	4	3 (75)	1.5×10^6
10^8	5	2 (40)	1180	0	8.5	5 (100)	2.4×10^7
10^{10}	5	4 (80)	802	0	6	5 (100)	4.9×10^7
N16961							
10^6	38	35 (92)	4227	10 (26)	15.2	38 (100)	3.0×10^7

[a]Number of *V. cholerae* per g of stool among positives.

occur, at each dose 25–80% of the volunteers passed one or more loose stools that met the definition of diarrhea. Table 8 shows the number of loose stools passed by each volunteer with diarrhea on each day of observation and the total diarrheal stool volume; in several instances loose stools were accompanied by abdominal cramps, anorexia, and low-grade fever. Total stool volumes were all below 2.0 liters and in 5 of the 7 individuals it did not exceed 1.0 liter.

JBK was recovered from coprocultures of all vaccinees and from duodenal cultures of 55% of them. As expected, no recipients of this A−B− strain showed rises in serum IgG antitoxin. However, their vibriocidal antibody responses were impressive, even when compared with individuals who ingested the fully toxigenic parent strain, N16961 (Table 9).

Although JBK 70 was associated with adverse reactions, it apparently colonized the intestine well and stimulated a prominent antibacterial immune response. Therefore, advantage was taken of the opportunity to determine whether this strain, which did not evoke a cholera antitoxin response, could provide significant protection; one month after vaccination, recipients of JBK 70 were challenged with wild toxigenic strain N16961 (Table 10). Diarrhea occurred in 7 of 8 controls but in only 1 of 10 JBK vaccinees (89% vaccine efficacy, $p < 0.003$). That antibacterial mechanisms were involved in the protection is demonstrated by the significantly lower yield of *V. cholerae* 01 by direct coproculture from vaccinees than from controls, as well as a thousandfold lower excretion of vibrios per gram of stool in vaccinees (Table 10).

CVD 101. The reason for the residual, albeit usually mild, diarrhea encountered in recipients of JBK 70 was not clear. It was important to determine whether this adverse reaction was related to the El Tor biotype origin of JBK 70 and whether genetically engineered nontoxigenic vaccine strains derived from the classical biotype of *V. cholerae* 01 might perhaps be better tolerated. An extensive dose/response evaluation of CVD 101, an A−B+ derivative of classical Ogawa 395, was carried out. As shown in Table 11, some diarrhea occurred in 40–67% of recipients at every dose but in no instance was it severe. The

TABLE 8
Clinical Spectrum of Adverse Reactions of Vaccinees Who Developed Diarrhea Following
Ingestion of Genetically Engineered *V. cholerae* 01 Vaccine Candidates, A−B− El Tor Inaba
Strain (JBK 70), or A−B+ Classical Inaba Strain (CVD 103)[a]

Volunteer	Dose	Total diarrheal stool volume	Loose stools on each day of observation					Abdominal cramps	Anorexia	Vomiting	Fever
			1	2	3	4	5				
JBK 70 vaccinees											
5012-2	10^6	543 ml	1	2	1	0	0	+	0	0	0
5012-5	10^8	710 ml	0	5	0	0	0	+	+	+	100°C
5012-21	10^8	1649 ml	0	4	6	2	0	+	0	0	0
5012-16	10^{10}	1878 ml	0	4	7	1	0	+	+	0	0
5012-15	10^{10}	499 ml	0	3	1	0	0	+	0	0	0
5012-7	10^{10}	596 ml	2	3	1	0	0	+	+	0	100°C
5012-9	10^{10}	235 ml	0	1	0	1	0	+	+	0	0
CVD 103 vaccinees											
5020-3	10^6	911 ml	0	1	1	1	1	0	0	0	0
5021-6	10^8	378 ml	0	2	3	1	0	+	0	0	0
5026-1	10^8	317 ml	0	1	1	0	0	0	0	0	0
5026-5	10^8	958 ml	3	2	0	1	0	0	0	0	0
5026-7	10^8	362 ml	0	0	1	0	1	0	0	0	0
5026-13	10^8	393 ml	0	1	1	0	0	0	0	0	0

[a]In the seven JBK 70 vaccinees who had diarrhea, all seven also had accompanying symptoms such as abdominal cramps, malaise, vomiting, or fever. In contrast, only one of the six CVD 103 vaccinees who manifested diarrhea also experienced these accompanying symptoms ($p < 0.005$).

total stool volumes, which were similar to those seen after ingestion of JBK 70, represented a mean reduction by 84% of the copious diarrhea (mean stool volume, 5.5 liters) that occurred in volunteers after ingestion of the wild type toxigenic parent strain Ogawa 395 (Table 11). CVD 101 was recovered in coprocultures from 23 of 24 volunteers (96%). Although severe cholera occurs more frequently in persons with blood group O,[164,165] the occurrence of diarrhea following ingestion of JBK 70 and CVD 101 was not seen more frequently in persons of this blood group.[75]

The serological responses of volunteers following ingestion of a single dose of CVD 101

TABLE 9
Comparison of Vibriocidal Antibody Responses of Volunteers Following Ingestion of Pathogenic
or Attenuated Vaccine Strains of *Vibrio cholerae* 01, Biotype El Tor

Strain	Dose ingested	N	Percent with fourfold or greater rises	Peak geometric mean titer	Percent with titers	
					≥2560	≥10,240
JBK 70, A−B− El Tor Inaba vaccine	10^6–10^{10}	14	100	7,608	86	79
	10^6	4	100	1,522	50	25
	10^8	5	100	11,763	100	100
	10^{10}	5	100	8,914	100	100
N16961, pathogenic El Tor Inaba	10^6	21	90	4,793	81	33
E7946, pathogenic El Tor Ogawa	10^6	21	95	3,674	81	43

TABLE 10
Study to Access the Efficacy of a Single Dose of JBK 70 Oral Attenuated *Vibrio cholerae*
El Tor Inaba Vaccine Strain Prepared by Recombinant DNA Techniques[a,b]

| Group | Diarrhea attack rate | Mean diarrheal stool volume per ill volunteer | Positive coprocultures | | Geometric mean excretion (vibrios per gm stool)[c] |
			Direct	After enrichment	
Controls	7/8[d]	4.5 (1.1–7.9)[e]	8/8	8/8	3.5 × 10[6]
	$p < 0.003$		$p = 0.001$		
Vaccinees	1/10	1.6	2/10	6/10	3.8 × 10[3]

[a] Volunteers were challenged with 10[6] pathogenic *V. cholerae* El Tor Inaba N16961 with $NaHCO_3$.
[b] Statistical comparisons by Fisher's Exact test.
[c] Geometric mean of positives only.
[d] No. positive/no. challenged.
[e] Range.

are shown in Table 11. Both the vibriocidal and IgG ELISA antitoxin responses resembled those that occurred following infection with the pathogenic parent strain, classical Ogawa 395; a single dose of CVD 101 induced a comparable geometric mean vibriocidal titer and the mean antitoxin response was approximately three-fourths of that seen after infection with Ogawa 395. Because of the adverse reactions that occurred with CVD 101, challenge studies to assess vaccine efficacy were not carried out.

Rationale for further clinical studies. At this point it appeared that, irrespective of biotype or serotype, deleting the genes that encode the ADP-ribosylating A subunit from pathogenic *V. cholerae* 01 was insufficient to render the strains completely nonreactogenic. However, the studies also showed that single doses of as few as 10[4] organisms of genetically engineered nontoxinogenic live *V. cholerae* 01 given orally readily colonized the intestine and elicited potent antibody responses (Table 11). Two hypotheses were proposed to explain the residual mild diarrhea observed in a proportion of vaccinees.[75] One was that colonization of the proximal small intestine by adherent vibrios perturbed intestinal function in some undefined manner, resulting in net intestinal secretion and mild diarrhea. The other hypothesis was that the *V. cholerae* 01 vaccine strains elaborated additional secretogenic products, distinct from cholera toxin, which caused mild diarrhea; suggested candidates for this effect were the hemolysins/cytotoxins, cytotoxins/proteases, or Shiga-like toxins.[166—172] The development of additional vaccine strains was undertaken to test these hypotheses.

CVD 104 and 105. In addition to cholera toxin, *V. cholerae* 01 can elaborate other products that might have a secretogenic effect on the intestinal mucosa.[166–170] For example, *V. cholerae* 01 El Tor elaborates a hemolysin[167] that destroys sheep and rabbit erythrocytes; a related hemolysin occurs in some non-01 *V. cholerae*.[166,171,172] The genes for the "El Tor hemolysin" are also found in classical biotype vibrios,[173] although classical organisms elaborate little, if any, hemolysin *in vitro*. Nevertheless, hemolysin genes cloned from classical Ogawa 395 are expressed in *E. coli* by the production of biologically active hemolysin.[173] Madden *et al.*[167] identified a cytotoxin in *V. cholerae* of both 01 and non-01 serogroups that stimulated secretion in rabbit ileal loops. This cytotoxin appeared to be identical to the El Tor hemolysin.[167] The genes encoding the El Tor hemolysin were deleted

TABLE 11

Clinical, Bacteriological, and Serological Responses Following Ingestion of A−B+ V. cholerae Vaccine Strain CVD 101 Prepared by Recombinant DNA Techniques or Its Virulent Parent, Classical Ogawa 395

Vaccine dose	Rate of diarrhea	Mean diarrheal stool volume	Mean number of loose stools	No. (%) with stool volume > 5.0 liter	Positive coprocultures	Vibriocidal antibody		Antitoxin	
						Seroconversion rate[a]	Peak GMT[b]	Seroconversion rate[c]	Peak GMT
CVD 101									
10^8	2/3[d]	1.3 liters (1.2–1.3)[e]	10 (9–11)	0	2/3	2/3	806	2/3	0.80[f]
10^7	3/5	1.2 (0.5–2.1)	8 (3–13)	0	5/5	5/5	3880	4/5	0.80
10^6	2/5	0.4 (0.38–0.42)	3	0	5/5	5/5	2560	4/5	0.89
10^5	2/5	1.1 (0.7–1.5)	9 (4–13)	0	5/5	5/5	3880	5/5	0.83
10^4	4/6	0.7 (0.3–1.1)	5 (2–7)	0	6/6	6/6	2032	4/6	0.73
Ogawa 395									
10^6	33/36	5.5 (0.3–17.5)	19.7 (1–60)	15 (45)	35/36	33/36	4223	26/28[g]	1.17

[a]Significant seroconversion refers to a fourfold or greater rise in titer after vaccination or challenge.
[b]Geometric mean titer.
[c]Significant seroconversion is defined as a rise of 0.15 or greater in IgG–ELISA net optical density units in the postvaccination or postchallenge sera over the prevaccination or prechallenge specimen tested at a single 1:50 dilution.
[d]No. positive/no. vaccinated.
[e]Range.
[f]ELISA net optical density units.
[g]Due to insufficient quantities of sera, serum antitoxin was not measured in eight volunteers.

from JBK 70 and from CVD 101, resulting in the further derivatives, CVD 104 and CVD 105, respectively. These were fed to volunteers in doses of 10^5 to 10^7. However, deletion of the genes encoding the El Tor hemolysin did not notably diminish the rate of adverse mild diarrheal reactions in the recipients. All vaccinees shed the vaccine strain and immune responses were quite satisfactory.

*O395-N1.*Mekalanos et al.[159] like Kaper et al.[76,158] prepared an A−B+ derivative of classical Ogawa 395, O395-N1, by deleting the genes encoding the A subunit of cholera toxin. One difference in the method of construction of these otherwise similar mutants was that Kaper et al. cloned the *ctxAB* genes from classical Ogawa 395 and deleted the A subunit genes *in vitro* by recombinant DNA methods before inserting the modified DNA back into Ogawa 395 by site-directed mutagenesis. In contrast, in the similar approach taken by Mekalanos et al., classical Inaba 569B was the source of the *ctxAB* genes that were cloned, deleted of the A subunit genes, and inserted into the chromosome of Ogawa 395 by site-directed mutagenesis to create A−B+ strain O395-N1. Mekalanos and co-workers then prepared a further derivative of O395-N1, strain TCP2,[104] by creating an internal deletion in the *tcpA* structural gene; as a consequence, TCP2 lacks TCP colonization factor pili. A group of 16 healthy, adult North American volunteers were randomized to receive a single 10^6 organism dose of either O395-N1 or TCP2 and were then observed in double-blind fashion for the occurrence of adverse reactions.[105] Only one of the eight volunteers who ingested TCP2 manifested adverse reactions; however, this strain failed to colonize any of the volunteers and, as would be expected, there was virtually no immune response detected. In contrast, O395-N1 was recovered in coprocultures of 6 of the 8 volunteers who ingested the strain; 7 of 8 volunteers manifested significant rises in vibriocidal antibody, and 6 of 8 had significant rises in serum antitoxin. However, O395-N1 caused adverse reactions in 7 of 8 recipients, including malaise, anorexia, fever, abdominal cramps, headache, or loose stools ($p=0.05$) versus volunteers who ingested TCP2. Although diarrhea was not a prominent symptom in volunteers who received O395-N1, the high frequency (88%) of other discomforting symptoms in a double-blind study discouraged further clinical studies with this vaccine candidate. Although strain TCP2 was well tolerated, it neither colonized the intestine nor induced serological responses; therefore, additional studies with this strain were also not pursued.

CVD 103. Attempts are in progress to delete the genes encoding the Shiga-like toxin from CVD 101 to determine whether in this manner the residual reactogenicity of live oral cholera vaccines can be diminished or eliminated. In the meantime, an A−B+ derivative has been prepared from a pathogenic strain, classical Inaba 569B, that does not elaborate Shiga-like toxin. This vaccine strain, CVD 103, has been extensively evaluated in volunteers.[174] Only 5 of 46 recipients of a dose of 10^8 organisms developed mild diarrhea, a highly significant reduction from the rate in CVD 101 and JBK 70 recipients (Table 12), where, even in doses as low as 10^4, the majority of vaccinees experienced mild diarrhea. Furthermore, the volume and number of stools passed by CVD 103 vaccinees who had diarrhea was modest and significantly reduced in comparison with the earlier vaccine strains. Of the five volunteers who developed diarrhea after ingesting 10^8 CVD 103 organisms, only one had a stool volume that exceeded 400 ml (958) (Table 8). In contrast with recipients of JBK 70, CVD 101, and O395-N1, who frequently experienced malaise, anorexia, and abdominal cramps, these symptoms were almost never recorded in individuals vaccinated with CVD 103, even among the few who experienced mild diarrhea (Table 8).

TABLE 12
Clinical and Bacteriological Responses of Volunteers Following Ingestion of A−B+ Classical Inaba Vaccine Strain CVD 103 and CVD 103-HgR Prepared by Recombinant DNA Techniques, of Their Virulent Parent, V. cholerae Classical Inaba 569B

Strain and dose ingested	No. of volunteers	No. (%) with diarrhea	No. (%) with stool volume		Coprocultures		Duodenal fluid cultures	
			> 5.0 liter	> 2.0 liter	No. (%) positive	Geometric mean excretion[a]	Proportion (%) positive[b]	Geometric mean titer[a]
CVD 103								
10^3	6	0 (0)	0 (0)	0 (0)	0 (0)	0	0/5 (0)	0
10^4	6	0 (0)	0 (0)	0 (0)	4 (67)	6.8×10^2	0/2 (0)	0
10^6	6	1 (17)	0 (0)	0 (0)	5 (83)	6.6×10^3	0/3 (0)	0
$2–3 \times 10^8$	46	5 (11)	0 (0)	0 (0)	40 (87)	3.4×10^3	23/42 (55)	1.2×10^2
CVD 103-HgR								
5×10^8	18	0 (0)	0 (0)	0 (0)	5 (28)	1.9×10^2	3/18 (17)	1.5×10^1
Classical Inaba 569B								
10^6	24	20 (83)	5 (21)	10 (42)	23 (96)	5.3×10^{4c}	3/10 (30)	1.0×10^1

[a] No. V. cholerae per g of stool or per ml of duodenal fluid among positives.
[b] No. positive/no. with duodenal fluid cultures.
[c] Geometric mean of 12 individuals who had quantitative coprocultures.

Although CVD 103 is significantly less reactogenic than CVD 101 and JBK 70, it evokes serum antibody responses nearly comparable (vibriocidal) or equal to (antitoxin) those induced by these earlier vaccine candidates (Tables 13 and 14). As expected, these immune responses were accompanied by significant protection against challenge with toxinogenic *V. cholerae* 01 of either serotype or biotype. To obtain this information, three separate challenge studies were carried out with CVD 103 vaccinees to assess the efficacy of the vaccine. As shown in Table 15, a single dose of CVD 103 provided significant protection against challenge with pathogenic *V. cholerae* 01 of both Inaba and Ogawa serotypes and both classical and El Tor biotypes.

CVD 103-HgR. The promising results obtained with CVD 103 in North American volunteers generated interest in determining how well such a vaccine might be tolerated in individuals in a cholera-endemic area, as well as how immunogenic it might be. However, before proceeding with such studies, genes encoding resistance to Hg^{2+}, a property not normally found in vibrios, were introduced into the CVD 103 chromosome in the hlyA locus, resulting in the further derivative, CVD 103-HgR. This was done so that the vaccine strain could be readily distinguished from wild *V. cholerae* 01 strains.

In the initial clinical study, a group of 18 North American volunteers ingested a single dose of 5×10^8 CVD 103-HgR organisms that had been reconstituted from a practical lyophilized formulation.[174] No adverse reactions occurred in any of the 18 vaccinees (Table 12). There was also significantly less recovery of vaccine organisms in coprocultures than had occurred with the CVD 103 parent (Table 12). Nevertheless, the CVD 103-HgR vaccine organisms apparently colonized the intestine sufficiently to evoke serum vibriocidal and antitoxin responses similar to those recorded after immunization with CVD 103 (Tables 13 and 14).

The practical formulation of CVD 103-HgR has since been extensively tested for safety and immunogenicity in 156 North American and 43 Swiss adults.[175] Table 14 summarizes

TABLE 13
Comparison of Vibriocidal Antibody Responses of Volunteers Following Ingestion
of Pathogenic or Attenuated Vaccine Strains of *Vibro cholerae* 01

Strain	Dose ingested	N	Vibriocidal antibody					Antitoxin	
			Percent with fourfold or greater rises	Peak geom. mean titer	Percent with titers		Percent with fourfold or greater rises	Peak mean titer[a]
					≥ 2560	$\geq 10,240$		
Attenuated								
CVD 103								
	$10^3, 10^4$	12	33	120	0	0	17	0.16
	10^6	6	100	2873	33	17	100	1.19
	10^8	46	98	1339	43	15	93	1.06
CVD 103-HgR	5×10^8	18	94	1810	50	17	83	1.17
Pathogenic								
Inaba 569B	10^6	24	100	2958	63	29	96	1.28

[a]Net optical density units.

TABLE 14
A Comparison of the Clinical and Immunologic Response of Volunteers Following Ingestion
of a Single Dose of Genetically Engineered Attenuated *V. Cholerae* Vaccine Strains or
after Three Oral Doses of the B Subunit/Killed Whole

	JBK 70 (10^{6-8})	CVD 101 (10^{6-8})	CVD 103 (10^{6-8})	CVD 103-HgR (10^8)	BS/WCV[a]
No vaccinated	9	13	52	144	19
Diarrhea attack rate	33%[c]	54%[d]	12%[e]	2.1%[f]	0%[g]
Mean diarrheal stool volume (ml)	967	1008	555	<400	0
Mean no. of loose stools	8	7.1	3.7	2.0	0
Positive coprocultures	89%	92%	81%	33%	NR[b]
Vibriocidal antibody response					
Significant rises	100%	92%	98%	91%	89%
Titers ≥ 2560	78%	54%	42%	50%	16%
Geometric mean peak titer	5940	2301	1410	1678[h]	595[i]
Serum antitoxin response					
Significant rises	NR	77%	94%	81%	100%
Mean titer	NR	0.81*	1.06	0.92	0.87
Significant protection in volunteers against					
El Tor Inaba	yes	NT	yes	yes	yes
Classical Inaba	NT	NT	yes	yes	NT
Classical Ogawa	NT	NT	yes	NT	NT

[a]Volunteers received a dose of vaccine on days 0, 14, and 28. Each dose contained 2×10^{11} inactivated *V. cholerae* and 5 mg of purified B subunit.
[b]NR, not relevant.
Statistical comparisons by Fisher's exact test or Student's test: $c + d$ vs e, $p = 0.0038$; $c + d$ vs f, p. 0.00081; $c + d$ vs g, $p = 0.0007$; e vs f, NS; e vs g, NS; h vs i, $p < 0.01$.
*Mean ELISA titer expressed in net optical density units.

the clinical and serological response of North American volunteers following ingestion of a single oral dose of 10^8 CVD 103-HgR organisms, in comparison with North Americans who received 10^{6-8} organisms of vaccine strains JBK 70, CVD 101, or CVD 103 or of volunteers who ingested three spaced doses of the B subunit/inactivated *V. cholerae* combination vaccine. Mild diarrhea was observed in only 2% of the CVD 103-HgR vaccinees. Ninety-one percent of the CVD 103-HgR vaccinees manifested significant rises in vibriocidal antibody (50% achieved titers of 1 : 2560 or greater) and 81% had significant rises in serum IgG antitoxin.

Beyond being well tolerated and highly immunogenic, a single oral dose of CVD 103-HgR was protective against experimental challenge with pathogenic *V. cholerae* 01 of either the homologous (classical) biotype or the heterologous (El Tor) biotype. Results of these challenge studies are summarized in Table 15.

Based on these encouraging observations in adult volunteers in industrialized countries, studies were initiated to evaluate the immunogenicity and reactogenicity of CVD 103-HgR in populations in less-developed countries where cholera is endemic. A single 5×10^8 organism dose of CVD 103-HgR, packaged in a formulation practical for immunizing children and adults, was well tolerated and highly immunogenic in Thai adults who participated in randomized, placebo-controlled, double-blind trials.[176] Large-scale safety/immunogenicity studies were subsequently initiated in several hundred 5- to 9-year-old children in Jakarta, Indonesia (Suhrayono, Simanjuntak C, Witham N, Levine MM, *et al.,* unpublished data) (see

TABLE 15
Experimental Challenge Studies to Assess the Efficacy of a Single Dose
of CVD 103 and CVD 103-HgR Oral Attenuated *Vibrio cholerae* Vaccine Strains
Prepared by Recombinant DNA Techniques[a]

Vaccine strain	Diarrhea attack rate	Mean diarrheal stool volume (ml) per ill volunteer	Direct coprocultures	Geometric mean excretion (vibrios per g stool)[b]
CVD 103				
Study 1[c]				
Controls	7/8[d]	1367 ± 1172	7/8	9.7×10^4
	p <0.003	p = not evaluable	p = 0.0004	p = 0.001
Vaccinees	1/9	519 ± 0	0/9	0
Study 2[e]				
Controls	8/8	8766 ± 5076	8/8	5.2×10^6
	p <0.001	p = 0.05	p = 0.017	p = 0.12
Vaccinees	2/11	1813 ± 1458	5/11	1.7×10^4
Study 3[f]				
Controls	9/9	2473 ± 1178	9/9	1.6×10^8
	p <0.01	p = 0.077	p = 0.40	p = 0.003
Vaccinees	2/6	306 ± 112	5/6	1.0×10^5
CVD 103-HgR				
Study 1[f]				
Controls	7/8	2972 ± 2059	7/8	1.3×10^8
	p = 0.06	p = 0.66	p = 0.69	p = 0.37
Vaccinees	2/6	1698 ± 801	5/6	9.5×10^6
Study 2[c]				
Controls	5/13	1100 ± 600	10/13	2.2×10^4
	p = 0.02		p = 0.02	p = 0.10
Vaccinees	0/14	—	4/14	3.7×10^2

[a]Statistical comparisons by Fisher's Exact test and Wilcoxon rank sum test
[b]Geometric mean of positives only.
[c]Volunteers were challenged with 10^6 pathogenic *V. cholerae* classical Inaba 569B with $NaHCO_3$.
[d]No. positive/no. challenged.
[e]Volunteers were challenged with 10^6 pathogenic *V. cholerae* classical Ogawa 395 with $NaHCO_3$.
[f]Volunteers were challenged with 10^6 pathogenic *V. cholerae* classical El Tor Inaba N16961 with $NaHCO_3$.

Fig. 2). The vaccine was well tolerated but a one log increase in dose (to 5×10^9 organisms) was necessary to elicit good immune responses with a single dose. Studies in Jakarta progressed to the 2- to 4-year-old age group. Results of these studies should determine whether a large-scale field trial of efficacy of CVD 103-HgR in a cholera-endemic area is warranted.

6.2.5.4b. Auxotrophic *V. cholerae* Strains

When initial experiences with chemically mutagenized vaccine strain Texas Star-SR and genetically engineered strains JBK 70 and CVD 101 showed that a notable proportion of the vaccinees developed mild diarrhea, one hypothesis put forth was that this might be an unavoidable response in some persons to any live vibrio that colonized the proximal small intestine and proliferated on the gut mucosa. A compromise that might combine some of the advantages of a live vaccine, while perhaps avoiding the problem of diarrhea, could be the use of auxotrophic mutants of *V. cholerae* as live oral vaccines. Such strains would have mutations making them dependent for growth on substrates unavailable in the human intes-

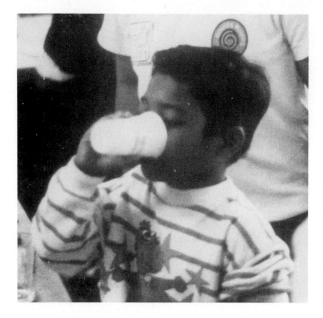

FIGURE 2. A Javanese child in North Jakarta, Indonesia, is shown ingesting a dose of live oral cholera vaccine strain CVD 103-HgR. This candidate vaccine, which is well tolerated and immunogenic after ingestion of just a single dose, is available in a practical formulation that is easy to administer to children. A sachet containing the dose of lyophilized vaccine and an accompanying sachet containing buffer and sweetener are mixed together in 100 ml of water; the suspension is then ingested by the child.

tine. Being unable to proliferate, they would probably have to be administered, like inactivated vibrio vaccines, in at least two spaced doses to adequately prime and boost the secretory immune system of the gut; this would represent a notable drawback. However, their inability to proliferate could render them very well tolerated. Moreover, since they would be living vibrios, they might interact quite effectively with the gut immune system to stimulate vigorous, protective immune responses. The only practical experience with auxotrophic strains of *V. cholerae* in humans has been obtained with attenuated *V. cholerae* vaccine candidate CVD 102.[75]

CVD 102. CVD 102 is a thymine-dependent auxotrophic mutant of CVD 101. It was given to five volunteers in a dose of 10^7 organisms, none of whom manifested adverse reactions. However, the absence of reactogenicity occurred at a great cost in immunogenicity; vaccine organisms could be recovered from only two of five individuals, only two of five had vibriocidal seroconversions (low titers) and none had antitoxin seroconversions.[75] Because of its greatly diminished immunogenicity, further studies with CVD 102 were not initiated, nor have there been reports of clinical studies with other auxotrophic mutants of *V. cholerae* 01.

6.2.5.4c. Attenuated *S. typhi* Vaccine Strains Expressing *V. cholerae* Antigens

Investigators in Australia have pioneered the use of attenuated *S. typhi* strains as carrier bacteria to express cloned genes of *V. cholerae* 01 antigens.[154,177] These scientists introduced into attenuated *S. typhi* vaccine strain Ty21a genes that encode the expression of Inaba O antigen from a classical Inaba strain. The safety, immunogenicity, and efficacy of Ty21a as an effective oral vaccine to prevent typhoid fever have been demonstrated; no specific adverse reactions have been attributed to Ty21a in either passive or active surveillance studies. Because of its established safety and its ability to elicit both humoral (circulating and secretory antibodies) and cell-mediated immune responses, Ty21a has been utilized as a carrier strain to express antigens of *Shigella sonnei*[178] and enterotoxigenic *Escherichia coli,*[179] as well as *V. cholerae* 01.

A plasmid encoding the genes necessary for expression of the Inaba O antigen of *V. cholerae* 01 was stabilized in Ty21a by making the Ty21a thymine-dependent and including the genes for thymine synthesis in the plasmid. Ty21a containing the stable plasmid encoding Inaba O antigen (strain EX645) was fed to 22 volunteers in a dose of 10^{11} viable organisms with buffer given on two occasions separated by one month; despite the extremely high dose, no notable adverse reactions were recorded.[177] All vaccinees manifested significant rises in serum antibody to Inaba LPS measured by ELISA. In contrast, the serum vibriocidal antibody responses were inconsistent and modest.

Subsequently, a group of 14 North American volunteers were given three 5×10^{10} organism doses of hybrid strain EX645 on days 0, 2, and 4.[180] The serological responses to the foreign (Inaba) O antigen were modest. Only 14% had significant rises in serum IgG or IgA Inaba O antibody and only 36% showed significant rises in serum vibriocidal antibody. In contrast, all vaccinees manifested significant rises in serum antibody to *S. typhi* O antigen and 86% showed rises in intestinal SIgA antibody to the typhi antigen. An experimental challenge study was carried out to determine if the Ty21a strain expressing Inaba O antigen could protect.[180] In the challenge study diarrhea occurred in 13 of 13 unvaccinated control volunteers and in six of eight vaccinees (25% vaccine efficacy, $p = 0.13$). While the hybrid vaccine did not provide protection overall against experimental cholera, the severity of diarrhea (as measured by total diarrheal stool volume) and excretion of the pathogen were significantly diminished ($p < 0.05$) in vaccinees compared with controls.[180]

7. SUMMARY

Parenteral killed whole-cell vaccines, first developed at the end of the 19th century and still available today, provide a moderate degree of protection in older children and adults in endemic areas but for only a few months; therefore vaccines of this type are of little practical use. Since *V. cholerae* is a noninvasive enteropathogen, local intestinal immunity mediated by SIgA is particularly critical. As a corollary, oral immunizing agents are more effective than parenteral vaccines in stimulating intestinal immunity.

In the 1980s, several new oral vaccines to prevent cholera were developed. Two oral vaccines, consisting of either a combination of purified B subunit and killed vibrios or of killed vibrios alone, have been the most extensively tested. These two vaccines were shown to be safe and to confer significant protection (51% vaccine efficacy for the combination and 52% for the whole-cell alone) for at least 36 months in a controlled field trial in Bangladesh. Notably, in the first six months of that trial, the combination vaccine conferred significantly higher protection (85% vaccine efficacy) than the oral whole-cell vaccine alone (58% vaccine efficacy); during this period the combination oral vaccine also provided significant protection in children less than six years of age; in the first three months after vaccination the combination vaccine conferred 75% protection against diarrhea due to LT-producing *E. coli*. The oral whole-cell vaccine and the B subunit/whole-cell combination vaccine are the best cholera vaccines, so far, to be evaluated in a large-scale field trial and represent a notable advance over all earlier vaccines. Possible drawbacks that may impede the ultimate widespread use of these vaccines include the requirement for multiple doses to prime and boost the intestinal immune system, relatively high cost of manufacture of the combination vaccine, and the short-lived protective effect (only six months) noted in young children less than six years of age (those at highest risk for cholera).

Attenuated strains of *V. cholerae* 01 prepared by recombinant DNA techniques that are deleted of genes encoding the A subunit of cholera toxin offer great promise for the future as live oral vaccines. These vaccine strains are highly immunogenic and protective in volunteer studies after ingestion of a single dose. Although the first two generations of genetically engineered vaccine candidates were greatly attenuated in comparison with the parent strains from which they were derived, they caused mild diarrhea in approximately one half of the recipients. Two later candidates, CVD 103 and CVD 103-HgR, were significantly better tolerated, while retaining the properties of appreciable immunogenicity and protectiveness after administration of a single oral dose. CVD 103-HgR, an A$-$B$+$ derivative of classical Inaba 569B that does not elaborate Shiga-like toxin and has Hg^{2+} resistance genes as a marker, has undergone extensive tests of safety and immunogenicity in North American, Swiss, and Thai adults and in Indonesian children. CVD 103-HgR has been remarkably well tolerated by all these groups in whom a single dose has been shown to elicit strong vibriocidal and antitoxin antibody responses in 80–95% of vaccinees. Results of further studies in younger children will determine whether a field trial should be undertaken to assess the protective efficacy of vaccine strain CVD 103-HgR.

REFERENCES

1. Diarrhoeal Diseases Control Programme: *Biomedical and Epidemiological Research Priorities of Global Scientific Working Groups.* WHO/CDD/86.8 Rev.1 (1987). Geneva, World Health Organization, 1987
2. Goodgame RW, Greenough WB: Cholera in Africa: a message for the West. *Ann Inter Med* 82:101–106, 1975
3. Umoh JU, Adesiyun AA, Adekeye JO, et al: Epidemiological features of an outbreak of gastroenteritis/cholera in Katsina, Northern Nigeria. *J Hyg (Camb.)* 91:101–111, 1983
4. Ferran J: Nota sobre la profilixas del colera por medio de inyecciones hipodermicas de cultivo puro del bacilo virgula. *Siglo Med* 32:480, 1885
5. Bornside GH: Jaime Ferran and preventive inoculation against cholera. *Bull Hist Med* 55:516–532, 1981
6. Koch R: Der zweite Bericht der deutschen Cholera-Commission. *Dtsch Med Wochschr* 9:743–744, 1883
7. Bornside: GH: Waldemar Haffkine's cholera vaccines and the Ferran-Haffkine priority dispute. *J Hist Med All Sci* 37:399–422, 1982
8. Kolle W: Die aktive Immunisierung des Menschen gegen Cholera nach Haffkine's Verfahren in Indien. *Zbl Bakt I Abt Orig* 19:217–221, 1896
9. Voges O: Die Cholera-Immunitat. *Zbl Bakt I Abt Orig* 19:325–241, 395–400, 444–470, 1896
10. Haffkine WM: Les vaccinations anticholeriques aux Indes. *Bull Inst Pasteur* 4:697–705, 737–747, 1906
11. Haffkine, WM: Protective inoculation against cholera, Calcutta. *C R Soc Biol (Paris)* 4: 635–671, 1985
12. Cvjetanovic B: Contribution of Haffkine to the concept and practice of controlled field trials. *Fortschr Arzneimittforsch* 19:481–489, 1975
13. Kolle W: Zur aktiven Immunisierung des Menschen gegen Cholera. *Zbl Bakt I Abt Orig* 19:97–104, 1896
14. Murata N: Uber die Schutzimpfung gegen Cholera. *Zbl Bakt I Abt Orig* 35:605–608, 1904
15. Sawtschenko J, Sabolotny DK: Versuch einer Immunisation des menschen gegen Cholera. *Zbl allg Path Path Anat* 4:625–636, 1893
16. Russell AJH: Besredka's cholera bilivaccin versus anti-cholera vaccine: a comparative field test, in: *Transactions of the Seventh Congress of the Far Eastern Association of Tropical Medicine, 1927, Calcutta,* Vol 1. p 253
17. Russell AJH: Le bilivaccin anticholerique et le vaccin anticholerique ordinaire. Essai de comparaison pratique, in: Graham JD, Recherhes sur le cholera et la vaccination anticholerique dans l'Inde Brittanique. *Bull Off Int Hyg Publ* 20:703–709, 1928
18. Russell AJH: Cholera in India, in: *Transactions of the Ninth Congress of the Far Eastern Association of Tropical Medicine, 1934, Nanking,* Vol 1. p 398

19. Sarramon: Sur l'emploi du vaccin anticholerique psr voie buccale. *Bull Soc Med-Chir Indochine* 8:180–183, 1930
20. Cash RA, Music SI, Libonati JP, et al: Response of man to infection with *Vibrio cholerae*. Protection from illness afforded by previous disease and vaccine. *J Infect Dis* 130:325–333, 1974
21. Levine MM, Nalin DR, Craig JP, et al: Immunity to cholera in man: relative role of antibacterial versus antitoxic immunity. *Trans Roy Soc Trop Med Hyg* 73:3–9, 1979
22. Levine MM: Immunity to cholera as evaluated in volunteers, in Ouchterlony O, Holmgren J (ed): *Cholera and Related Diarrheas*. Basel, S. Karger, 1980, pp 195–203
23. Levine MM, Black RE, Clements ML, et al: Volunteer studies in development of vaccines against cholera and enterotoxigenic *Escherichia coli:* a review, in Holme T, Holmgren J, Merson M, Mollby R (eds): *Acute Enteric Infections in Children: New Prospects for Treatment and Prevention*. Amsterdam, Elsevier/North Holland, 1981
24. Levine MM, Black RE, Clements ML, et al: The quality and duration of infection-derived immunity to cholera. *J Infect Dis* 143:818–820, 1981
25. Levine, MM, Kaper JB, Black RE, et al: New knowledge on pathogenesis of bacterial enteric infections as applied to vaccine development. *Microbiol Rev* 47:510–550, 1983
26. Shedlofsky S, Freter R: Synergism between ecologic and immunologic control mechanism. *J Infect Dis* 129:296–303, 1974
27. Woodward WE: Cholera reinfection in man. *J Infect Dis* 123:61–66, 1971
28. Glass RI, Becker S, Huq MI, et al: Endemic cholera in rural Bangladesh, 1966–1980. *Am J Epidemiol* 116:959–970, 1982
29. Glass RI, Svennerholm A-M, Stoll B, et al: Protection against cholera in breast-fed children by antibodies in breast milk. *N Eng J Med* 308:1389–1392, 1983
30. Glass RI, Svennerholm A-M, Khan RN, et al: Seroepidemiological studies of El Tor cholera in Bangladesh: association of serum antibody levels with protection. *J Infect Dis* 151:236–242, 1985
31. Benenson AS: Review of experience with whole-cell and somatic antigen cholera vaccines, in: *Symposium on Cholera, Sapporo, 1976*. US–Japan Cooperative Medical Science Program, National Institute of Health, Tokyo, 1977, pp 228–252
32. Feeley JC, Gangarosa EJ: Field trials of cholera vaccine, in *Cholera and Related Diarrheas, 43rd Nobel Symposium, Stockholm, 1978*. Basel, Karger, 1980, pp 204–210
33. Joo I: Cholera vacines, in Barua D, Burrows W (eds): *Cholera*. Philadelphia, WB Saunders, 1974, pp 333–335
34. Oseasohn RO, Benenson AS, Fahimuddin Md: Field trial of cholera vaccine in rural East Pakistan. *Lancet* i:450–453, 1965
35. Benenson AS, Mosley WH, Fahimuddin M, et al: Cholera vaccine field trials in East Pakistan. 2. Effectiveness in the field. *Bull WHO* 38:359–372, 1968
36. Mosley WH, McCormack WM, Ahmed A, et al: Report of the 1966–67 cholera field trial in rural East Pakistan. 2. Results of the serological surveys in the study population—the relationship of case rate to antibody titre and an estimate of the inapparent infection rate with *Vibrio cholerae*. *Bull WHO* 40:187–197, 1969
37. Mosley WH: The role of immunity in cholera. A review of epidemiological and serological studies. *Texas Rep Biol Med* 27(1):227–244, 1969
38. Mosley WH, McCormack WM, Ahmed A, et al: Report of the 1966–67 cholera vaccine field trial in rural East Pakistan. 1. Study design and results of the first year of observation. *Bull WHO* 40:177–185, 1969
39. Mosley WH, Woodward WE, Aziz KMS, et al: The 1968–1969 cholera vaccine field trial in rural East Pakistan. Effectiveness of monovalent Ogawa and Inaba vaccines and a purified Inaba antigen, with comparative results of serological and animal protection tests. *J Infect Dis* 121:S1–S9, 1970
40. Mosley, WH, Aziz KMS, Mizanur Rahman ASM, et al: Report of the 1966–67 cholera vaccine trial in rural East Pakistan. *Bull WHO* 47:229–238, 1972
41. Mosley WH, Aziz KMS, Mizanur Rahman ASM, et al: Field trials of monovalent Ogawa and Inaba cholera vaccines in rural Bangladesh—three years of observation. *Bull WHO* 49:381–387, 1973
42. Philippines Cholera Committee: A controlled field trial of the effectiveness of cholera and cholera El Tor vaccines in the Philippines. *Bull WHO* 32:603–625, 1965
43. Azurin JC, Cruz A, Pesigan TP, et al: A controlled field trial of the effectiveness of cholera and cholera El Tor vaccines in the Philippines. *Bull WHO* 37:703–727, 1967
44. Philippines Cholera Committee: A controlled field trial of the effectiveness of various doses of cholera El Tor Vaccine in the Philippines. *Bull WHO* 38:917–923, 1968
45. Das Gupta A, Sinha R, Shrivastava DL, et al: Controlled field trial of the effectiveness of cholera and cholera El Tor vaccines in Calcutta. *Bull WHO* 37:371–385, 1967

46. Pal SC, Deb BC, Sen Gupta PG, et al: A controlled field trial of an aluminum phosphate-adsorbed cholera vaccine in Calcutta. *Bull WHO* 58:741–745, 1980

47. Saroso JS, Bahrawi W, Witjaksono H, et al: A controlled field trial of plain and aluminum hydroxide-adsorbed cholera vaccines in Surabaya, Indonesia, during 1973–75. *Bull WHO* 56:619–627, 1978

48. Clemens JD, Sack DA, Harris JR, et al: Field trial of oral cholera vaccines in Bangladesh. *Lancet* ii:124–127, 1986

49. Freter R: Studies on the mechanism of action of intestinal antibody in experimental cholera. *Texas Rep Exp Biol Med* 27:299–316, 1969

50. Neoh SH, Rowley D: Protection of infant mice against cholera by antibodies to three *Vibrio cholerae* antigens. *J Infect Dis* 126:41–47, 1972

51. Fubara ES, Freter R: Protection against enteric infection by secretory antibodies. *J Immunol* 111:395–403, 1973

52. Bellamy JEC, Knop EJ, Steele EJ, et al: Antibody cross-linking as a factor in immunity to cholera in infant mice. *J Infect Dis* 132:181–188, 1975

53. Steele EJ, Chaicumpa W, Rowley D: Further evidence for cross-linking as a protective factor in experimental cholera: properties of antibody fragments. *J Infect Dis* 132:175–180, 1975

54. Guentzel MN, Field LH, Eubanks ER, et al: Use of flourescent antibody in studies of immunity to cholera in infant mice. *Infect Immun* 15:539–548, 1977

55. Eubanks ER, Guentzel MN, Berry LJ: Evaluation of surface components of *Vibrio cholerae* as protective immunogens. *Infect Immun* 15:533–538, 1977

56. Yancey RJ, Willis DL, Berry LJ: Flagella-induced immunity against experimental cholera in adult rabbits. *Infect Immun* 25:220–228, 1979

57. Hranitsky KW, Mulholland A, Larson AD, et al: Characterization of a flagellar sheath protein of *Vibrio cholerae*. *Infect Immun* 27:597–603, 1980

58. Chaicumpa W, Atthasisishta N: Study of intestinal immunity against *V. cholerae:* role of antibody to *V. cholerae* haemagglutinin in intestinal immunity. *SE Asian J Trop Med Publ Hlth* 8:13–18, 1977

59. Fujita K, Finkelstein RA: Antitoxic immunity in experimental cholera: comparison of immunity induced perorally and parenterally in mice. *J Infect Dis* 125:647–655, 1972

60. Holmgren J, Svennerholm A-M, Ouchterlony O, et al: Antitoxic immunity in experimental cholera: protection and serum and local antibody responses in rabbits after enteric and parenteral immunization. *Infect Immun* 12:463–470, 1975

61. Pierce, NF, Sack RB, Sircar BK: Immunity to experimental cholera. III. Enhanced duration of protection after sequential parenteral–oral toxoid administration to dogs. *J Infect Dis* 135:888–896, 1977

62. Pierce NF, Reynolds HY: Immunity to experimental cholera. I. Protective effect of humoral IgG antitoxin demonstrated by passive immunization. *J Immunol* 113:1017–1023, 1974

63. Pierce NF, Cray WC Jr, Sircar BK: Induction of a mucosal antitoxin response and its role in immunity to experimental canine cholera. *Infect Immun* 21:185–193, 1978

64. Lange S, Hansson H-A, Molin S-O, et al: Local cholera immunity in mice: intestinal antitoxin-containing cells and their correlation with protective immunity. *Infect Immun* 23:743–750, 1979

65. Svennerholm A-M, Lange S, Holmgren J: Correlation between intestinal synthesis of specific immunoglobulin A and protection against experimental cholera in mice. *Infect Immun* 21:1–6, 1978

66. Pierce NF, Cray WC Jr, Engel PF: Antitoxic immunity to cholera in dogs immunized orally with cholera toxin. *Infect Immun* 27:632–637, 1980

67. Pierce NF, Cray WC Jr, Sacci JB Jr: Oral immunization of dogs with purified cholera toxin, crude cholera toxin, or B subunit: evidence for synergistic protection by antitoxic and antibacterial mechanisms. *Infect Immun* 37:687–694, 1982

68. Peterson JW: Protection against experimental cholera by oral or parenteral immunization. *Infect Immun* 26:594–598, 1979

69. Pierce, NF, Cray WC Jr, Sacci JB Jr, et al: Procholeragenoid: a safe and effective antigen for oral immunization against experimental cholera. *Infect Immun* 40:1112–1118, 1983

70. Svennerholm A-M, Holmgren J: Synergistic protective effect in rabbits of immunization with *Vibrio cholerae* lipopolysaccharide and toxin/toxoid. *Infect Immun* 13:735–740, 1976

71. Holmgren J, Svennerholm A-M: Mechanisms of disease and immunity in cholera: a review. *J Infect Dis* 136:S105–S112, 1977

72. Peterson JW: Synergistic protection against experimental cholera by immunization with cholera toxoid and vaccine. *Infect Immun* 26:528–533, 1979

73. Resnick IG, Ford CW, Shackleford GM, et al: Improved protection against cholera in adult rabbits with a combined flagellar–toxoid vaccine. *Infect Immun* 30:375–380, 1980

74. Chaicumpa W, Boonthum A, Kalumbaheti T, et al. Cell-bound haemagglutinin (CHA) of *V. cholerae* 01 as protective antigen. *SE Asian J Trop Med Publ Hlth* 15:407–413, 1984

75. Levine MM, Kaper JB, Herrington D, et al: Deletion mutants of *Vibrio cholerae* 01 prepared by recombinant techniques: insights on pathogenesis and immunity. *Infect Immun* 1988: in press

76. Black RE, Levine MM, Clements ML, et al: Protective efficacy in humans of killed whole-vibrio oral cholera vaccine with and without the B subunit of cholera toxin. *Infect Immun* 55:1116–1120, 1987

77. Kaper JB, Lockman H, Baldini M, et al: Recombinant nontoxigenic *Vibrio cholerae* strains as attenuated cholera vaccine candidates. *Nature* 308:655–658, 1984

78. Curlin G, Levine R, Aziz KMS, et al: Field trial of cholera toxoid, in: *Proceedings of the 11th Joint Conference on Cholera*. U.S.–Japan Cooperative Medical Science Program, 1975, pp 314–329

79. Noriki H: Evaluation of toxic field trial on the Philippines, in Fukumi H, Zinnaka Y (eds): *Proceedings of the 12th Joint Conference on Cholera,* U.S.–Japan Cooperative Medical Science Program. Sapporo. Fuji, Tokyo, 1976, pp 302–310

80. Clemens JD, Harris JR, Sack DA, et al: Field trial of oral cholera vaccines in Bangladesh: results of one year follow-up. *J Infect Dis* 158:60–69, 1988

81. Clemens JD, Sack DA, Harris Jr, et al: Field trial of oral cholera vaccines in Bangladesh: results from three year follow-up. *Lancet* 335:270–273, 1990

82. Clemens JD, Sack DA, Harris JR, et al: Cross-protection by B subunit-whole cell cholera vaccine against diarrhoea associated with heat-labile toxin-producing enterotoxigenic *Escherichia coli:* results of a large-scale field trial. *J Infect Dis* 158:372–377, 1988

83. Neoh SE, Rowley D: The antigens of *Vibrio cholerae* involved in the vibriocidal action of antibody and complement. *J Infect Dis* 121:505–513, 1970

84. Kaur J, Burrows W: Immunity to cholera: relation of fraction II of type 2 cholera toxin to vibriocidal. *J Bacteriol* 98:467–474

85. Attridge SR, Rowley D: Prophylactic significance of the nonpolysaccharide antigens of *Vibrio cholerae*. *J Infect Dis* 148:931–939, 1983

86. Ahmad A, Bhattacharjee AK, Mosley WH: Characteristics of the serum vibriocidal and agglutinating antibodies in cholera cases and normal residents of the endemic and non-endemic cholera areas. *J Immunol* 105:431–441, 1970

87. Merritt CB, Sack RB: Sensitivity of agglutinating and vibriocidal antibodies to 2-mercaptoethanol in human cholera. *J Infect Dis* 121:S25–S30

88. Majumdar AS, Ghose AC: Evaluation of the biological properties of different classes of human antibodies in relation to cholera. *Infect Immun* 32:9–14, 1981

89. Clements ML, Levine MM, Young CR, Black RE, Lim Y-L, Robins-Browne RM: Magnitude, kinetics and duration of vibriocidal antibody response in North Americans after ingestion of *Vibrio cholerae*. *J Infect Dis* 145:465–473, 1982

90. Tomasi TB: *The Immune System of Secretions.* Englewood Cliffs, NJ, Prentice-Hall, 1976

91. Waldman RH, Bencic Z, Sakazaki R, et al: Cholera immunology. II. Serum and intestinal secretion antibody response after naturally-occurring cholera. *J Infect Dis* 126:401–407, 1972

92. Champsur H, Iscaki S, Bernard, et al: Induction of *Vibrio cholerae* specific biliary antibodies after oral immunization with a cholera cell wall fraction. *Lancet* i:1276–1277, 1985

93. Estavoyer JM, Panouse-Perrin J, Dodin A, et al: La maladie cholerique: etude serologiques d'un cas. *Bull Soc Path Ex* 75:242–247, 1982

94. Chaicumpa W, Rowley D: Experimental cholera in infant mice: protective effects of antibody. *J Infect Dis* 125:480–485, 1972

95. Freter R, Jones GW: Adhesive properties of *Vibrio cholerae:* nature of the interaction with intact mucosal surfaces. *Infect Immun* 14:246–256, 1976

96. Chitnis DS, Sharma KD, Kamat RS: Role of somatic antigen of *Vibrio cholerae* in adhesion to intestinal mucosa. *J Med Microbiol* 5:53–61, 1982

97. Benenson AS, Saad A, Mosley WH, et al: Serological studies in cholera. 3. Serum toxin neutralization—Rise in titre in response to infection with *Vibrio cholerae,* and the level in the "normal" population of East Pakistan. *Bull WHO* 38:287–295, 1968

98. Levine MM, Young CR, Hughes TP, et al: Duration of serum antitoxin response following Vibrio cholerae infection in North Americans: relevance for seroepidemiology. *Am J Epidemiol* 114:348–354, 1981

99. Levine MM, Young CR, Black RE, et al: Enzyme-linked immunosorbent assay to measure antibodies to purified heat-labile enterotoxins from human and porcine strains of *Escherichia coli* and to cholera toxin: application in serodiagnosis and seroepidemiology. *J Clin Microbiol* 21:174–179, 1985

100. Svennerholm A-M, Jertborn M, Gothefors L, et al: Mucosal antitoxic and antibacterial immunity after cholera disease and after immunization with a combined B subunit whole cell vaccine. *J Infect Dis* 149:884–893, 1984

101. Taylor R, Miller VL, Furlong DB, et al: Use of phoA gene fusions to identity a pilus colonization factor coordinately regulated with cholera toxin. *Proc Nat Acad Sci USA* 84:2833–2837, 1987

102. Miller VL, Mekalanos JJ: Synthesis of cholera toxin is positively regulated at the transcriptional level by toxR. *Proc Nat Acad Sci USA* 81:3471–3475, 1984

103. Hall R, Vial PA, Kaper JB, et al: Morphological studies on fimbriae expressed by *Vibrio cholerae* 01. *Microbial Path* 4:257–265, 1988

104. Herrington DA, Hall RH, Losonsky G, et al: Toxin, toxin-coregulated pili, and the *toxR* regulon are essential for *Vibrio cholerae* pathogenesis in humans. *J Exp Med* 168:1487–1492, 1988

105. Taylor RK, Shaw C, Peterson K, et al: Safe, live *Vibrio cholerae* vaccines? *Vaccines* 6:151–154, 1988

106. Mestecky J, McGhee JR: Immunoglobulin A (IgA) molecular and cellular interaction involved in IgA biosynthesis and immune response. *Adv Immunol* 40:153–245, 1987

107. Pierce NF, Gowans: Cellular kinetics of the intestinal immune response to cholera toxoid in rats. *J Exp Med* 142:1550–1563, 1975

108. Weisz-Carrington P, Roux ME, McWilliams M, et al: Organ and isotype distribution of plasma cells producing specific antibody after oral immunization: evidence for a generalized secretory immune system. *J Immunol* 123:1705–1708

109. Strober W, Hanson LA, Sell KW: *Recent Advances in Mucosal Immunity*. New York, Raven Press, 1982

110. Jertborn M, Svennerholm A-M, Holmgren J: Gut mucosal, salivary and serum antitoxic and antibacterial antibody responses in Swedes after oral immunization with B subunit-whole cell cholera vaccine. *Int Archs Allergy Appl Immun* 75:38–43, 1984

111. Jertborn M, Svennerholm A-M, Holmgren J: Saliva, breast milk, and serum antibody responses as indirect measures of intestinal immunity after oral cholera vaccination or natural disease. *J Clin Microbiol* 24:203–209, 1986

112. Majumdar AS, Dutta P, Dutta D, et al: Antibacterial and antitoxin responses in the serum and milk of cholera patients. *Infect Immun* 32:1–8, 1981

113. Lange S, Vygren H, Svennerholm A-M, et al: Antitoxic cholera immunity in mice. Influence of antigen deposition on antitoxin-containing cells and protective immunity in different parts of intestine. *Infect Immun* 28:17–23, 1980

114. Pierce NF: The role of antigen form and function in the primary and secondary intestinal immune responses to cholera toxin and toxoid in rats. *J Exp Med* 148:195–206, 1978

115. Lycke N, Holmgren J: Intestinal mucosal memory and presence of memory cells in lamina proporia and Peyer's patches in mice 2 years after oral immunization with cholera toxin. *Scand J Immunol* 23:611–616, 1986

116. Svennerholm A-M, Gothefors L, Sack DA, et al: Local and systemic antibody responses and immunological memory in humans after immunization with cholera B subunit by different routes. *Bull WHO* 62:909–918, 1984

117. Svennerholm A-M, Hanson LA, Holmgren J, et al: Different secretory immunoglobulin A antibody responses to cholera vaccination in Swedish and Pakistani women. *Infect Immun* 30:427–430, 1980

118. Levine MM, Black RE, Clements ML, et al: Prevention of enterotoxigenic *Escherichia coli* diarrheal infection by vaccines that stimulate anti-adhesion (anti-pili) immunity, in Boedeker EC (ed): *Attachment of Organisms to the Gut Mucosa,* Boca Raton, CRC Press, 1984, pp 223–244

119. Yardley JM, Keren DF, Hamilton SR, et al: Local (immunoglobulin A) immune responses by the intestine to cholera toxin and its partial suppression by combined systemic and intra-intestinal immunization. *Infect Immun* 19:589–597, 1978

120. Pierce NF, Koster FT: Priming and suppression of the intestinal immune response to cholera toxoid/toxin by parenteral toxoid in rats. *J Immunol* 124:307–311, 1980

121. Philippines Cholera Committee: A controlled field trial of the effectiveness of monovalent classical and El Tor cholera vaccines in the Philippines. *Bull WHO* 49:13–19, 1973

122. Northrup RS, Chisari FV: Response of monkeys to immunization with cholera toxoid, toxin, and vaccine: reversion of cholera toxoid. *J Infect Dis* 125:471–479, 1972

123. Black RE, Yunus Md, Eusof A, et al: Report and immunogenicity of Wellcome cholera toxoids in Bangladeshi

volunteers. International Centre for Diarrhoeal Disease Research, Bangladesh, Scientific Report No. 29, Dacca, 1979

124. Merson MN, Black RE, Sack DA, et al: Maternal cholera immunisation and secretory IgA in breast milk. *Lancet* i:931–932, 1980

125. Ohtomo N: Safety and potency tests of cholera toxoid lot 11 in animals and volunteers, in Fukumi H, Zinnaka Y (eds): *Proceedings of the 12th Joint Conference on Cholera*. US–Japan Cooperative Medical Science Program, Sapporo, Fuji, Tokyo, 1976, pp 286–296

126. Rappaport RS, Pierzchala WA, Bonde G, et al: Development of a purified cholera toxin. III. Refinements in purification of toxin and methods for the determination of residual somatic antigen. *Infect Immun* 14:687–693, 1976

127. Finkelstein RA, Fujita K, Lospallutto JJ: Procholeragenoid: an aggregated intermediate in the formation of choleragenoid. *J Immunol* 107:1043–1051, 1971

128. Germanier R, Furer E, Varallyay S, et al: Preparation of a purified antigenic cholera toxoid. *Infect Immun* 13:1692–1698, 1976

129. Germanier R, Furer E, Varallyay S, et al: Antigenicity of cholera toxoid in humans. *J Infect Dis* 135:512–516, 1977

130. Holmgrem J, Svennerholm A-M, Lonnroth I, et al: Development of an improved cholera vaccine based on subunit toxoid. *Nature* 269;602–604, 1977

131. Holmgren J: Actions of cholera toxin and the prevention and treatment of cholera. *Nature* 292:413–417, 1981

132. Svennerholm A-M, Sack DA, Holmgren J, et al: Intestinal antibody responses after immunisation with cholera B subunit. *Lancet* i:305–308, 1982

133. Freter R: Detection of coproantibody and its formation after parenteral and oral immunization of human volunteers. *J Infect Dis* 111:37–48, 1962

134. Freter R, Gangarosa EJ: Oral immunization and production of coproantibody in human volunteers. *J Immunol* 91:724–729, 1963

135. Ganguly R, Clem LW, Benck Z, et al: Antibody response in the intestinal secretions of volunteers immunized with various cholera vaccines. *Bull WHO* 52:323–330, 1975

136. Denchev V, Jeleva M, Duncheve St: Human immunization with killed cholera vaccine. *Acta Microbiol Acad Sci Hung* 21:209–212, 1974

137. Oberdoerster F, Thilo W: A new inactivated oral cholera vaccine. *Acta Microbiol Acad Sci Hung* 21:213–215, 1974

138. Clemens JD, Jertborn M, Sack DA, et al: Effect of neutralization of gastric acid on immune responses to an oral B subunit, killed whole cell cholera vaccine. *J Infect Dis* 154:175–178, 1986

139. Dodin A, Plawecki M: Étude sur l'animal de fractions antigeniques radio-actives isoless de *V. cholerae*. I. La fraction de Ch 1 + 2. *Bull Soc Path Ex* 71:22–33, 1977

140. Dodin A: Les antigenes vaccinants. *Bordeaux Medical* 2:299–301, 1979

141. Dodin A: Un vaccin oral contre le cholera. *A Recherche* 110:468–469, 1980

142. Gateff C, Dodin A, Wiart J: Comparaison des reactions serologiques induites par un vaccin anticholerique classique et une fraction vaccinante purifiée associés ou non au vaccin anti-amaril. *Ann Microbiol* 126A:231–246, 1975

143. Dodin A, Masengo B, Loucq C: Resultats controles du vaccin anticholerique oral de l'Institut Pasteur au cours de l'épidemie du Shaba-Zaire en 1983. *C.R. Acad Sci Paris serie III* 299:205–207, 1984

144. Levine MM, Hughes, TP, Young CR, et al: Antigenicity of purified glutaraldehyde-treated cholera toxoid administered orally. *Infect Immun* 21:158–162, 1978

145. Sanyal S, Mukerjee S: Live oral cholera vaccine: report of a trial on human volunteer subjects. *Bull WHO* 40:503–511, 1969

146. Cash RA, Music SI, Libonati JP, et al: Live oral cholera vaccine: evaluation of the clinical effectiveness of two strains in humans. *Infect Immun* 10:762–764, 1974

147. Levine MM, Black RE, Clements ML, et al: The pathogenicity of nonenterotoxigenic *Vibrio cholerae* serogroup 01 biotype El Tor isolated from sewage water in Brazil. *J Infect Dis* 145:296–299, 1982

148. Finkelstein RA, Vasil ML, Holmes RD: Studies on toxigenesis in *Vibrio cholerae*. 1. Isolation of mutants with altered toxigenicity. *J Infect Dis* 129:117–123, 1974

149. Holmes RK, Vasil ML, Finkelstein RA: Studies on toxigenesis in *Vibrio cholerae*. III. Characterization of nontoxigenic mutants in vitro and in experimental animals. *J Clin Invest* 55:551–560, 1975

150. Woodward WE, Gilman RH, Hornick RB, et al: Efficacy of a live oral cholera vaccine in human volunteers. *Dev Biol Stand* 33:108–112, 1976

151. Honda T, Finkelstein RA: Selection and characteristics of a *Vibrio cholerae* mutant lacking the A (ADP-ribosylating) portion of the cholera enterotoxin. *Proc Natl Acad Sci USA* 76:2052–2056, 1979

152. Levine MM, Black RE, Clements ML, et al: Evaluation in man of attenuated *Vibrio cholerae* El Tor Ogawa strain Texas-Star SR as live oral vaccine. *Infect Immun* 43:515–522, 1984

153. Mekelanos JJ, Moseley SL, Murphy JR, et al: Isolation of enterotoxin structural gene deletion mutations in *Vibrio cholerae* induced by two mutagenic vibriophages. *Proc Natl Acad Sci USA* 79:151–155, 1982

154. Manning PA, Heuzenroeder MW, Yeadon J, et al: Molecular cloning and expression in *Escherichia coli* K-12 of the O antigens of the Inaba and Ogawa serotypes of the *Vibrio cholerae* 01 lipolysaccharides and their potential for vaccine development. *Infect Immun* 53:272–277, 1986

155. Wahdan MH, Serie C, Germanier R, et al: A controlled field trial of live oral typhoid vaccine Ty21a. *Bull WHO* 58:469–474, 1980

156. Levine MM, Ferreccio C, Black RE, et al: Large-scale field trial of Ty21a typhoid vaccine in enteric-coated capsule formulation. *Lancet* i:1049–1052, 1987

157. Levine MM, Herrington D, Murphy J, et al: Safety, infectivity, immunogenicity, and in vivo stability of two attenuated auxotrophic mutant strains of *Salmonella typhi,* 541 Ty and 543 Ty, as live oral vaccines in human. *J Clin Invest* 79:888–902, 1987

158. Kaper JB, Lockman H, Baldini MM, et al: Recombinant live oral cholera vaccine. *Biotechnology* 2:345–349, 1984

159. Mekalanos JJ, Swartz DJ, Pearson GDN, et al: Cholera toxin genes: nucleotide sequence, deletion analysis and vaccine development. *Nature* 306:551–557, 1983

160. Levine MM, Black RE, Clements ML, et al: Present status of cholera vaccines. *Biochem Soc Trans* 12:200–202, 1984

161. Levine MM, Kaper JB, Black RE, et al: Landmarks on the road toward a live oral attenuated cholera vaccine, in Takeda Y (ed): *Vibrio cholerae and Cholera.* Tokyo, KTK Scientific Publishers, 1988 pg 155–161

162. Levine MM, Kaper JB, Herrington D, et al: Volunteer studies of deletion mutants of *Vibrio cholerae* 01 prepared by recombinant techniques. *Infect Immun* 56:161–167, 1988

163. Kaper JB, Levine MM, Lockman H, et al: Development and testing of recombinant live oral cholera vaccine, in: *Vaccines 85. Molecular and Chemical Basis of Resistance to Parasitic, Bacterial and Viral Diseases.* Cold Spring Harbor Laboratories, 1985, pp 107–111

164. Glass RI, Holmgren J, Haley CE, et al: Predisposition for cholera of individuals with O blood group. *Am J Epidemiol* 121:791–796, 1985

165. Levine MM, Nalin DR, Rennels MB, et al: Genetic susceptibility to cholera. *Ann Human Biol* 6:369–374, 1979

166. Ichinose Y, Yamomoto K, Nakasone N, et al: Enterotoxicity of El Tor-like hemolysin of non-01 *Vibrio cholerae.* *Infect Immun* 55:1090–1093

167. Madden JM, McCardell BA, Shah DB: Cytotoxin production by members of genus *Vibrio. Lancet* i:1217–1218, 1984

168. Nishibuchi M, Seidler RJ, Rollins DM, et al: Vibrio factors cause rapid fluid accumulation in suckling mice. *Appl Environ Microbiol* 45:228–231, 1983

169. O'Brien AD, Chen ME, Holmes RK, et al: Environmental and human isolates of *Vibrio cholerae* and *Vibrio parahaemolyticus* produce a *Shigella dysenteriae* 1 (Shiga-like) cytotoxin. *Lancet* i:77–78, 1984

170. Sanyal SC, Neogi PKB, Alam K, et al: A new enterotoxin produced by *Vibrio cholerae* 01. *J Diar Dis Res* 2:3–12, 1984

171. Yamamoto K, Ichinose Y, Nakasone N, et al: Identity of hemolysins produced by *Vibrio cholerae* non-01 and *V. cholerae* 01, biotype El Tor. *Infect Immun* 51:927–931, 1986

172. Yamamoto K, Maliha A-O, Honda T, et al: Non-01 *Vibrio cholerae* hemolysin: purification, partial characterization, and immunological relatedness to El Tor hemolysin. *Infect Immun* 45:192–196

173. Richardson K, Michalski J, Kaper JB: Hemolysin production and cloning of two hemolysin determinants from classical *Vibrio cholerae. Infect Immun* 54:415–420, 1986

174. Levine MM, Kaper JB, Herrington D, et al: Safety, immunogenicity and efficacy of recombinant live oral cholera vaccines, CVD 103 and CVD 103-HgR. *Lancet* ii:467–470, 1988

175. Cryz SJ, Levine MM, Kaper JB, et al: Randomized, double-blind placebo-controlled trial to evaluate the safety and immunogenicity of the live oral cholera vaccine strain CVD 103-HgR in Swiss adults. *Vaccine* in press, 1990

176. Migasena S, Pitisuttitham P, Prayurahong B, et al: Preliminary assessment of the safety and immunogenicity of live oral cholera vaccine strain CVD 103-HgR in healthy Thai adults. *Infect Immun* 57:3261–3264, 1989

177. Forrest BD, LaBrooy JR, Attridge SR, et al: Immunogenicity of a candidate live oral typhoid/cholera hybrid vaccine in humans. *J Infect Dis* 159:145–146, 189

178. Formal SB, Baron LS, Kopecko DJ, et al: Construction of a potential bivalent vaccine strain: introduction of *Shigella sonnei* form I antigen genes into the *galE Salmonella typhi* Ty21a typhoid vaccine strain. *Infect Immun* 34:746–750, 1981

179. Clements JD, El-Morshidy S: Construction of a potential live oral bivalent vaccine for typhoid fever and cholera-*Escherichia coli*-related diarrheas. *Infect Immun* 46:564–569, 1984

180. Tacket CO, Forrest B, Morona R, et al: Safety, immunogenicity and efficacy against cholera challenge in humans of a typhoid-cholera hybrid vaccine derived from *Salmonella typhi*. *Infect Immun* 58:1620–1627, 1990

15

Prevention and Control of Cholera

Dhiman Barua and Michael H. Merson

1. INTRODUCTION

Chapter 1, on the history of the disease, concluded that the quirks of cholera are likely to continue to cause concern and despair as this pestiferous disease continues to menace much of the developing world, where at least 65% of the world's population lives. Since 1991 Latin America has been affected and North America may be at risk. The word "cholera" still provokes considerable fear because, although measures exist for its prevention, control, and treatment, they are not available where they are most needed. Platitude or not, cholera continues to harass the developing world because of the underlying social and economic predicaments.

Early in the 19th century, long before the discovery of the microbial origin of cholera and recognition of its contagiousness, cholera control began with quarantine measures, which had been devised to protect against the importation of plague. Cordons for cholera control were probably first used in 1823 by the Astrakhan health authorities within the Russian territories.[1] When a new wave of infection approached Russia in 1829, the threatened frontiers were fortified with a double line of troops, quarantine stations were established on all major roads for surveillance, washing, airing, and fumigation of everything that arrived from the infected countries and quarantine (the Italian word for forty) restrictions were imposed on all ships for up to 40 days; yet cholera reached Moscow in 1830. Countries to the west of Russia posted guard houses at intervals of 3000 paces along their frontiers, with mounted officers and armed patrols, to ensure that persons and goods passed through quarantine stations where purification was carried out. When such cordons failed, even more draconian measures were enforced; cordons were doubled and drastic penalties, including capital punishment, were imposed for any transgressions. Cholera, however, paid no heed and continued to spread.

Cholera, edited by Dhiman Barua and William B. Greenough III. Plenum Medical Book Company, New York, 1992.

Liebermeister[2] in 1896, realizing the difficulties of implementing a *cordon sanitaire,* favored segregation or local quarantine measures. He recommended restriction of traffic "as much as can be done without detriment to important interests."

During the 1830s, when cholera was devastating most of Europe and the different quarantine requirements imposed by different countries were causing innumerable difficulties to traffic and trade, the French Government took the initiative of calling an international meeting to standardize protective measures against the importation of exotic diseases; the first meeting was held in Paris in 1852.[3] This meeting of seven countries was the beginning of international cooperation in health and was followed by a series of 14 International Sanitary Conferences that ultimately led to the founding of the World Health Organization (WHO) in 1948 and to the development of the International Health (originally "Sanitary") Regulations (IHR).[4]

The purpose of these regulations, which were adopted by the fourth World Health Assembly in 1951, is to ensure maximum security against the international spread of diseases with a minimum of interference with world traffic. According to the IHR, every member nation is required to notify WHO as soon as a case of cholera is detected within its territory. Notification has remained very deficient, however, partly because of the inadequacies of national surveillance systems, but especially for fear of the imposition of restrictions far in excess of the regulations on traffic and trade. In any case, the premise of protection by the IHR is built around sea and air travel by regular traffic, whereas cholera travels frequently by unscheduled routes and by clandestine travelers, boat dwellers, fishermen, nomads, and smugglers, whose itineraries generally elude control. Moreover, the large number of imported cases detected in the industrialized countries during recent years indicates that measures at sea- and airports under the regulations do not prevent the introduction of cholera.

The 26th World Health Assembly in 1973 amended the regulations, in particular the provisions for cholera, by abolishing the need for a valid cholera vaccination certificate for international travel. This was done because it was realized that the current vaccine was ineffective in preventing asymptomatic infections and the introduction of the infection into a country. A small number of countries, however, still continue to demand the certificate. During 1961–1964, the Japanese quarantine authorities found 51 confirmed carriers among travellers carrying a valid vaccination certificate, which is one of many instances that demonstrate the ineffectiveness of this certificate.

The limited measures permitted by the regulations concern certain foodstuffs carried as cargo onboard transports in which a case of cholera has been detected during the journey; hence, they are of very little practical importance. Stool examination of healthy persons is not permitted by the regulations, but is often carried out at border posts at great cost, although it is well known that it is not possible to detect all carriers by a single stool examination and that not all carriers pass through border posts.

It is therefore not inappropriate to conclude that the IHR have not succeeded in affording security against the international spread of cholera and are not respected. While notification, however deficient it may be, has provided a picture of the global epidemiological trend, the imposition of illogical and excessive restrictions on traffic and trade originating in cholera-affected countries continues to hinder compliance with this provision of the regulations.

As national experiences accumulated during the seventh pandemic, it became clear that cholera could be best controlled through national programs for the control of all diarrheal diseases.

2. STRATEGIES APPLIED IN DIARRHEAL DISEASE CONTROL (CDD) PROGRAMS AND THEIR RELEVANCE FOR CHOLERA CONTROL

The objectives of national CDD programs are to reduce diarrhea-related mortality and malnutrition, and diarrheal morbidity. The strategy for achieving the first objective is to ensure appropriate clinical management of diarrhea including cholera, with emphasis on oral rehydration therapy (ORT). For the second objective the strategies include the following, which are important and effective in cholera control:

1. Good personal and domestic hygiene
2. Construction and proper maintenance of hygienic excreta disposal facilities, and their regular use by all
3. Identification or provision and protection of safe, convenient, and plentiful water sources and proper storage and use of the water at home
4. Hand-washing with soap and sufficient water, after defecation and before preparing and eating food
5. Improving weaning practices and the safety of food—care in the preparation and protection of food from contamination, and consumption of cooked food while still hot
6. Proper disposal of refuse and waste water

National CDD programs, as an integral part of national primary health-care activities, train health workers and provide logistical support for the treatment of cases of diarrhea at hospitals, health centers, and in the community; this treatment is also effective for cholera. Instances of trained community health workers/volunteers successfully treating cases of cholera have been recorded in Bangladesh[5,6] and the Philippines (unpublished observation) and this experience is undoubtedly being repeated in many other countries. Health centers and community health workers in countries with properly implemented CDD programs should have no problem in treating mild and moderately severe cases of cholera with ORT, using available resources and, with additional manpower and supplies of intravenous fluids and antibiotics, in taking care of severe cases as well; the ready availability of treatment avoids the need for long-distance travel by patients and their contacts and thus limits the spread of the disease and prevents panic.[7]

Health workers providing diarrhea treatment are in a very good position to detect an epidemic at a very early stage (see Section 3.2). Early detection of an epidemic is a key factor for prompt containment and is feasible wherever a national CDD program is functioning effectively.

The above-mentioned strategies for morbidity reduction can reduce endemic cholera, and with strengthening, will help in epidemic control. Health education provided by health workers while treating diarrhea cases is apt to be more effective in improving personal and domestic hygiene and care of food and in promoting awareness and self-reliance with regard to improvement in sanitation and water supply.

The Diarrheal Diseases Control (CDD) Program of the World Health Organization has prepared materials for training in clinical management and laboratory diagnosis and guidelines for cholera control, which can be used by health workers to detect and treat cases and also to control an outbreak.

It has been suggested that the control of cholera epidemics is too big a task for a national CDD program. Although this may be true when an epidemic is extensive, it is often forgotten that such large outbreaks are a result of initial delay in their detection and of failure to contain them where they began. A properly organized CDD program provides the framework for quick detection and prompt containment; some strengthening of existing human and material resources may be required, but this is much easier than fighting epidemics on an *ad hoc* basis after they have become a widespread problem.

3. PREPAREDNESS FOR CHOLERA CONTROL

Making preparations to control cholera epidemics when indicated by international surveillance and notification has not been found to work. Therefore, cholera-receptive areas or countries with high diarrhea rates should be in a constant state of preparedness, which can best be achieved by developing a national CDD program. Within such a program the following activities are most important; they may need to be reinforced before the cholera season or when there is a risk of introduction of cholera.

3.1. National Epidemic Control Committee

The implementation of a national CDD program frequently entails the formation of an interministerial advisory committee and the designation of a national program manager to be responsible for all program activities, including cholera control. The same committee, with the national program manager as its secretary, may also function as a National Cholera Epidemic Control Committee. This Committee should be responsible for bilateral, regional, and international collaboration, collection and reporting of information, organization of necessary training, procurement, storage, and distribution of supplies, and coordination of implementation, monitoring, and evaluation activities. Depending on the size and structure of the health service, similar committees may be created at a provincial or state level. In countries that do not have a national committee, similar bodies (e.g., a special task force) may be established to perform these functions when an outbreak occurs or is threatening.

As an alternative, there may exist in some countries an Epidemic Control Committee with responsibility for the control of all epidemics and emergencies created by natural disasters. In such cases, the manager of the CDD program should be a member of the Committee, so that he can coordinate the activities required for cholera control.

3.2. Surveillance

Continuous surveillance of diarrheal diseases is the basis for early recognition of outbreaks of cholera, whether newly introduced or recrudescent. As called for in the CDD program, treatment facilities and village health workers should maintain a record of the diarrhea cases seen daily. Any significant and unusual increase in the number of cases or change in their age or severity, e.g., higher incidence in older children and adults, particularly when associated with severe dehydration or death from dehydrating diarrhea and a clustering of cases in time and place, may indicate the beginning of an outbreak of cholera. Health workers should be trained to note such changes in the pattern of diarrhea and to notify their supervisors immediately, giving the names, addresses, and ages of the patients, and the dates of onset. The supervisors should then, on receipt of such information, be able to arrange for rapid bacteriological and case investigations and inform the national CDD program manager so that he or she may take appropriate action for control and for notification according to the IHR. This clinic-based surveillance is practical and effective.

Surveillance in receptive areas and along possible routes of introduction should be strengthened by altering health facilities/workers there during cholera seasons and when there is a threat of cholera from outside. Community leaders and persons in contact with travelers (e.g., air- and seaport health officers, hotel managers, pharmacists) should also be alerted to look for and report cases of severe diarrhea to public health officials.

3.3. Environmental Sanitation and Water Supply

Reinforcement of good sanitation and hygienic practices pertaining to the use of safe water, human waste disposal, personal hygiene, and care of food should be given highest priority. Particular care must be taken with regard to these aspects where large groups of people congregate, e.g., fairs, markets, and religious festivals.

3.4. Communication of Health Information

Through communication activities, information on the prevention of diarrheal diseases, including cholera, is exchanged between health workers and the people or among the people themselves to reach common understanding and agreement. Communication should go beyond attempts to educate by didactic methods and use a two-way approach to involve and motivate people. While the provision of water supplies and latrines is essential, without public cooperation in their proper use and maintenance the impact of these facilities will be insignificant.

It is important to inform the population about the ways in which diarrheal diseases like cholera spread and how these means can be interrupted. When there is a risk of epidemics, it is particularly important to explain that cholera need no longer be a fatal disease, since most cases can be treated with simple measures and that vaccine is not a substitute for good domestic and personal hygiene. Ideally, all members of the health team should provide information on preventive measures, while giving service to the community, e.g., while providing treatment, supplying soap and disinfectants, digging latrines, and improving water supply. It is also very important that the religious and political leaders, teachers, students, and the media are motivated and involved in transmitting these messages, as they are most effective in influencing public behavior.

3.5. Training in Clinical Management

In a national CDD program, medical and paramedical personnel should receive "hands-on" training to ensure that they are familiar with up-to-date techniques for the clinical management of diarrheal diseases, including cholera. Their training should be reinforced by refresher courses, drawing attention to special features of cholera and supported by the provision of adequate supplies during preparations for cholera control (see Chapter 13).

3.6. Laboratory Services

Microbiology laboratories at the district level or large health centers should be capable of isolating and identifying *V. cholerae* 01. They should stock the necessary supplies of media and antisera, and be able to provide transport media, rectal swabs, etc., to trained field workers for the collection of specimens. Biotype and serotype determinations need not be done as they are of no significance for the control and treatment of cases.

In areas at risk, national reference laboratories should assume responsibility for the provision of culture media and diagnostic antisera, the training of workers in peripheral and regional laboratories on appropriate isolation techniques, and the conducting of proficiency testing to determine laboratory competence and training needs. National, regional, and university laboratories should have the competence to identify and biotype *V. cholerae* 01 and perform antibiotic resistance testing. For more complicated procedures (e.g., phage-typing, toxin testing), appropriate international assistance may be required (see Chapter 12).

3.7. Mobile Teams

In areas with very poor peripheral health services, mobile teams, while more costly and less effective than a static facility, may have to be formed and sent in the case of an outbreak. The team members should have had the training and experience to enable them to:

1. Establish a temporary treatment center and treat cases
2. Apply appropriate environmental sanitary measures and disinfection
3. Carry out communication activities to disseminate information to the public, allay panic, and secure community participation
4. Identify and, if necessary, treat close contacts
5. Carry out simple case investigations to determine, if possible, the mode of transmission involved in the outbreak
6. Collect stool and environmental specimens, as indicated by the epidemiological trend, for submission to a bacteriology laboratory

All these functions are described in detail in Section 4.

In the interest of cost-effectiveness, team members should be drawn from among the workers in a laboratory, hospital, or elsewhere. They should be brought together for briefing on their individual responsibilities, the location of their supplies, the situations in which their services will be needed, and the sources to contact for further technical and logistical support.

3.8. Logistics

Based on the planned strategies for dealing with an epidemic, supply requirements for treatment, laboratory investigations, and control measures should be established and, if necessary, procurement initiated. Guidelines prepared by WHO[8] and UNICEF[9] may help in preparing the list. The need for international assistance should be assessed and requested at this time. Warehouses should be designated to facilitate distribution. The surface or air transport needed for moving mobile teams and supplies should be identified and arranged.

4. CONTROL ACTIVITIES DURING THE EPIDEMIC

When a cholera outbreak occurs, its management should essentially consist of intensification of the following activities, which should already be in operation as part of the national CDD program and the preparatory activities described in Section 3. If needed, the mobile control team should be brought promptly into the area. The prime objectives should be to treat cases properly and confine the disease to the site of the outbreak and control it there.

4.1. Treatment and Investigation

4.1.1. Surveillance and Case-Finding

Aggressive case-finding is necessary in order to isolate the cases to limit environmental contamination and initiate treatment before patients go into shock. Early discovery of cases also permits the detection of infected household contacts and helps the epidemiologist in investigating the means of spread so that a specific intervention can be applied. Members of voluntary or other local rural or urban organizations, religious leaders, teachers, students, etc., should be encouraged to help by providing information on the occurrence of cases.

4.1.2. Establishing Treatment Centers

The most important advance that has been made in recent years in cholera control is the simplification of treatment, which has made it possible to bring it within the immediate reach of patients and thus to prevent deaths. Most cases can be treated at the community level or in health centers if rehydration materials, intravenous fluid and Oral Rehydration Salts (ORS),* and antibiotics are available, and health workers are trained in the management of cases. In countries with an efficient CDD program, both of these elements should already be in place, though there may be a need for additional staff and supplies. Otherwise, it will be necessary to bring a mobile team or make other arrangements to establish treatment facilities in or near the affected communities, using, for example, huts, school buildings, or tents. The grouping of patients close to their domicile facilitates treatment, reduces deaths, panic, and environmental contamination, and generates community participation.[5-7] Overcrowding and poor hygiene have led to some outbreaks in hospitals,[10,11] which should be prevented.

4.1.3. Treatment

Most cholera cases can be adequately treated by the oral administration of ORS, which is used widely for the treatment of dehydration from all acute diarrheas. Intravenous saline solutions containing alkali and potassium salts, e.g., lactated Ringer, are usually required only for the initial rehydration of severely dehydrated patients who are in shock or unable to drink, after the correction of which they can be treated with ORS. ORS can also be administered through a nasogastric tube when intravenous fluid is unavailable (see Chapter 13).

---

* ORS consists of sodium chloride, 3.5 g; trisodium citrate, dihydrate, 2.9 g (or sodium bicarbonate, 2.5 g); potassium chloride, 1.5 g; and glucose, anhydrous, 20.0 g (or sucrose, 40.0 g); to be dissolved in one liter of drinking water.

Antibiotics are useful adjuncts and should be given orally. Vomiting usually stops within a few hours of beginning rehydration, making this possible. It is neither urgent nor of additional benefit to use injectable antibiotics, which are expensive. Tetracycline is the antibiotic of choice. Tetracycline is usually withheld from children under 8 years of age and pregnant women because of its potential to cause permanent tooth staining. However, its use for the treatment of cholera in children appears to be justified because effective alternatives like chloramphenicol and trimethoprim-sulfamethoxazole occasionally have fatal side-effects and because the evidence that treatment with tetracycline for only 2–3 days causes tooth staining is minimal; use of oxytetracycline or possibly doxycline may cause less tooth staining[12,13] (see Chapter 13).

A single dose of sulfadoxine (fanasil) has also been used for the treatment of cholera. As resistance to it has been found in a few countries in Africa[14] and potentially serious and fatal adverse reactions (e.g., Stevens–Johnson syndrome) can occur following even a single dose,[15,16] its use should be avoided.

4.1.4. Case Investigation

The general control measures described in other parts of this section must be applied from the onset of an outbreak. At the same time, attempts should be made to define the extent of the outbreak and, if possible, to determine the mode of transmission by examining the recent journeys of cases, the consumption of particular foods, beverages, etc., so that more specific control measures can be applied. While such studies have helped to identify the means of transmission and to apply specific control measures in some newly infected areas,[17,18] outbreaks in endemic areas are often multifactoral, making it difficult to find a single mode of transmission.[19,20] Therefore, arrangements should be made to follow contacts and remedy the hygienic deficiencies observed in home environments, by disinfection and other measures.

Close liaison between the epidemiologists stationed in an area or attached to a mobile team and the clinicians, sanitarians, and laboratory staff is important. This will permit the identification and recording of cholera cases by time and place, preferably on a spot map, and facilitate laboratory examination of epidemiologically implicated water sources, sewage, and foods.

In newly affected areas, the disease may be observed in all age groups, but with a higher attack rate among the more mobile population groups (usually young adults) who are exposed to a greater variety of sources of infection, particularly water and food outside the home. A preponderance of cases among children under 5 years of age indicates that the disease is endemic in the area.

The epidemiologist or responsible health officer or a member of the mobile team should alert and maintain contact with all health workers and community civic leaders in his area to ensure the prompt detection of new foci of disease and to try to determine the factors favoring spread. He should also keep the CDD program manager informed of the situation in his area. Working with health communicators, he should ensure that pertinent factual information is disseminated to the population to prevent panic and to obtain their support for control activities.

4.1.5. Laboratory Support

Successful treatment of cholera does not depend on the results of laboratory examinations. However, bacteriological diagnosis is essential to confirm the presence of an outbreak of cholera in order to mobilize national and international resources, and determine the epidemiological features. Once the presence of cholera has been proven, it is not necessary to culture stools from all cases or their contacts; in fact, this should be discouraged to avoid unnecessary laboratory work. Cases should be treated on a clinical basis, but those used for epidemiological investigation must be bacteriologically confirmed. Antibiotic susceptibility patterns should be tested if resistance is suspected on clinical or epidemiological grounds or, if possible, as a routine on representative isolates. Environmental sampling should be limited to items indicated by epidemiological investigation; Moore swabs for sewage sampling[21-23] may help to define the extent of spread, the persistence, and also the disappearance of infection from a community. The laboratory should make available fresh transport media for the collection of samples and keep hospital clinicians and epidemiologists informed of all results, using the most rapid means of communication.

4.2. Control and Prevention

Cholera is usually acquired by the ingestion of water or food contaminated with cholera vibrios. Food and beverages, particularly when consumed outside the home[18,19] and at feasts during festivals and funerals, have often been the source of infection; food-borne spread is facilitated by the growth of *V.cholerae* 01 in foods kept at ambient temperature after cooking.[24] Person-to-person transmission has been observed to occur in hospitals[10,11] institutions,[25] and families[26-28] with poor hygiene and overcrowding; these conditions also prevail in refugee camps. Food- and water-borne outbreaks may continue to linger on a small scale due to intrafamilial transmission through complex interaction of contaminated food, water, clothes, fomites, etc., common in homes of endemic areas; it is difficult to study their roles separately. Feachem[29] has ably pointed out the difficulties in interpreting the findings of studies in Bangladesh on the roles of tube-well and surface water without considering the possibilities of nonwaterborne transmission (see Chapter 7).

Unless a definite mode of transmission is known, prevention should be based on reducing all these means of transmission. When cholera appears in a community, the following control measures must be adopted or intensified, keeping this principle in mind.

4.2.1. Communication of Health Information

Arrangements must be made, and maintained, for the dissemination of appropriate information that will motivate the members of the community to participate in control activities. All health workers engaged in cholera control should be prepared to communicate. During an epidemic, exaggerated rumors create fear and panic in the populace. Carefully designed messages delivered through multiple channels (media, home visits, schools, religious leaders, etc.) should be used to keep the public informed about the extent and severity of the outbreak, the effectiveness and simplicity of the present methods of treatment, the benefits of early reporting for prompt treatment, and the usefulness of simple preventive measures. The public should be advised of the possible vehicles of transmission and the best available ways of avoiding infection. Communication and technical experts should work together to determine how to educate and to develop materials containing correct messages that are based on the beliefs and practices of the people. Emphasis should be placed on the proper disposal of excreta, personal hygiene, safe food, and safe water. The need for proper hand washing[30] after defecation and before eating or preparing food deserves special emphasis. The distribution of soap for hand washing,[30] chlorine preparations to disinfect water, and narrow-mouthed water containers to protect water at home[31] have been shown to be very effective for interrupting transmission; it also helps to secure community participation (see Sections 3.4, 4.2.3, 4.2.4, and 4.6.2).

4.2.2. Disposal of Human Waste

Appropriate facilities for human waste disposal are a basic need of all human settlements; in many areas the threat of cholera has hastened their development. When cholera threatens or appears in a community, the need for these facilities becomes vital. Various sanitary systems suitable for rural and urban communities have been described.[32,33] With the cooperation of the community, an appropriate sanitary system should be selected and constructed, after taking into consideration the customs and practices of the population, the existing terrain and geology, and available resources. A pit latrine may be a practical solution in rural areas; it must be at least 10 m away from the living quarters and 20–30 m away from any surface or underground water source; marshy areas are not suitable. For one family the pit should be at least 2 m deep with a 1 m^2 opening, while a trench for a community should be 1 m wide, 2 m deep, and 6–10 m long. The edges of the pit or trench must be higher than ground level to prevent rain or other water from draining into it. The latrines should have a concrete or wooden cover supported by beams, leaving openings with properly fitting lids that can be closed after use.

Simultaneous health education should stress the proper use by all and the maintenance of such facilities, the dangers involved in depositing feces on the ground and in or near water, and of ablutions in rivers and ponds, and the importance of hand washing with soap or ash after defecation.

4.2.3. Water Supply

Access to safe water is also a basic requirement. The need becomes more urgent and is obligatory for the prevention and control of cholera. The role of water in the transmission of cholera was clearly demonstrated in the mid-19th century by John Snow and has since been repeatedly confirmed. Recently, a brand of commercially bottled water—possibly from a contaminated source and noncarbonated—has also been incriminated in an outbreak.[17]

Various methods have been described[32,33] for supplying safe water with limited resources. Facilities should be selected and installed that will be appropriate for and acceptable to the community. In urban areas, properly treated, piped drinking water containing free residual chlorine should be made available to all families. In rural areas where tube-well or closed dug-well water is not available and untreated surface water from rivers, ponds, or open wells (which are extremely difficult to treat) has to be used, special efforts should be made to protect these sources from contamination, if necessary, by providing the community with alternative facilities for bathing and washing of various articles. In case of doubt about the safety of water, an attempt should be made to make the water safe at home by an appropriate method. Boiling is generally advised, but it is easier said than done, because firewood is generally scarce and about 1 kg is needed to bring 1 liter of water to a "rolling" boil for 1 or 2 min (the time required to achieve sterilization). Boiled water needs to be protected from recontamination by proper storage. Alum potash (500 mg/liter) has been claimed[34] to kill vibrios by acidification of water in addition to flocculation, but the taste may be unacceptable to some and experience with its use is limited.

There is no doubt about the effectiveness of a chlorine-releasing preparation, such as high-test calcium hypochlorite, bleaching powder, or iodine. For large water-supply systems, the dosage should be based on the breakpoint of the water. For domestic or small-scale chlorination,[35] the following simple procedure can be used: A 1% stock solution is prepared by adding enough water to 4 teaspoons (16 g) of high-test hypochlorite (70% available chlorine), or 10 teaspoons (40 g) of bleaching powder (30% available chlorine), to make up one liter of solution. After mixing thoroughly, the solution should be kept tightly stoppered; fresh solution should be prepared daily as it loses strength rapidly when exposed to sunlight.

Three drops of the stock solution for one liter, or 1 teaspoon (4–5 ml) for 30 liters of water should be used—the addition of water to the stock solution helps proper mixing. The chlorinated water should be allowed to stand for 20–30 min before use.

Commercial antiseptic solutions such as Zonite and Milton contain about 1% chlorine. Household and laundry bleaches, available as liquids under a variety of trade names, may contain 3–15% available chlorine; they should be diluted to contain 1% chlorine before use.

Water purification tablets and liquid preparations containing chlorine are also commercially available under different trade names. Attention has to be given to their stability and cost. Combination tablets containing chlorine and thiosulfate, the latter to neutralize any excess of chlorine and remove the taste, are sometimes used, but they are costly; all the tablets required to treat a given volume of water must be added at the same time.[35]

Iodine is also an excellent disinfectant for water—2 drops of 2% tincture of iodine are sufficient for 1 liter of water. Cloudy or turbid water should be filtered and the filtrate treated with iodine in the same way. Iodine-containing preparations such as "Globaline" and "Potable aqua" are commercially available.

The supply of suitable chemicals for treatment of water at the domestic level and the provision of narrow-mouthed earthen jars,[31] with covers for water storage within the household, have been shown to reduce transmission within the family. Supplying water by tanker can help only if a regular supply of adequate volume is assured.

The possibility of acquiring infection from swimming in contaminated public bathing places, such as beaches and pools, must be considered. If bacteriological testing of such waters reveals the presence of vibrios or gross fecal contamination is suspected, appropriate measures should be taken, including closure.

4.2.4. Care of Food

Since food may be an important vehicle of infection, special care should be taken to cook food properly and to prevent contamination of cooked food in the home, at feasts, festivals, and fairs, in eating places and in mass catering establishments. Food should not be allowed at the funerals of cholera cases. Health communication messages must explain the reasons and stress the importance of (1) eating cooked food while it is still hot, (2) proper kitchen hygiene, (3) food handling practices to prevent cross contamination, and (4) washing hands with soap (see Section 4.2.1).

The housefly probably plays a relatively small role in the spread of cholera, but its prevalence is an indicator of the level of sanitation; the breeding of flies should be controlled by burying or incinerating refuse.

Vibrios do not survive for long on dry food surfaces; very rarely have foods like bananas and potatoes been found with vibrios on their surface. Even when such foods have been deliberately contaminated, the organisms have persisted only for 1–2 days. However, leafy vegetables must be individually washed or chemically treated if they are to be eaten uncooked, as they may provide moisture and a nidus for vibrios to survive. All suspicious and leftover food should be discarded or properly reheated to more than 60°C for a few minutes (rewarming is not enough) before eating. Where facilities exist, leftover food should be refrigerated. Seafood is an important vehicle—any seafood that may have come from suspected waters or is likely to have been contaminated after harvesting must be cooked thoroughly. Cooking utensils should be cleaned and dried after use; this is particularly important for wooden chopping boards and utensils used for handling foods after cooking.

4.2.5 Disinfection of Patients' Belongings and Disposal of Dead Bodies

As contamination of the surroundings of a case of cholera living in an unhygienic environment is almost inevitable, concurrent and terminal disinfection of the patient's room, clothing, used articles, and surroundings should be encouraged and disinfectants provided. Several effective disinfectants are available, but 2% chlorine solution or 1–2% phenolic preparations like Lysol are cheap and practical. Thorough sun drying is also effective. Washing contaminated articles, particularly clothes in rivers, ponds, and near wells has led to many outbreaks. The funerals of persons dying from cholera should take place quickly, near the place of death; efforts should be made to restrict funeral gatherings, ritual washing and touching of the dead, and especially feasting, by intensive health education or by legislation, as appropriate.

4.2.6. Chemoprophylaxis

Mass treatment of members of a community with antimicrobials is theoretically an attractive strategy to control an epidemic, as the drugs, when administered properly, have been shown to reduce vibrio excretion in close contacts of cases.[36–40] During the last two decades, workers in several countries and refugee camps have tried this approach, but their claims of success have not been substantiated, as protracted outbreaks have continued in most of these situations.

The reasons for this disappointing outcome are not wholly unexpected and include the following:

1. It usually takes longer to organize the distribution and administration of the drug and for the drug to act than for the infection to spread.
2. The effect of the drug persists only for a few days.
3. The total population of the area therefore needs to be treated simultaneously under supervision, otherwise reinfection of the treated from the untreated occurs.[37] However, the logistics involved in administering a drug to a large number of supposedly infected but healthy people under supervision are overwhelming. Supervision should also include screening for contraindications, ensuring administration of the drug in full dosage, and follow-up for untoward reactions.

The strategy has not only failed to achieve the objective, but has often diverted attention and resources from important measures. In addition, side-effects of the drugs have largely remained undetected in the absence of surveillance under supervision. In several countries, it has also contributed to the emergence of multiple drug-resistant strains[14,41] depriving the severely ill cases of a valuable tool for treatment.

In view of the above constraints, mass treatment or chemoprophylaxis may be justified only when cholera breaks out with a high attack rate (e.g., more than 2%) in a closed group, e.g., aboard ship or in a refugee camp of moderate size, where everyone can be treated with full dosage of the drug simultaneously under supervision.

Selective chemoprophylaxis for close household contacts sharing the same food and shelter as a cholera case is often considered to be more useful than mass chemoprophylaxis, as 7–25% of these contacts may become vibrio excretors in contrast to less than 1% of community contacts and because in some communities secondary cases in a family are common. The use of such selective treatment therefore depends on the local situation, and can probably be justified only when the secondary case rate among close household contacts is high, e.g.,>20%.

The definition of a close contact, however, is difficult in societies where intimate social mixing and the exchange of food between families are common. In addition, as a majority of those infected with *V. cholerae* 01 of El Tor biotype suffer only from a mild disease, many index cases escape detection and, thus, their close contacts remain untreated.

Tetracycline is generally used in such situations, except where the organism is resistant. It must be given over a period of at least 2 days, in 2 daily doses of 500 mg each for adults and 125 mg for children aged 8–13 years. For chemoprophylaxis, tetracycline should be avoided in children below 8 years of age, pregnant women, and persons with kidney disease for fear of side-effects and risk–benefit considerations. Chloramphenicol has also been used in a similar dosage, but it carries a greater risk of severe adverse reactions. For young children, liquid preparations of erythromycin or trimethoprim-sulfamethoxazole may be used in the same dosages as those recommended for the treatment of cases (see Chapter 13). However, their efficacy in chemoprophylaxis has not been evaluated.

Doxycycline[40] may also be used in a single dose of 300 mg in adults (smaller dosages have not been tested). This dosage may cause low rates of nausea and vomiting. However, as the drug is well absorbed in the intestine, even in the presence of food, it may be given soon after a meal to reduce these side effects. As it is excreted through the kidneys, liver, and directly across the intestinal mucosa, accumulation of the drug to toxic levels is rare. With the expiration of patent rights, the price of this drug is now declining in most countries. In view of the advantages of single-dose treatment and its decreasing cost, doxycycline may be the drug of choice for selective chemoprophylaxis. Its use in children may be of less concern than use of tetracycline as it is possibly less likely to cause tooth staining (see Section 4.1.3.).

Long-acting sulfonamides (e.g., fanasil), which have been claimed to make carriers vibrio-free when given in a single dose,[38] are slow in action[39] and have a high potential for serious adverse reactions like the Stevens–Johnson syndrome, even after a single dose.[15,16] Moreover, resistant strains have been isolated in Africa.[15] They should not be used.

In summary, mass chemoprophylaxis with antimicrobials is difficult to implement properly and has not been found effective. It may be justified only for closed groups when the incidence of cholera is more than 2%, all individuals can be treated simultaneously, and administration is well supervised. Selective chemoprophylaxis may be useful in families with a high (e.g., >20%) attack rate. For this purpose, doxycycline is preferable because it can be given in a single dose under supervision.

4.2.7. Vaccination

As mentioned earlier, although the currently available whole-cell parenteral vaccine has been in use since the last decade of the 19th century, controlled field trials and intensive laboratory studies of this type of vaccine began only in the 1960s (see Chapter 14). The relevant findings and experiences may be recapitulated here:

1. The efficacy of the vaccine in controlled field trials in endemic areas was around 60% for the first 2–3 months, declining to around 30% during the next 3 months, and is generally expressed as 50% for 6 months.[42] To reach this efficacy in children in an endemic area and to be effective in a nonendemic area, the vaccine has to be given in 2 doses at 7- to 28-day intervals.

2. This degree of efficacy was found only when the potency of the vaccines was good, as determined by an active mouse protection test.[42] This test has been shown to be a more sensitive indicator of type-specific immunity than serum antibody titers,[43] but it is expensive and difficult to perform. Most vaccine producers nowadays produce vaccine of low potency and do not perform proper potency testing.

3. Vaccination does not alter the course or severity of the disease.[44]

4. The vaccine also does not significantly reduce the rate of asymptomatic infection or the carrier rate among family contacts[44,45] and thus cannot prevent the spread of infection by carriers.[44]

5. In an endemic community it takes about 6 to 8 days for the vaccine to induce immunity and in volunteer studies the peak antibody titer is observed 2 weeks after the initial vaccination,[43] while the usual incubation period of cholera is very often less than 5 days. In a study in family contacts in Bangladesh, even a potent cholera vaccine failed to prevent new cases.[45]

6. A cost–benefit comparison of vaccination and treatment for cholera in Bangladesh showed distinct advantages of the latter and led to the conclusion that health administrators ought to concentrate their limited resources on providing therapy and gradually upgrade sanitation.[44,46]

7. By the time vaccination campaigns are organized and implemented, epidemics are usually on their decline, giving an impression of vaccine effectiveness.

Although there are some uncertain and anecdotal reports on the successful termination of epidemics by vaccination, in not a single situation has it been possible to demonstrate clearly that the termination was truly due to vaccination. Health administrators are in fact gradually realizing the limitations of the vaccine and are fighting epidemics without vaccination. In the early 1970s there was a considerable public demand for vaccine, but national and international efforts have, to a great extent, succeeded in reducing this pressure on governments. It is now recognized that persons coming forward to receive vaccine are usually those who are less likely to become ill with cholera; also vaccination gives a false sense of security to those vaccinated, who consequently neglect more effective precautions, and rouses feelings of accomplishment and complacency among health authorities. However, vaccination campaigns are still sometimes undertaken for reasons other than technical ones. Such campaigns, even with vaccines obtained free of charge (most of which do not have the required potency), divert resources, attention, and manpower from more useful activities. Donations of vaccines may thus do more harm than good and would be better replaced by support for the more effective measures described above. Moreover, there have been anecdotal reports of outbreaks of serum hepatitis, a more serious problem, following mass vaccination campaigns. The risk of acquired immune deficiency syndrome (AIDS) should also be considered when one syringe and needle is used for multiple vaccinations without sterilization between injections; one type of jet-gun has also been found to transfer serum hepatitis.

Despite its doubtful benefit, vaccination is still sought by some travelers for personal prophylaxis. There is hardly any justification for this, as the incidence of cholera among travelers to endemic area, including those returning to their home country, has been estimated after very careful reviews to be only about one per 500,000 journeys.[47,48]

4.2.8. Restrictions on Travel and Trade

The history of quarantine measures in cholera control mentioned earlier shows that the imposition of restrictions on travel and trade between countries or different areas within a country has never succeeded in preventing spread of cholera, because it is extremely difficult to control the movements of people. Similarly, no outbreak in a developed country has yet been convincingly traced to an imported contaminated food. On the other hand, the imposition of restrictions on travel and trade encourages the suppression of information, which impeded bilateral and international collaboration and preparatory efforts for cholera control in neighboring countries. The use of check-posts at borders to detect asymptomatic infected persons by laboratory examination is a mere cost-intensive and less effective exercise. A *cordon sanitaire* of any kind hinders community cooperation and diverts manpower and resources from more effective activities.

It may, however, be possible to reduce population movements between infected and noninfected areas on a voluntary basis if the risk is properly explained to the people; this approach may be more successful than coercion.

5. ACTIVITIES AFTER THE EPIDEMIC

The problem of cholera will ultimately be solved only when water supplies, sanitation, and hygienic practices attain such a level that fecal–oral transmission of *V. cholerae* 01 becomes an improbable event. This cannot be expected to happen without a marked amelioration in social and economic conditions in the developing world. Therefore, the emergency epidemic control measures should not be relaxed in a nonendemic area until careful surveillance of diarrhea cases and environmental sources (particularly sewage), indicates that *V. cholerae* 01 is no longer present in the community. In endemic areas, the emergency cholera control measures should be continued until the incidence decreases to preepidemic levels. Ideally, they should lead to an intensification of national CDD program activities and to the further development of long-term control measures directed towards improving surveillance and developing essential water supply and sanitation facilities.

In urban areas, a water-supply system should ideally provide potable water under constant positive pressure through a piped system into individual homes. The water supplied should be plentiful and contain a residual antibacterial agent to prevent recontamination by dirty hands or unhygienic practices. This ideal may be difficult to attain, but efforts over time should be directed towards this goal. In rural areas, water sources should be deep tube-wells or dug wells properly built and covered and protected from surface contamination; latrines should always be sited so that they drain away from the water sources. If surface water like a river, a pond, or shallow wells are to be used, they should be protected from contamination. The public should be indoctrinated in the concept that no untreated surface water, regardless of its apparent clarity, is safe to drink.

In urban and peri-urban areas, properly operated sewage-treatment plants to which all households are connected by a water-borne system are the ideal towards which all communities should strive. In rural areas, latrine facilities should be provided that prevent human wastes from polluting the surface of the ground and contaminating water sources; such facilities will also prevent fly breeding. If the cost of such facilities exceeds the resources available to the community, it is nevertheless possible progressively to reduce the risk of spread of cholera by increasing the number of simpler but appropriate facilities.[32,33] It is also very important to persuade the population to maintain and utilize the facilities properly, and, if necessary, to change their customs and practices. This can best be achieved by communicating realistic messages and at the same time providing some support that will motivate the community to adopt the measures advised.

6. REASONS FOR FAILURE TO CONTROL CHOLERA EPIDEMICS

Despite the accumulated knowledge and experience, cholera epidemics often continue to spread and cause high case fatality particularly when they first strike an area. There are several reasons for this:

1. Inadequate national surveillance. Surveillance requires systematic detection and reporting of cholera cases, which is extremely difficult for the health authorities in countries most affected by the problem, as they lack the necessary infrastructure, manpower, and other resources. Only by developing an appropriate surveillance system will it be possible to detect epidemics in their earliest stages (see Section 3.2).

2. Reliance on quarantine measures. Despite the lack of success of quarantine measures since they were first introduced in the 19th century, restrictions such as *cordons sanitaires* to stop road traffic, laboratory examinations of rectal swabs from travelers to detect carriers at border check-posts, closure of airports to aircraft from infected countries, prevention of trains to pass frontiers, prohibition of imports of mineral ores, timber, cement, and foodstuffs and compulsory disinfection of mail and printed matter were frequently imposed during the 1960s and 1970s, causing substantial economic losses and hassles to many countries. Although international efforts have partly succeeded in reducing the number of such incidents, they continue to be sufficiently common to discourage notification by affected countries, which in turn encourages the imposition of restrictive measures based on media reports, rumors, and suspicion. Thus is created a vicious circle which is difficult to interrupt.

3. Delay in information exchange within the country. When cholera breaks out in remote areas, the information often does not reach the health authorities without considerable delay. The nomadic life-style of segments of the population, particularly in Africa, can contribute further to late detection and containment.

4. Poor access to treatment. A case-fatality rate of 50% or more has not been unusual when a cholera epidemic appears in an unprepared community, and when there are no trained community health workers or health center staff to provide treatment. Moreover, in such circumstances, cases and their contacts may travel long distances by land or river to seek treatment, spreading infection along the route and causing panic.

5. Inappropriate treatment. Use of the wrong kind of intravenous fluid (e.g., 5% glucose in water, normal saline or glucose–saline as the only fluid) or of the right fluid in an inadequate volume have been responsible for unnecessary deaths in many instances. These have been mainly due to inadequate training and inappropriate supplies, the latter often coming as donations.

6. Drought and inadequate hygienic improvements. Overcrowding and poor sanitary conditions, particularly in refugee camps and urban slums, favor rapid and wide dissemination of infection. Drought in particular has led to large outbreaks because of associated mass movements of populations, scarcity of water and food, and prevailing malnutrition. Attempts to improve water supplies, sanitation facilities, domestic and personal hygiene, and food safety are usually inadequate for various reasons. Even the provision of a temporary water supply in tankers has failed because of irregularity in supply and distribution.

7. Traditional practices. The custom of gathering around the sick and funeral rites such as the washing of dead bodies and feasting have led to outbreaks in many areas in Africa.

8. Shortage of supplies, equipment, and transport. Lack of preparedness has often resulted in shortages of rehydration fluids, antibiotics, and disinfectants, and transportation for patients, supplies, and health workers. Sometimes supplies have remained unused in a central store in the capital city, while epidemics were raging in remote areas due to inadequate planning for distribution and lack or misuse of transport for less important activities.

9. Reliance on inappropriate control measures. As mentioned earlier (Section 4.2.8), there is little justification for diverting resources to the control of external or internal traffic and trade because this never succeeds. The reasons for not relying on mass chemoprophylaxis can be found from studying the epidemiology of the disease and the mode of action of the available drugs (see Section 4.2.6). The limitations of vaccination with the currently available vaccine have been discussed in Section 4.2.7.

It may be noted that most of these deficiencies can be prevented or avoided, particularly if there is a properly managed national diarrheal diseases control program.

7. CHOLERA CONTROL IN A REFUGEE CAMP

Outbreaks of cholera in refugee camps have become a rather common feature in recent years, particularly in Africa. Many of the factors favoring transmission of V. *cholerae* 01 are usually present in these camps. Attack rates as high as 15/1000 have been found in large camps in Africa, although insufficient information is available on this aspect as well as on the clinical spectrum of illness. In contrast, in a small refugee camp in Bangladesh,[49] the rate was only 4.3/1000 and in a transit center for Indo-Chinese refugees in Thailand, the rate of all diarrheas was about 2.8 and 3.2/1000 during two small cholera outbreaks.[50]

The organization of well-coordinated cholera control measures at administrative, social, and technical levels is often difficult. Important contributory factors include the lack of trained and experienced physicians and nurses, poorly planned physical layout of the camps, with inadequate water supply, sanitation, and lighting, and irregular supplies of intravenous and oral fluids, antibiotics, disinfectants, and equipment for setting up temporary hospitals. Relatively larger volumes of intravenous fluid are often used, which may be a reflection of a greater number of severe cases and their delayed arrival for treatment and/or a lack of staff with experience/confidence in the use of oral rehydration. A scarcity of appropriate rehydration fluids (intravenous and oral) might have contributed to the high case–fatality rates sometimes reported in the media.

When refugee camps are established in cholera-endemic areas, it is desirable to make provision for supplies and personnel for the management of cholera outbreaks. It is essential to ensure the availability of sufficient safe water and latrines, and if possible, enough soap for distribution. It may be useful to divide the camp into different sectors and to assign a health volunteer to each to provide primary health-care services, under supervision, and help in the surveillance of common infectious diseases, including cholera. The volunteers should be given some basic training and supplies to help them in carrying out their work.

Vaccination and mass chemoprophylaxis deserve special consideration in these situations, though it is difficult to provide a general recommendation as the decision on their use will depend on local circumstances. Theoretically, vaccination using a vaccine of proven potency to reduce the number of cases in overcrowded camps with very poor sanitation, water supply, and hygiene may be considered a useful measure, but in practice the results have not been encouraging for the reasons mentioned in Section 4.2.7. It may be considered in exceptional situations where the population in the camp is large, the attack rate is high (e.g., more than 2%), the vaccine is potent, and it can be delivered without disrupting other services.

The use of mass chemoprophylaxis should only be considered in special circumstances (see Section 4.2.6). Regular monitoring of antibiotic resistance patterns in a camp is difficult. The administration of an antibiotic even in a single dose to a large number of people simultaneously is a major undertaking. If not taken by all individuals in the camp at the same time, the chances of reinfection of the treated from the untreated persist and a protracted epidemic results. Selected chemoprophylaxis of close contacts in a camp is not justified because of the difficulty in identifying them in such situations.

For personal protection of health personnel, proper hygienic practices, particularly washing of hands with soap and disinfectants, should be adequate. Administration of anti-microbials and vaccination are not necessary. All eating, drinking, and smoking should be prohibited on the hospital ward or in the area where cholera cases are being treated. Wearing of aprons should be obligatory, but gloves, masks, caps, and boots are not necessary.

8. CHOLERA PREVENTION AT FAIRS AND PILGRIMAGES

As has been mentioned in Chapter 1, health authorities, particularly those concerned with the Mecca pilgrimage, have learned by experience that, for the control and prevention of cholera, good surveillance for rapid detection of any suspicious case, prompt isolation and treatment of cases, and provision of sufficient chlorinated water and facilities for the disposal of excreta and refuse are adequate. The distribution of responsibilities to medical teams of different national groups appears to have helped. The experience of the Mecca pilgrimage is worth emulating. In India, pilgrims are also offered safe water and sanitation along their routes. There have been no large outbreaks at any of the many religious gatherings there in the last 3–4 decades; mass chemoprophylaxis has never been used and compulsory vaccination has recently been stopped (see seventh pandemic in Chapter 1).

9. CONCLUSIONS

Of all the pestilential diseases, only cholera is still causing so much human suffering in Africa, Asia, and South America. The industrialized countries also are not entirely secure. Given the speed and volume of travel today, and the many endemic foci in the world, no part of the globe is beyond the reach of an incubating case of cholera. The chances of such a person arriving, falling ill, and causing a problem in a place where sanitation is less than ideal and surveillance is lax have now increased considerably.

However, cholera is no longer the deadly disease it used to be; when properly treated it does not kill. The presence of endemic foci and of indigenous cases of *V. cholerae* 01 in the USA and Australia indicates that such foci can exist anywhere and are not necessarily a sign of an insalubrious environment. What is important is not to allow the infection to become a large public health problem.

The battle can only be won if there is a global political will to accept cholera as one of the acute diarrheal diseases and an agreement not to impose restrictions on trade and traffic against countries affected by the disease. Such restrictions hinder frank notifications and international cooperation and, thus, prevent the handling of cholera control as a purely technical problem.

Countries with a high incidence of diarrheal diseases should develop or strengthen their national program for the control of these diseases, which alone can provide the infrastructure to contain cholera wherever and whenever it breaks out. Cooperation between industrialized and developing countries in this effort and also in long-term endeavors to improve water supply and sanitation should be very rewarding in reducing the menace of this last remaining ancient disease.

ACKNOWLEDGMENT. We should like to acknowledge the able editorial assistance of Mrs. C.A. Martinez, Technical Officer, Diarrhoeal Diseases Control Programme, World Health Organization, Geneva.

REFERENCES

1. Pollitzer R: *Cholera*. Geneva, World Health Organization, 1959
2. Liebermeister C: Cholera Asiatica and Cholera nostras, in Nothnagel H (ed): *Spezielle Pathologie und Therapie, Wien*, Vol 4, Part 1, 1896, p 1
3. Howard-Jones N: The scientific background of the International Sanitary Conferences, 1851–1938.1 *Who Chron* 28:159–179, 1974
4. World Health Organization: *International Health Regulations (1969)*, second annotated edition. Geneva, World Health Organization, 1974
5. Baqui AH, Yunus M, Zaman K: Community-operated Treatment Centres prevented many cholera deaths. *J Diar Dis Res* 2:92–98, 1984
6. Faruque ASG, Eusof A, Islam ABMQ, et al: Community participation in a Diarrhoeal Outbreak: A Case Study. *Trop Geogr Med* 37:216–222, 1985
7. Mandara MP, Mhalu FS: Cholera in an inaccessible district in Tanzania: Importance of temporary rural centres. *Med J Zambia* 15:10–13, 1980–1981
8. World Health Organization: *Guidelines for Cholera Control* WHO/CDD/SER 80.4 Rev.1, Geneva, 1986
9. *Assisting in Emergencies. A resource handbook for UNICEF field staff*, New York, UNICEF, 1986
10. Mhalu FS, Mtango FDE, Msengi AE: Hospital outbreaks of cholera transmitted through close person-to-person contact. *Lancet* ii:82–84, 1984
11. Cliff JL, Zinkin P, Marteli A: A hospital outbreak of cholera in Maputo, Mozambique. *R Soc Trop Med Hyg* 80:473–476, 1986
12. Grossman ER, Walchek A, Freedman H: Tetracycline and permanent teeth: The relation between dose and tooth colour. *Pediatr* 47:567–570, 1971
13. Stewart DT: Prevalence of tetracyclines in children's teeth—Study II: A resurvey after 5 years. *Br Med J* 2:320–322, 1973
14. Garrigue GP, Ndayo M, Sigard JM, et al: Resistance aux Antibiotique des Souches de Vibrio cholerae El Tor Isoléea à Douala (Cameroun). *Bull Soc Pathol Exot Filiales* 79:305–312, 1986

15. Bergoend H, Loffler A, Malville J: Reactions Cutanées Survennues au Cour de la Prophylaxie de Masse de la Meningite Cerebrospinale par un Sulfamide Long-retard. *Ann Dermatol* 95:481–490, 1968

16. Hernborg A: Stevens Johnson syndrome after mass prophylaxis with sulphadoxine for cholera in Mozambique. *Lancet* ii: 1072–1073, 1985

17. Blake PA, Rosenberg ML, Costa JB, et al: Cholera in Portugal, 1974. 1. Modes of transmission. *Am J Epidemiol* 105:337–343, 1977

18. MacKenzie DJM: Cholera: Whither Prevention? *Med Clin North Am* 51:625–635, 1967

19. Gunn RA, Kimball AM, Matthew PP, et al: Cholera in Bahrain: Epidemiological characteristics of an outbreak. *Bull WHO* 59:61–66, 1981

20. Glass RI, Alim ARMA, Eusof A, et al: Cholera in Indonesia: Epidemiologic studies of transmission in Aceh province. *Am J Trop Med Hyg* 33:933–939, 1984

21. Moore BE, Perry L, Chard ST, A survey by the sewage swab method of latent enteric infections in an urban area. *J Hyg (Lond)* 50:357–364, 1952

22. Barrett TJ, Blake PA, Morris GK, et al: Use of Moore Swabs for isolating Vibrio cholerae from sewage. *J Clin Microbiol* 11:385–388, 1980

23. Isaacson M: Practical aspects of cholera surveillance program. *S Afr Med J* 49:1699–1702, 1975

24. Kolvin JL, Roberts D: Studies on growth of *Vibrio cholerae* biotype El Tor and biotype classical in foods. *J Hyg (Lond)* 89:243–252, 1982

25. Goh KT, Lam S, Ling MK: Epidemiological characteristics of an institutional outbreak of cholera. *Trans R Soc Trop Med Hyg* 81:230–232, 1987

26. Felix H, Dodin A: Epidémiologie mondiale du choléra: Evolution entre 1970 et 1980. *Bull Soc Pathol Exot Filiales* 74:17–30, 1981

27. Stock RF: *Cholera in Africa (African Environment Special Report 3)*. London; International African Institute, 1976

28. Sitas F: Some observations on a cholera outbreak at the Umvoti Mission Reserve, Natal. *S Afr Med J* 70:215–218, 1986

29. Feachem RG: Environmental aspects of cholera epidemiology. III. Transmission and Control. *Trop Dis Bull* 79:1–47, 1982

30. Khan MU: Interruption of shigellosis by hand washing. *Trans R Soc Trop Med Hyg* 76:164–168, 1982

31. Deb BC, Sircar BK, Sengupta PG, et al: Studies on interventions to prevent El Tor cholera transmission in urban slums. *Bull WHO* 64:127–131, 1986

32. Rajagopalan S, Shiffman MA: *Guide to Simple Sanitary Measures for the Control of Enteric Diseases*. Geneva, World Health Organization, 1974

33. Technical Advisory Group, UNDP Interregional Project: *Series of Publications on Water Supply and Sanitation*. Washington, D.C., WUD Publications Group, The World Bank

34. Khan MU, Khan MR, Hossain BR, et al: Alum potash in water to prevent cholera. *Lancet* ii: 1032, 1984

35. Clark RN: The purification of water on a small scale. *Bull WHO* 14:820–826, 1956

36. MacCormack WM, Chowhury AM, Jahangir M, et al: Tetracycline prophylaxis in families of cholera patients. *Bull WHO* 38:787–792, 1968

37. Joint ICMR–GWB–WHO Cholera Study Group: Effect of tetracycline on cholera carriers in households of cholera patients. *Bull WHO* 45:451–455, 1971

38. Lapeysonnie L: Chémioprophylaxie de l'infection cholérique: Interet, Espoirs et Limites. *Méd Trop (Mars)* 31:127–132, 1971

39. Deb BC, Sengupta PG, De SP, et al: Effect of sulfadoxine on transmission of *Vibrio cholerae* infection among family contacts of cholera patients in Calcutta. *Bull WHO* 54:171–175, 1976

40. Sengupta PC, Sircar BK, Mondal S, et al: Effect of doxycycline on transmission of *Vibrio cholerae* infection among family contacts of cholera patients in Calcutta. *Bull WHO* 56:323–326, 1978

41. Mhalu FS, Mmari PW, Ijumba J: Rapid emergence of El Tor *Vibrio cholerae* Resistant to antimicrobial agents during first 6 months of fourth cholera epidemic in Tanzania. *Lancet* i:345–347, 1979

42. Joo I: Cholera vaccines, in Barua D, Burrows W (eds): *Cholera*. Philadelphia, WB Saunders, 1974, p 339

43. Watanabe Y: Antibacterial immunity in cholera, in Barua D, Burrows W (eds): *Cholera*. Philadelphia, WB Saunders, 1974, p 298

44. Mosley WH, Aziz KMA, Rahman ASMM, et al: Report of the 1966–67 cholera vaccine trial in rural East Pakistan. 4. Five years of observation with practical assessment of the role of a cholera vaccine in cholera control programmes. *Bull WHO* 47:229–238, 1972

45. Sommer A, Khan M. Mosley WH: Efficacy of vaccination of family contacts of cholera cases. *Lancet* i:1230–1232, 1973

46. Sommer A, Mosley WH: Ineffectiveness of cholera vaccination as an epidemic control measure. *Lancet* i:1232–1235, 1973

47. Steffen R: Epidemiologic studies of traveler's diarrhea, severe gastrointestinal infections, and cholera. *Rev Infect Dis* 8 (Suppl 2):S122–S130, 1986

48. Snyder JD, Blake PA: Is cholera a problem for US travelers. *JAMA* 247:2268–2269, 1982

49. Khan MU, Shahidullah M: Role of water and sanitation in the incidence of cholera in refugee camps. *Trans R Soc Trop Med Hyg* 76:373–377, 1982

50. Morris JG, West GR, Holck SE, et al: Cholera among refugees in Rangsit, Thailand. *J Infect Dis* 145:131–133, 1982

Epilogue
The Latin American Cholera Epidemic

Eugene J. Gangarosa and Robert V. Tauxe

In January 1991, epidemic cholera appeared explosively in villages, towns, and cities along the Peruvian coast. In the following year, the epidemic spread swiftly throughout Latin America, challenging the health infrastructure of the entire Western Hemisphere. It resembles the great urban epidemics of nineteenth century Europe and the United States in its intensity, and is spreading with late twentieth century velocity. Mortality rates have been low because of widespread use of fluid replacement therapy, including oral rehydration solutions (ORS). The extraordinary numbers of patients needing emergency treatment, however, have strained the resources of many Ministries of Health. The economic impact of many countries has been substantial. Tourists hesitate to visit areas affected by epidemic cholera, and exporters encounter concern that foodstuffs in international trade could transport cholera. We confront this new cholera epidemic with tools to understand and control it that have been under development for many years. The epidemic brings new challenges and the opportunity for rapid advances in knowledge of the organism and in the means to limit the number of infections it causes.

SUCCESS AND FAILURE

In 1961, the so-called seventh pandemic of cholera appeared in Indonesia and Southeast Asia and was associated with a biotype of *Vibrio cholerae* 01 not previously recognized to have pandemic potential. Epidemics caused by this El Tor biotype spread rapidly across the Asian continent, and its introduction into Africa in 1970 led to considerable concern that it would next appear in Latin America, where some preparations were made in anticipation of this introduction. For reasons that still defy explanation, cholera did not then appear in Latin America. In the following years, programs to produce and distribute oral rehydration solutions for the treatment of diarrheal diseases were introduced in the Americas. When epidemic

Cholera, edited by Dhiman Barua and William B. Greenough III. Plenum Medical Book Company, New York, 1992.

cholera did appear in 1991, it reached a continent that was far more prepared than it had been 20 years before. Peru benefited from these recent efforts and had in place an extensive oral rehydration program to treat cases, an epidemic field investigation service to investigate outbreaks, and laboratory resources to identify the cholera organism early in the epidemic. A case fatality rate of 1.2%, one of the lowest rates recorded in the first year in a newly infected developing country, attests to the efficacy of these preparations. The course of events in Peru, where a diarrheal diseases control program was established before the epidemic, is a tribute to the health authorities of that country, because as bad as the situation was, it could have been far worse.

The Latin American epidemic also signals a major failure. The year 1990 marked the culmination of the "Water and Sanitation Decade," a global effort during the 1980s to provide "safe water for all" by the end of the decade. These efforts notwithstanding, the rapid spread of epidemic cholera in the Western Hemisphere and the large number of cases reported have been staggering. At the time of writing, the World Health Organization (WHO) had received reports of more than 570,000 cholera cases and nearly 17,000 deaths from cholera worldwide in 1991. Latin American countries reported 391,171 (68%) cases and 3,871 (23%) deaths. In the meantime, cholera has become even more entrenched in the developing countries of Africa and Asia. In many African countries, epidemic cholera continues to be reported every year since it was introduced in the 1970s. The reported cases worldwide for 1991, representing the tip of the iceberg, are more than double the cumulative number of cases reported in the previous five-year period (263,117). Thus, we start the 1990s with the worst year on record since the current pandemic began 30 years ago. What went wrong? What are the lessons for decision makers as we cope with the continued challenge of pandemic cholera? To answer these questions, we will need to analyze the current Latin American epidemic and compare it with previous experience to determine the implications for prevention and control.

THE NEW EPIDEMIC

Epidemiologic investigations conducted in the first year of the Latin American epidemic suggest that in many respects it is all too similar to previous epidemics in Asia and Africa. The highest attack rates occurred in large periurban slums, where safe water supplies and sewage disposal are limited or nonexistent. All age groups and both sexes are affected, and serologic surveys in some areas suggest that as many as half of the population may have been affected in the first three months. Not surprisingly, microbiologic culture surveys showed that at the height of the epidemic, nearly all acute watery diarrhea could be correctly presumed to be cholera, whether the group sampled was adult or pediatric, inpatient or outpatient. The case mortality rate was less than 1% in most age groups, though higher in the elderly and the extremely young. Extension of the epidemic to remote Andean mountain communities or villages in the Amazon jungle was also associated with higher mortality.

Before this epidemic, cholera had not been reported from South America since 1895. In the intervening years, especially during the period of heightened concern in the 1970s, local surveys failed to identify toxigenic *V. cholerae* 01 in samples from diarrhea patients or from the environment. A small number of nontoxigenic strains of biotype El Tor were identified, which are only distantly related to strains from the current Latin American epidemic or elsewhere. This shows that methods used could have identified toxigenic strains if they were present.

The source of the 1991 introduction of cholera into Peru has not been clarified. It may have been a ship discharging contaminated ballast water or human sewage into a harbor, or feces of a returning traveler that contaminated a shellfish bed. Less likely is the possibility that a preexisting but undetected focus of nontoxigenic *V. cholerae* 01 suddenly acquired both the ability to produce toxin and epidemic potential. Available microbiologic data have not resolved which of these different possibilities is correct.

Following its appearance on the Peruvian coast in January 1991, the epidemic rapidly spread to contiguous areas, crossing the Andes mountains to reach the source waters of the Amazon River and spreading to contiguous areas of Ecuador, Columbia, and Brazil within a few months. It also spread in discontinuous leaps, appearing suddenly in Santiago, Chile, 1000 miles to the south and in central Mexico 1500 miles to the north. These appearances warned the rest of the hemisphere that sudden introductions could be expected. In general, spread followed the trade and transportation routes that move people rapidly throughout the hemisphere. Anecdotes of introduction show how easily cholera can spread from area to area when the circumstances permit transmission. Migrant shrimp farm workers are said to have introduced cholera to Ecuador from Peru, itinerant preachers to have brought it from El Salvador into Honduras, and drug-smugglers flying from Amazon jungle bases have brought it, as well as cocaine, to airstrips in Mexico. The extraordinary spread also underscores the mystery of why cholera did not appear in the 1970s, when its arrival on the east coast of South America or in the Caribbean was anticipated.

By February 1992, after the first year of the epidemic, 18 countries in the Western Hemisphere had reported cholera cases, including all countries in Central America and most in South America (see Figure 1). Of particular concern, the brief lull in the epidemic that occurred during winter in the Southern Hemisphere ended, and 62,039 cases were reported in the first two months of 1992. Widespread epidemic cholera was resurgent in many of the same countries and cities where it had been most intense in the first year of the epidemic. Each country that reported cases in 1991 has also reported cases by February 1992. In Africa, many countries affected in the early 1970s are still reporting cholera epidemics now. It seems likely that in parts of Latin America, epidemic cholera may persist for years to come. Hopes that the epidemic will end spontaneously are likely to be in vain as long as the circumstances for transmission are ripe.

TRANSMISSION BY WATER AND FOOD

Detailed epidemiologic investigations in Latin America have shown that several different beverages and foods could serve as important sources of infection. Because the sources vary by location, local epidemiologic investigations are needed to target control measures to specific vehicles when generic control measures fail. One cannot assume what the vehicle of transmission is in any particular outbreak. The personnel necessary to conduct appropriate case-control investigations should be seen as an integral part of the public health infrastructure.

As in the large urban cholera epidemics in nineteenth century Europe and elsewhere since, one major source of cholera in Latin America has been contaminated drinking water. Large urban water systems may function as efficient distributors of contaminated water unless they are adequately maintained and water is appropriately disinfected. Further compounding the challenge, most people store drinking water in their homes, where water that is clean at the tap may be subsequently contaminated. Street vendors use tap water to prepare

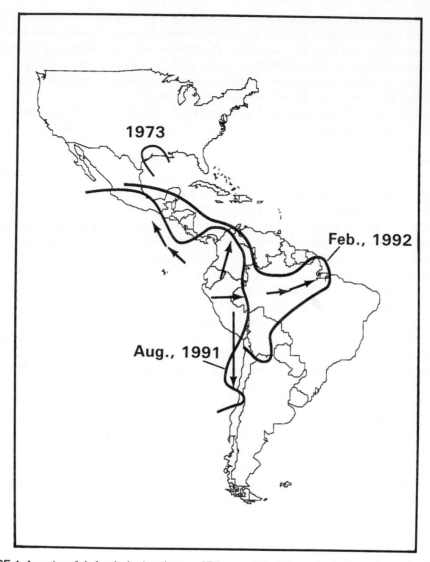

FIGURE 1. Location of cholera in the Americas as of February 1992. A focus of endemic cholera on the Gulf Coast of the United States was first demonstrated in 1973. Epidemic cholera in Latin America appeared in Peru in January 1991, spread to neighboring countries and Central America by August, and affected all of Central America and descended the Amazon by February 1992. The 1973 and 1991 strains were quite different.

beverages, and icemakers freeze it to ship perishable foods. Although it is relatively easy to begin educating a population that water from a river or stream is unsafe and needs further treatment, it can be politically explosive to tell them that municipal water at the tap is not to be trusted.

As has been demonstrated repeatedly elsewhere in the world in the last two decades, epidemic cholera in Latin America has been associated with unsafe foods. At ambient temperatures, *Vibrio cholerae* 01 can grow rapidly to high counts on a variety of foods after they are contaminated. In some epidemic investigations, food purchased from street vendors has been an important source of cholera; in others, rice left out for hours and eaten without reheating has been associated with disease. Fresh fruit and vegetables grown in raw sewage and eaten raw have been suspected, although not yet documented, as sources of cholera.

Seafood has been a particular concern. It was suspected, although not confirmed, as a source of cholera at the outset of the Peruvian epidemic, and as a result, the Peruvian public temporarily stopped eating raw seafood. In other Latin American settings, seafood was proven to transmit cholera; sources include souvenir seafood brought back to the United States in travelers' luggage, seafood salad served to passengers on an airliner in early 1992, and local seafoods implicated in investigations outside of Peru, where the public had not been specifically warned. Seafood may be contaminated before harvest if it lives in waters harboring *V. cholerae* 01 or after harvest if contaminated water is used either to "freshen" the catch or as part of further processing. Less contamination would occur if raw sewage were not discharged into harbors near shellfish beds, fishing docks, and seafood processing plants. Again, it is ironic that the incomplete development of sanitation projects, which results in sewage collection without sewage treatment, may actually promote contamination of the food supply.

The epidemic has also demonstrated the great rarity of transmission other than by food and waterborne routes. Nosocomial spread has not yet been reported, and there is no evidence of direct person-to-person spread by contact without intervening contamination of food or water. Importantly, to date no transmission has been related to any of the extensive exports from affected countries, although they have been monitored closely in many importing countries.

NEW CHALLENGES

Despite many broad similarities, the current epidemic in Latin America differs from previous epidemics in several ways. These differences mark gaps in our understanding of cholera. First, the organism is definably different from the relatively homogenous biotype El Tor strains of *V. cholerae* 01 that are part of the pandemic spread of cholera in the last 30 years. The detected differences are small and of uncertain significance, but they indicate that the Latin American epidemic may be more than the simple appearance of the seventh pandemic in the Western Hemisphere. Whether this represents the beginning of a new pandemic, or represents a simple offshoot of the current pandemic, remains to be clarified.

The people of Latin America and the circumstances in which they live differ in important ways from Europeans in the nineteenth century or Asians or Africans in the 1970s. One difference is genetic. For unclear reasons, blood group O is associated with a marked increase in susceptibility to severe cholera. This is the dominant blood group in Latin America, but is much less frequent in Asia or Africa. This means that the Latin American epidemic may cause proportionately more severe illness than previous epidemics. The population of Latin America tripled between 1950 and 1990, and vast periurban slums now exist in many of these countries. The sheer mass of humanity crowded into these slums is enormous; individual cities in Latin America have greater populations than entire European nations did a century ago. Modern means of transportation now connect slums and city centers, regions, and entire countries with each other, and large numbers of people regularly travel seeking work, profit, or pleasure. The international trade ties between countries of Latin America and other parts of the world are extensive and swift and include commerce in perishable foods and other commodities that could conceivably be contaminated with tox- igenic *V. cholerae* 01.

Perhaps the biggest gaps in our understanding of the transmission of cholera are the factors contributing to the establishment and persistence of the cholera vibrio in environmen- tal reservoirs. Identification of unique strains of toxigenic *V. cholerae* 01 that persist on the Gulf Coast of the United States and in rivers of Northeastern Australia has proved that this can occur without repeated contamination by human sewage. The ecologic relationships, seasonal determinants, and microbiologic adaptations that make this persistence possible need further clarification. We assume that such reservoirs may also exist for the pandemic and Latin American strains. The existence of natural environmental reservoirs implies that the organism cannot be eradicated. We can, however, limit its epidemic potential.

The risk of epidemic cholera in industrialized nations has been extremely low during this century. General availability of safe water and sewage collection and treatment make sustained transmission extremely unlikely. Developed countries have already been affected by the Latin American epidemic, however, and we can expect future introductions. Some ways that cholera has affected the United States are relatively simple to prevent, while others are novel and more challenging. Travelers infected in countries with epidemic cholera have returned to the United States with the illness. On two occasions, healthy travelers returned with contaminated crabs in their luggage that caused cholera in family members who later ate them. Educating travelers in simple preventive measures may prevent most such infections. Early in 1992, a large outbreak of cholera affected passengers debarking in Los Angeles, after they ate cold seafood salad prepared in Peru while flying on an Argentine airliner. The recommendations for international travelers do not necessarily end when the passenger boards the plane for the trip home. Although secondary transmission following introductions into the United States has not yet been documented, limited transmission may be possible if cholera is introduced into destitute populations that are not well served by water and sewer systems. There is also a risk that the epidemic strain could contaminate fresh foods shipped on ice from affected areas or could contaminate local food supplies. At the height of the initial expansion of epidemic cholera into Africa in the 1970s, epidemics in several European countries occurred as a result of contamination of shellfish or of inadequately protected water supplies. In 1991, detection of the Latin American strain of *V. cholerae* 01 in oysters from a closed commercial oyster bed and from ballast water discharged in U.S. ports from freighters arriving from Latin America shows that similar introductions are possible in this hemisphere.

To date, efforts to develop and test cholera vaccines have given us substantial insight into the difficulties of inducing reliable immunity. Extensive trials of the parenteral cholera vaccine conducted early in the seventh pandemic demonstrated that it was of limited benefit to the individual and was of little use in protecting the public health. More recent trials with killed oral vaccine in Bangladesh demonstrated somewhat longer protection but indicate that the degree of protection varies widely, depending on the type of *V. cholerae* 01 that is causing illness, the previous cholera experience of the recipient, and even his or her blood group. The vaccine was least effective in young children with no previous cholera experi- ence, who were blood group O, and who were challenged with El Tor biotype of *V. cholerae* 01. Unfortunately, this describes the Latin American situation. Efforts to test live oral vaccines are accelerating under the stimulus of the Latin American epidemic. Perhaps the most interesting result of the recent Bangladesh trials was the observation that even natural infection is not necessarily protective and was distinctly limited following infection with El Tor strains. That is of concern to Latin America in general, as well as to the developers of live vaccines. It suggests that more needs to be learned about the determinants of mucosal immunity to cholera.

THE TREATMENT BREAKTHROUGH

The development of modern treatment methods means that cholera should no longer be perceived as the dread disease it once was. Basic research in the pathophysiology of cholera has reaped rich dividends. Modern treatment methods based on rapid volume replacement evolved from research conducted during the 1960s and 1970s and have transformed this disease from a highly malignant one to one that is easily managed. Especially significant was the introduction of oral rehydration therapy, the application of which encompasses the wide spectrum of diarrheal diseases of which cholera is the prototype. Perhaps the most prophetic comments relative to this breakthrough were made in a Lancet editorial in 1978, which heralded ORT as perhaps the most significant breakthrough in this century. This statement recognized the universal acceptance of ORT as a generic treatment for many diarrheal diseases, a low-cost and highly efficacious technology that many rank second only to the discovery of antibiotics in terms of lives saved. The ORT breakthrough makes it possible for all acute noninvasive secretory diarrheas to be dealt with therapeutically as a single clinical entity regardless of etiology. Anyone arriving alive at a treatment center or hospital with dehydrating diarrhea should survive. The transformation of cholera from a malignant to an easily managed disease permits the clinician to shift from treating cholera as a single clinical entity to a broader focus on the generic group of acute secretory diarrheas. This is because most patients afflicted with these diseases can now be treated in the same way, with intravenous fluids for those initially seen with cardiovascular collapse and ORT as the mainstay of therapy.

This clinical transformation is only one facet of our modern understanding of this group of diseases. Because many share the same root causes—poverty and unsafe water and foods—a common approach to the control of transmission is possible. The public health practitioner can also think of these diseases in a more generic way. The benefits that will come from investments made to correct the root deficiencies will provide an analogous "cure" by preventing all fecal transmitted diseases.

PREPARATION AND PREVENTION

Great strides have been made in provision of primary care for acute watery diarrhea throughout the world. The development of national training programs for treatment of diarrheal disease, under the auspices of the WHO Diarrheal Diseases Control Programme, has been the fruit of the labor of many over the last twenty years. Cholera has been the impetus that established or expanded this program in many countries, and establishing such programs may be one of the most immediate and productive responses possible in a country threatened by cholera. The strategy to control cholera as outlined by WHO and practiced by virtually every country in Latin America avoids the excesses of the past and focuses resources on the most essential areas. Dr. Gangarosa, who began his career at the onset of the current global pandemic, has seen repeatedly the futility of the *cordon sanitaire*, the inappropriate use of antimicrobial drugs for "community prophylaxis," the senseless embargoes of commodities, the misconceived efforts to control person-to-person transmission, and the misuse of cholera vaccine.

Instead, many Latin American countries followed the practical strategy for management of cholera epidemics outlined by WHO. Care providers were educated in proper treatment methods, and the availability of ORS was expanded. Laboratory capacity to identify the organism in patient and environmental samples has been improved. Surveillance systems were developed to efficiently identify the beginning of epidemics, direct the distribution of treatment and disinfection materials, and monitor the success of control measures. Such critical preparations depend on a functioning public health infrastructure. This is never more obvious than in a cholera epidemic, and resources of central governments and foreign donors should be made available to support them.

In many areas, preventing cholera starts with public education to promote home treatment of water by the most propitious means, the selection of safe foods from street vendors, and the need for cooking seafoods thoroughly. Such measures are likely to be temporary, and their efficacy depends in part on the faith the population has in the source of the advice. While such short-term preparations are important, and are likely to limit morbidity, they are by themselves insufficient where epidemic cholera is likely to persist or reoccur.

A long-term solution is also needed. Epidemic cholera has come to be a metaphor for underdevelopment. Experience has shown that communities that have made the investments necessary to ensure its citizens a safe water supply, safe disposal of human wastes, and safe food handling practices have been spared the onslaught of cholera. The benefits of these investments go well beyond cholera. Cholera is a surrogate, the tip of the iceberg, for many diseases that are transmitted by bad water and contaminated food. The solution lies in a "Sanitary Reform" revolution in each affected country, like the efforts made in European countries and the United States at the end of the last century and the first few decades of this century. This means investments in the maintenance and improvement of existing water systems, the development of water systems in communities where none now exist, widespread installation of sewage systems, implementation of shellfish safety programs, and programs to ensure safe food handling practices.

The argument is made that there is a lack of resources necessary to correct these problems. In fact, some Latin American countries have accelerated their water and sewage system construction programs and may soon be at low risk for epidemic cholera. In the future, the priority given to these issues in many countries may depend largely on the economic consequences of the disease. Economic policies that defer investments in infrastructure because of the appeal of short-term gains from investments in vertical development programs, such as the development of tourism and fisheries, may need to be reworked. The economic disasters created by cholera underscore how tenuous vertical investments can be when they are built on weak infrastructures.

Thus, cholera should be seen as both a challenge and an opportunity for the public health practitioner. It provides leverage to persuade decision makers who control purse strings to reorder priorities and make the commitment of resources needed to correct the root problems. The disease is also a challenge to the decision makers outside the traditional health arena who have a critical role in correcting the root problems. The experiences in many countries, including those of Peru, underscore the importance of the multisectorial approach in the control of cholera. The epidemic of cholera in Latin America, and its persistence in Africa and parts of Asia, emphasize the continued need for an international response to a common threat. Short-term strategies to prepare for epidemic cholera and long-term strategies to prevent it offer the most rational recipe for control. This book will have its most useful application for clinicians, public health practitioners, and laboratory workers entrusted with the implementation of these strategies and for students destined for leadership in the twenty-first century.

Index